theclinics.com

HEART FAILURE CLINICS

Neurohumoral Modulators in Heart Failure

GUEST EDITOR
Gregg C. Fonarow, MD

CONSULTING EDITORS
Jagat Narula, MD, PhD
James B. Young, MD

April 2005 • Volume 1 • Number 1

SAUNDERS

An Imprint of Elsevier, Inc.
PHILADELPHIA LONDON TORONTO MONTREAL SYDNEY TOKYO

W.B. SAUNDERS COMPANY
A Division of Elsevier Inc.

The Curtis Center • Independence Square West • Philadelphia, Pennsylvania 19106

http://www.theclinics.com

HEART FAILURE CLINICS **Volume 1, Number 1**
April 2005 **ISSN 1551-7136**
Editor: Heather Cullen **ISBN 1-4160-2664-9**

Heart Failure Clinics (ISSN 1551-7136) is published three times a year by W.B. Saunders Company (quarterly beginning in 2006). Corporate and editorial offices: 170 S Independence Mall W 300 E, Philadelphia, PA 19106-3399. Accounting and circulation offices: 6277 Sea Harbor Drive, Orlando, FL 32887-4800. Subscription prices are USD 99 per year for US individuals, USD 149 per year for US institutions, USD 49 per year for US students and residents, USD 109 per year for Canadian individuals, USD 169 per year for Canadian institutions, USD 119 per year for international individuals, USD 169 per year for international institutions and USD 59 per year for Canadian and foreign students/residents. To receive student and resident rate, orders must be accompanied by name of affiliated institution, date of term, and the *signature* of program/residency coordinator on institution letterhead. Orders will be billed at individual rate until proof of status is received. Foreign air speed delivery is included in all *Clinics* subscription prices. All prices are subject to change without notice. POSTMASTER: Send address changes to *Heart Failure Clinics*, W.B. Saunders Company, Periodicals Fulfillment, Orlando, FL 32887-4800. **Customer Service: 1-800-654-2452 (US). From outside of the US, call 1-407-345-4000.**

Printed in the United States of America.

FORTHCOMING ISSUES

July 2005

Pathogenesis of Heart Failure
Roger Hajjar, MD, and
Federica del Monte, MD, *Guest Editors*

October 2005

Myocarditis
G. William Dec, MD, *Guest Editor*

January 2006

Diabetic and Hypertensive Pre–Heart Failure Patient
David Bell, MD, *Guest Editor*

April 2006

Imaging Heart Failure
Vasken Dilsizian, MD, David Bello, MD, and
Mario Garcia, MD, *Guest Editors*

July 2006

Biomarkers in Heart Failure
Vasan Ramachandran, MD, *Guest Editor*

October 2006

Stage D Heart Failure
Clyde W. Yancy, MD, *Guest Editor*

CONSULTING EDITORS

JAGAT NARULA, MD, PhD, Professor, Medicine; Chief, Division of Cardiology; and Associate Dean, College of Medicine, University of California at Irvine, University of California Medical Center, Orange, California

JAMES B. YOUNG, MD, Chairman and Professor, Department of Medicine, Lerner College of Medicine; and George and Linda Kaufman Chair, Cleveland Clinic Foundation, Case Western Reserve University, Cleveland, Ohio

GUEST EDITOR

GREGG C. FONAROW, MD, Eliot Corday Professor of Cardiovascular Medicine and Science; Director, Ahmanson–University of California at Los Angeles Cardiomyopathy Center; and Division of Cardiology, University of California at Los Angeles Medical Center, Los Angeles, California

CONTRIBUTORS

WILLIAM T. ABRAHAM, MD, FACP, FACC, Professor, Medicine; and Chief, Division of Cardiovascular Medicine, The Ohio State University, Columbus, Ohio

JOHAN ÄRNLÖV, MD, PhD, National Heart, Lung, and Blood Institute's Framingham Heart Study, Framingham, Massachusetts; and Section of Geriatrics, Department of Public Health and Caring Sciences, Uppsala University, Uppsala, Sweden

JOHN C. BURNETT, Jr, MD, Professor, Medicine and Physiology, Mayo Clinic College of Medicine; and Director, Cardiorenal Research Laboratory, Division of Cardiovascular Diseases, Department of Internal Medicine, Mayo Clinic and Foundation, Rochester, Minnesota

JOHN G.F. CLELAND, MD, Professor, Department of Cardiology, University of Hull, Castle Hill Hospital, Kingston-upon-Hull, UK

ANITA DESWAL, MD, MPH, Assistant Professor, Medicine, Winters Center for Heart Failure Research and Houston Center of Quality of Care and Utilization Services, Michael E. DeBakey Veterans Affairs Medical Center and Baylor College of Medicine, Houston, Texas

JOHN FINLEY, MD, Instructor, Medicine, Department of Medicine, Tufts–New England Medical Center and Tufts University School of Medicine, Boston, Massachusetts

GARY S. FRANCIS, MD, Professor, Medicine, Cleveland Clinic Lerner College of Medicine, Case Western Reserve University; and Head, Section of Clinical Cardiology, Department of Cardiovascular Medicine, Cleveland Clinic Foundation, Cleveland, Ohio

MIHAI GHEORGHIADE, MD, Feinberg Cardiovascular Research Institute, Northwestern University Feinberg School of Medicine, Chicago, Illinois

OLAF HEDRICH, MD, Instructor, Medicine, Division of Cardiology, Department of Medicine, Tufts–New England Medical Center and Tufts University School of Medicine, Boston, Massachusetts

SRINIVAS IYENGAR, MD, Fellow, Division of Cardiovascular Medicine, The Ohio State University, Columbus, Ohio

DHRUV KAZI, MD, Department of Medicine, Baylor College of Medicine, Houston, Texas

MARVIN A. KONSTAM, MD, Chief, Division of Cardiology, Department of Medicine, Tufts–New England Medical Center and Tufts University School of Medicine, Boston, Massachusetts

HUAN LOH, MBChB, B Med Sci, Research Fellow, Department of Cardiology, University of Hull, Castle Hill Hospital, Kingston-upon-Hull, UK

DENNIS M. McNAMARA, MD, Associate Professor, Medicine; and Director, Heart Failure/Transplantation Program, University of Pittsburgh Medical Center, Pittsburgh, Pennsylvania

BERTRAM PITT, MD, Professor, Medicine, Division of Cardiology, Department of Internal Medicine, University of Michigan School of Medicine, Ann Arbor, Michigan

JONATHAN A. RAPP, MD, Department of Medicine, Northwestern University, Chicago, Illinois

WILLEM J. REMME, MD, PhD, Professor, Medicine, Sticares Cardiovascular Research Foundation, "Albrandssate", Rhoon, The Netherlands

W.H. WILSON TANG, MD, Assistant Professor, Medicine, Lerner College of Medicine, Case Western Reserve University; Associate Staff, Section of Heart Failure and Cardiac Transplantation Medicine, Department of Cardiovascular Medicine; and Assistant Program Director, General Clinical Research Center, Cleveland Clinic Foundation, Cleveland, Ohio

JAMES E. UDELSON, MD, Associate Chief, Division of Cardiology, Department of Medicine, Tufts–New England Medical Center and Tufts University School of Medicine, Boston, Massachusetts

RAMACHANDRAN S. VASAN, MD, Senior Investigator, National Heart, Lung, and Blood Institute's Framingham Heart Study, Framingham; and Associate Professor, Cardiology Section, Preventive Medicine and Epidemiology, Department of Medicine, Boston University School of Medicine, Boston, Massachusetts

JONATHAN WINDRAM, MBChB, BSc, Research Fellow, Department of Cardiology, University of Hull, Castle Hill Hospital, Kingston-upon-Hull, UK

JAMES B. YOUNG, MD, Chairman and Professor, Department of Medicine, Lerner College of Medicine; and George and Linda Kaufman Chair, Cleveland Clinic Foundation, Case Western Reserve University, Cleveland, Ohio

CONTENTS

ELSEVIER
SAUNDERS

Heart Failure Clin 1 (2005) xi – xii

HEART
FAILURE
CLINICS

Editorial

Heart Failure Clinics: Arrival of Gen-3

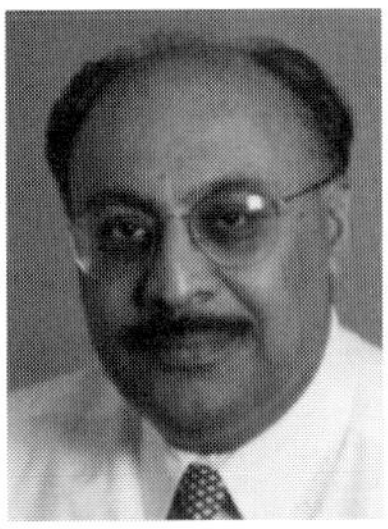
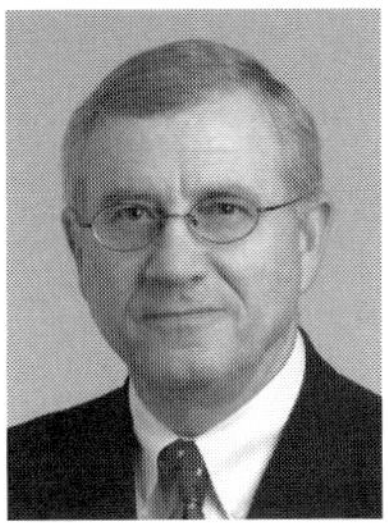

Jagat Narula, MD, PhD James B. Young, MD
Consulting Editors

The concept of *Clinics of North America* was introduced 90 years ago with the sole objective of integrating the established and current literature on a selected disease entity and then disseminating an evidence-based consensus regarding practice guidelines for optimizing diagnostic and management strategies. The *Clinics* issues were guest edited by acclaimed clinicians and investigators, and in the ensuing years, incorporated the gamut of important medical specialties. *Clinics* became instantly popular with training and community physicians and paved the way for subsequent subspecialty *Clinics* in over 50 disciplines. Among the many subspecialities represented, *Cardiology Clinics* has enjoyed an extensive readership. Enormous advances in the field of subspecialty medicine have necessitated the initiation of *Generation 3 Clinics,* and *Heart Failure Clinics* happens to be the first of this generation. This is so because of the enormous burden of heart failure (HF) and the rapid advances made in our understanding and approach. *Heart Failure Clinics* does not in any way pretend to simulate a HF journal and will not produce original research manuscripts; rather it will present clinical practices and clinically-relevant basic research in the field of HF and cardiac transplantation, including related topics such as device-based therapies for HF. The sole objective remains the same as that of the 90-year-old *Medical Clinics of North America*: reaching out to clinicians-in-training and community-based physicians.

We do not think justification of such a focus on HF is necessary, as this syndrome has become the foremost cardiovascular health problem worldwide. It is believed that at least 20% of the global population suffers from diseases that predispose it to HF. We need to martial efforts to better prevent and manage this scourge. Since HF is the only non-procedural subspecialty of cardiology, dissemination of knowledge to grass-roots levels promises to be effective. For the 3 years of our initial assignment as Consulting Editors of *Heart Failure Clinics,* we have developed 12 issues for you that cater to various tastes. The inaugural issue "Neurohumoral Modulation in Heart Failure" is guest edited by Gregg C. Fonarow, MD. The next two issues for the year 2005 include "Pathogenesis of Heart Failure" guest edited by Roger Hajjar, MD and Frederica del Monte, MD, and "Myocarditis" guest edited by G. William Dec, MD.

The current issue focuses on the use of neurohormonal antagonists in day-to-day practice: which agent, what sequence, what dose, how to up-titrate and how far to go, and who deserves these drugs and who might not. These nuances have been captured in this inaugural issue. Neurohumoral modulation constitutes the most important management strategy

1551-7136/05/$ – see front matter
doi:10.1016/j.hfc.2005.03.001

in HF that has enormously improved survival in devastatingly-ill patients. Paradoxically, population studies suggest that only a small proportion of eligible patients receive antiangiotensin and -adrenergic therapy (perhaps 50% of patients that should be treated). This unacceptably low utilization rate is a challenge to physicians committed to care of HF patients. We believe that the purpose of this issue will be fulfilled if we are able to convert some and reinforce the commitment of a few others to utilizing neuro-hormonal antagonism in HF.

We congratulate the guest editor and authors for their valuable contributions. We would also like to thank the team at Elsevier, especially Ms. Heather Cullen, for her leadership in making *Generation 3* a reality.

Jagat Narula, MD, PhD
Professor, Medicine
Chief, Division of Cardiology
Associate Dean, College of Medicine
University of California at Irvine
University of California Medical Center
101 The City Drive
Building 53, Mail Route 81
Orange, CA 92868-4080, USA

E-mail address: narula@uci.edu

James B. Young, MD
Chairman, Department of Medicine
Professor, Medicine
Lerner College of Medicine
Case Western Reserve University
Cleveland Clinic Foundation
9500 Euclid Avenue
Desk T-13
Cleveland, OH 44195, USA

E-mail address: youngj@ccf.org

ELSEVIER
SAUNDERS

Heart Failure Clin 1 (2005) xiii – xiv

HEART
FAILURE
CLINICS

Preface

Neurohumoral Modulators in Heart Failure

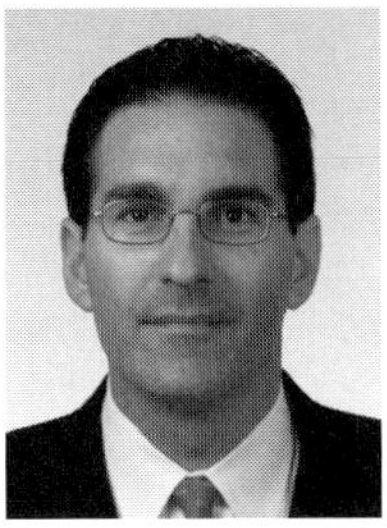

Gregg C. Fonarow, MD
Guest Editor

There has been intensive research into the pathophysiology of heart failure. Neurohormonal activation is now thought to play a key role in the initiation and progression of heart failure. Neurohormonal activation plays a major role in the cardiac remodeling process. Increased tissue and plasma levels of neurohormones occur in patients with left ventricular dysfunction even when they are at an asymptomatic stage without overt heart failure, with activation increasing further as symptomatic heart failure develops. The renin–angiotensin–aldosterone system, sympathetic nervous system, endothelin system, arginine vasopressin, and naturietic peptides contribute significantly to the pathogenesis of heart failure.

Researchers have conducted many clinical trials to assess the impact of medical therapies on patient outcomes. As a result, many therapeutic options are available to manage heart failure. The most important therapeutic advance during the past decade has been the recognition that agents inhibiting neurohormonal activation relieve symptoms, reduce hospitalizations, and prolong survival in patients with heart failure from left ventricular systolic dysfunction. Neurohormonal inhibition has also been shown to prevent the development of heart failure in patients at risk. There is compelling clinical trial evidence that medical therapies including angiotensin-converting enzyme inhibitors, aldosterone antagonists, and beta-blockers reduce the risk of hospitalization and substantially improve survival in patients with heart failure. Recent clinical trials have helped to further define the role of these agents as well as the angiotensin receptor antagonists. The single most effective medical therapy for chronic heart failure has proven to be beta-blockers. Despite the demonstration of marked benefits in numerous clinical trials, there has been significant variability in the extent to which neurohormonal inhibitors are used and the patient populations in which they are employed. There have been questions regarding which patient populations benefit, how patients should receive the medications, the most appropriate doses, and the most effective combination of agents. In the course of their development, several types of beta-blockers have emerged and have proved to be a diverse class of agents in terms of their pharmacology, effect on important clinical outcomes, and tolerability. A number of recent trials have helped to address many of these questions and to better define the extent of therapeutic benefits of neurohormonal inhibition in preventing and treating heart failure.

This first issue of the *Heart Failure Clinics* is focused on neurohumoral modulators in heart failure. The role of neurohormonal activation in populations susceptible to heart failure and in the pathophysiology of this disease are reviewed. The role of angiotensin-converting enzyme inhibitors, angiotensin receptor antagonists, aldosterone antagonists, and

1551-7136/05/$ – see front matter
doi:10.1016/j.hfc.2005.01.001

beta-blockers are presented. Articles on novel neurohumoral antagonists and natriuretic peptides are included. Current knowledge regarding the pharmacogenomics for neurohormonal intervention in heart failure is presented. In addition, the role of neurohumoral modulators in heart failure with preserved systolic function is discussed. It is our hope that this information will prove useful in advancing the understanding of the pathophysiology of this complex disease, guide future research, and further promote the use of evidenced-based, guideline-recommended neurohumoral antagonists in the treatment of heart failure.

Gregg C. Fonarow, MD
Eliot Corday Professor of Cardiovascular Medicine and Science
Director, Ahmanson–UCLA, Cardiomyopathy Center
Division of Cardiology
University of California at Los Angeles Medical Center
10833 Le Conte Avenue, CHS 47-123
Los Angeles, CA 90095, USA

E-mail address: gfonarow@mednet.ucla.edu

ELSEVIER
SAUNDERS

Heart Failure Clin 1 (2005) 1 – 9

HEART
FAILURE
CLINICS

Neurohormonal Upregulation in Heart Failure

W.H. Wilson Tang, MD[a,b,*], Gary S. Francis, MD[a,b]

[a]*Case Western Reserve University, Cleveland, OH, USA*
[b]*Cleveland Clinic Foundation, Cleveland, OH, USA*

There has been a major shift in the conceptual framework of the understanding of heart failure, from the simple notion of impairment of heart pump function to a more complex interplay between the inciting or predisposing events and the body's compensatory and defense mechanisms. The "neurohormonal hypothesis" began as a risky idea that could be tested thoroughly only in the field (ie, in the treatment of patients who have heart failure). The neurohormonal hypothesis has evolved partly from the remarkable clinical benefits of angiotensin-converting enzyme (ACE) inhibitors and beta-adrenergic antagonists observed in patients who have heart failure [1]. Many so-called "neurohormones" circulate in abnormal quantities in such patients (Box 1), but not all play a key role in heart failure. Moreover, most clinical studies of neurohormonal upregulation have focused on associations between the heart failure phenotype and peripheral blood neurohormonal levels that have highly variable concentrations. One could argue that the neurohormonal hypothesis has been too descriptive or more akin to phenomenology than science.

Although there is no direct proof of causality, the principles of "Koch's postulates" can be applied to several neurohormonal systems: (1) neurohormonal activation may occur early in the course of the illness, even at the asymptomatic stages, and upregulation may be caused by either pathogenic or counter-regulatory response; (2) infusion of some neurohormones (such as angiotensin II or epinephrine), at least in animal models, may lead to progression of the heart failure syndrome and cardiac dysfunction; (3) although the extent and clinical significance of neurohormonal activation varies widely from patient to patient, the overall trend of gradual activation occurs in several major neurohormonal pathways across the natural history of heart failure; and (4) therapies designed to block neurohormonal activation, such as ACE inhibitors and beta-adrenergic blockers, have had consistent favorable effects on the natural history of heart failure.

Complex neurohormonal systems that modulate vascular tone and salt and water retention are initially adaptive responses to cardiac insufficiency, possibly designed to preserve perfusion pressures. Although some systems may provide transient support to the failing heart by protecting blood pressure and blood volume by promoting sodium and water retention (eg, the adrenergic, renin–angiotensin–aldosterone, vasopressin, and endothelin systems), prolonged activation of neurohormones in most cases promotes disease progression by production of myocardial and vascular remodeling and maladaptive loading conditions (Fig. 1). Some neurohormones, such as natriuretic peptides, may offset excessive vasopressive/volume-retaining effects to maintain cardiac homeostasis (so-called "counterregulatory hormones"). This balance is dynamic, and perhaps unique to each patient at a particular clinical setting, thus providing an endless permutation of neuroendocrine upregulation as detected in patients who

* Corresponding author. Section of Heart Failure and Cardiac Transplantation Medicine, Department of Cardiovascular Medicine, Cleveland Clinic Foundation, 9500 Euclid Avenue, Desk F25, Cleveland, OH 44195.
E-mail address: tangw@ccf.org (W.H.W. Tang).

1551-7136/05/$ – see front matter
doi:10.1016/j.hfc.2004.11.002

Box 1. Neurohormonal changes in heart failure

Norepinephrine
Epinephrine
Dopamine
Endothelin
Arginine vasopressin
Renin
Angiotensin II
Aldosterone
Neuropeptide Y
Atrial natriuretic peptide
B-type natriuretic peptide
C-type natriuretic peptide
Adrenomedullin
Urodilantin
Urotensin II
Cardiotropin I
Bradykinin
Apelin
Periostin

have acute and chronic heart failure. Nevertheless, prolonged activation of neurohormones is associated often with adverse clinical outcomes in patients who have heart failure [2].

This article provides a brief overview of the major neurohormonal systems (excluding inflammatory cytokines) that are involved in the pathophysiology of heart failure and cardiomyopathy.

The adrenergic nervous system

It has been recognized since the days of Starling that patients who have heart failure often manifest signs and symptoms of hyperadrenergic states, such as tachycardia, vascular constriction, diaphoresis, and oliguria. Increased central sympathetic nerve outflow occurs in such patients, and is associated with an increase in plasma norepinephrine [3]. The relationships between sympathetic overactivation and other neurohormonal systems are complex. In patients who have heart failure, several processes may lead to excessive sympathetic activity and progression of cardiac dysfunction: (1) increased neuronal release of norepinephrine [4], (2) decreased efficiency of neuronal norepinephrine reuptake [4], (3) chronically increased central norepinephrine turnover [5], (4) excessive sympathetic nerve firing (as measured by increased cardiac norepinephrine spillover rate) [6], and (5) increased adrenal medullary activity leading to increase in epinephrine production (excessive epinephrine release usually occurs only in the setting of acute stress, as in acute pulmonary edema or severe end-stage heart failure).

Furthermore, excessive local sympathetic drive to the heart in patients who have heart failure is likely responsible for downregulation of the β_1-adrenocep-

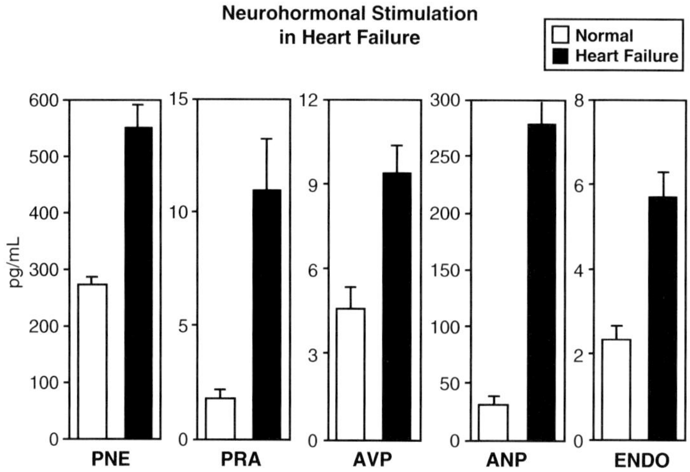

Fig. 1. Neurohormal stimulation in heart failure. (*From* Francis GS, Benedict C, Johnstone DE, et al. Comparison of neuroendocrine activation in patients with left ventricular dysfunction with and without congestive heart failure. A substudy of the Studies of Left Ventricular Dysfunction (SOLVD). Circulation 1990;82:1724–9; with permission.)

tor and perhaps uncoupling of the β_2-adrenoceptor, often without affecting the myocytes' response to calcium [7]. This presumably "protective" receptor-downregulation process of the failing myocardium may prevent toxic adrenergic stimulation.

Research studies have suggested consistently that resting plasma levels of norepinephrine [8] and cardiac norepinephrine spillover rates [9] provide prognostic information. Clinically, surrogate measures such as heart rate, sweating, and skin temperature are relied upon to determine the adrenergic state [8,10]. Nevertheless, there is a wide spectrum of adrenergic overactivation in heart failure, and up to 70% of patients may tolerate some degree of antiadrenergic therapy [11]. Autonomic dysfunction such as impaired sympathetic response to vasodilation or orthostatic stress is common in heart failure, and is also indicative of a poor prognosis [12]. The circulating norepinephrine is enhanced, whereas the myocardial norepinephrine content is depleted and the β_1-adrenoceptor density diminished.

The advent of β-adrenergic blocker therapy has provided new ideas opposed to the old doctrine that any interference with the circulatory and inotropic support provided by the upregulated adrenergic drive would lead to devastating consequences. Several large-scale clinical studies have confirmed the clinical benefits of antiadrenergic therapy across the spectrum of chronic heart failure [13–16].

Nevertheless, there are several unresolved questions regarding the potential differences between comprehensive (β_1-, β_2-, and α_1-) versus selective (β_1-adrenoreceptor) antiadrenergic blockade [17]. Theoretically, blockade of β_2-adrenoceptors may facilitate peripheral vasoconstriction and bronchoconstriction and could be deleterious. On the other hand, β_2-adrenoceptor blockade could be advantageous either by more effectively protecting the cardiac myocyte from catecholamine excess and reducing neuronal exocytosis, or by preventing catecholamine-induced hypokalemia.

Nevertheless, the β_1- and not the β_2 -adrenoceptors subserve most toxic effects of catecholamine excess. Additional blockade of α_1-adrenoceptors may provide further peripheral vasodilator actions, thereby providing optimal myocardial, metabolic, and hemodynamic benefits. This hypothesis is supported by the recent results from the Carvedilol or Metoprolol European Trial (COMET), showing a significant clinical benefit when patients were treated with carvedilol (β_1-, β_2-, and α_1-) versus metoprolol tartrate (β_1-specific) [18]. The quantitative contribution of β_2- and α_1-blockade to clinical improvement is not entirely understood, however.

The renin–angiotensin–aldosterone system

As with the sympathetic nervous system, the renin–angiotensin–aldosterone system (RAAS) is activated in patients who have heart failure. It is often difficult to detect RAAS upregulation in patients who have minimal symptoms, however [10]. As heart failure progresses, there are profound incremental changes in circulating renin, angiotensin II, and aldosterone. Furthermore, it is beginning to be understood that this is a dynamic system, and pharmacologic inhibition at one point of the pathway may not deter the evolution of "escape" pathways within the system, leading to persistent activation of angiotensin II and aldosterone receptors despite the "blockade" [19].

Renin release is stimulated by processes commonly found in patients who have heart failure: (1) decreased perfusion to the kidney sensed by a reduction in the renal tubular concentrations of sodium and chloride ions in the macula densa, (2) increased activity of the sympathetic nervous system, (3) chronic diuretic use, and (4) restricted dietary sodium. Renin interacts with the conversion of angiotensinogen to produce angiotensin I in the brain, the liver, and the blood vessels. Angiotensin II is then produced from local and systemic conversion from angiotensin I by way of the ACE that is the target for pharmacologic inhibition. Angiotensin II is a potent vasoconstrictor through its action on type-1 (AT_1) receptors, and also can act on the adrenal cortex to release aldosterone, a mineralocorticoid with potent sodium-retentive properties. Furthermore, investigators recently have uncovered several non-ACE pathways in the RAAS that may affect the balance between these different peptides at different times of treatment. Although the concept of tissue-specific angiotensin-II and aldosterone expression in the pathophysiology of heart failure is attractive, direct evidence that tissue activity is important in clinical disease has been difficult to prove.

Clinical observations regarding RAAS facilitation are complex. Serum ACE activity often is heightened in patients who have heart failure [20]. In a subset of patients, however, systemic RAAS activation cannot be detected by neurohormonal levels. In general, excessive adrenergic nervous system activity and increased RAAS activity are believed to contribute to progressive remodeling of the left ventricle, and may facilitate the transformation from hypertrophy to failure. The effectiveness of ACE inhibitors is related partly to their ability to block excessive angiotensin-II activity, thus reducing some of the pathoexcitatory drive and diminishing the hypokalemic and hypomagnesemic effects of aldosterone in the kidney. ACE-inhibitor therapy also increases local concentrations of bradykinin, which may have antiremodeling effects in the heart and contributes to vasodilation. Sustained dose-dependent reductions of serum ACE activity can be measured in patients who have heart failure treated with ACE inhibitors [20].

Despite reductions in plasma aldosterone and serum angiotensin-II levels following ACE inhibitor initiation, however, levels may rise slowly in some patients, presumably as a result of the production of angiotensin II through non-ACE pathways (kinins and chymases) (Fig. 2) [20]. This "escape" phenomenon has been the basis for the development of therapy using direct AT_1-receptor blockers (ARBs) and selective aldosterone antagonists [19]. ARBs are used primarily in ACE inhibitor–intolerant patients [21,22]. Adding an ARB to an ACE inhibitor in persistently symptomatic patients, however, may derive additional benefit. For example, in the CHARM-Added study, the addition of candesartan to standard ACE-inhibitor therapy has provided additional cardiovascular morbidity and mortality benefit in some patients who have heart failure [23].

There also has been a renewed interest in the role of aldosterone in the pathophysiology of heart failure. Since its discovery 50 years ago, the various actions of aldosterone in the cardiovascular system are understood better; many are involved intricately in the progression of heart failure and cardiomyopathy [24]. Although most aldosterone actions involve binding to minerocorticoid receptors that exert genomic effects on myocyte hypertrophy, myocardial metabolism, collagen turnover, and sodium homeostasis, nongenomic effects of aldosterone may exert vascular effects such as endothelial dysfunction [25–27]. This is evident in the recently published neurohormonal analysis from the Val-HeFT study, where treatment with the ARB valsartan resulted in the sustained reduction of plasma aldosterone levels, whereas the placebo group had a rising plasma aldosterone trend [28]. In patients who have heart failure or hypertensive heart disease, direct inhibition by spironolactone or eplerenone of the effects of aldosterone through its receptors leads to further regression of left ventricular mass [29], reduction in collagen turnover (leading to reduced myocardial fibrosis) [30], as well as improvement in clinical outcomes [31,32]. These effects are often synergistic with background ACE-inhibitor therapy, suggesting the importance of direct aldosterone blockade in the treatment of heart failure.

The vasopressin system

Vasopressin is released by the hypothalamus as a result of baroreceptor, osmotic, and neurohormonal stimuli. This hormone normally maintains body fluid balance, vascular tone, and regulates contractility

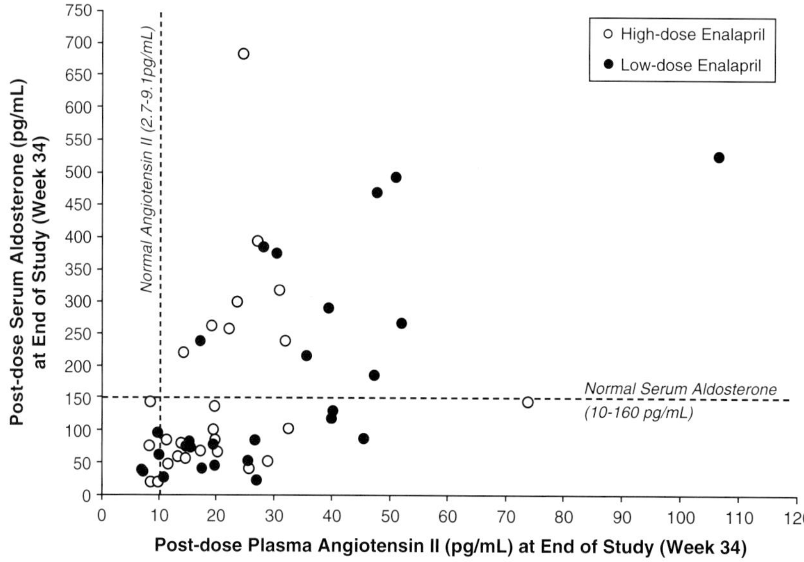

Fig. 2. Angiotensin II and aldosterone escape in patients who have heart failure treated with long-term ACE inhibitors. (*From* Tang WH, Vagelos RH, Yee YG, et al. Neurohormonal and clinical responses to high- versus low-dose enalapril therapy in chronic heart failure. J Am Coll Cardiol 2002;39:70–8; with permission.)

[33,34]. Although enhancement of vasopressin activity has not been found consistently in patients who have heart failure, there is a general trend for a gradual, incremental rise in plasma vasopressin levels as patients develop progressive cardiac dysfunction and overt heart failure [35].

The primary osmotic stimulus to vasopressin release is hyponatremia, whereas excessive diuresis, hypotension, and angiotensin II, as well as certain reflex control mechanisms, can act as important nonosmotic stimuli [36]. The nonosmotic stimulation of vasopressin release is probably more important in heart failure. Therefore, vasopressin levels do not correlate necessarily with serum sodium, plasma norepinephrine, or hemodynamic variables, and the role of this system in the pathogenesis of heart failure is not well understood [37].

Vasopressin upregulation is involved intricately as a response to volume-overloaded states and diuretic use [36]. Vasopressin promotes water retention as well as vasoconstriction by activating V_2 and V_{1A} receptors [34]. Activation of the V_{1A} receptors causes vasoconstriction of the peripheral vessels, enhancing platelet aggregation, and promotes adrenocorticotrophic-hormone stimulation. Activation of the V_2 receptors within the renal collecting duct promotes free-water retention by reducing clearance of free water. V_2 receptors also can be found in vascular tissue, where they subserve vasodilation in response to vasopressin. Experimental studies indicate that blockade of these receptors, alone or in combination, results in a beneficial hemodynamic profile [38]. Only V_{1A}-receptor blockade in animal models prevents remodeling, however [39]. For hyponatremic patients presenting with acute decompensated heart failure, pharmacologic blockade with tolvaptan (a selective V_2-receptor antagonist) after stabilization resulted in correction of hyponatremia and significant weight reduction from water loss compared with placebo [38,40,41]. Similar results have been observed with dual V_{1A}/V_2-receptor blockers [38]. Hyponatremia improves as well. Several drugs in this class are being tested as adjunctive therapy in patients admitted for decompensated heart failure or who have hyponatremia [37,42].

The endothelin system

Endothelin is a family of 21–amino acid peptides that arise from multiple sources within the cardiovascular system. These peptides promote vasoconstriction, inflammation, fibrosis, and hypertrophy in the pulmonary and systemic vasculature. There are three known isoforms that share common receptors with different affinities: endothelin 1 (ET-1), endothelin 2 (ET-2), and endothelin 3 (ET-3). Only ET-1 is synthesized by vascular endothelial cells. There are at least two endothelin receptors, ET_A and ET_B, that mediate biologic actions. ET_A receptors bind ET-1 and ET-2 with higher affinity than ET-3. ET_A stimulation leads primarily to vasoconstriction. In contrast, ET_B receptors bind all three endothelin peptides with relatively equal affinities, and mediate vasodilation as well as clearance of circulating ET-1. Both receptors may mediate pathologic hypertrophy and fibrosis.

In addition to potent vasoconstrictive and mitogenic effects on vascular smooth muscle cells, ET-1 acts on endothelial cells in an autocrine fashion to induce the release of nitric oxide and prostacyclin. Furthermore, ET-1 has numerous effects on various tissues, including stimulation of the secretion of natriuretic peptides and aldosterone, as well as inhibition of renin release and potent positive inotropic effects on the heart. Therefore, mice deficient in ET-1 often developed elevated blood pressures. Based on these findings, it has been suggested that endothelin has a role in maintaining the homeostasis of the circulatory system and may be important in the pathogenesis of various cardiovascular disorders, such as hypertension, heart failure, vasospasm, and atherosclerosis. In addition to its effects on circulatory homeostasis, endothelin may have important functions in the regulation of contractility when released from the endothelial lining of the heart.

Plasma ET-1 levels are elevated in patients who have cardiomyopathy or chronic heart failure, and correlate with severity and prognosis. In particular, the degree of plasma elevation of endothelin correlates with the magnitude of alterations in cardiac hemodynamics and functional class. Because endothelin is associated with pressure-overload hypertrophy, it may be important in the development of progressive left ventricular remodeling. ET_A-receptor blockers prevent cardiac hypertrophy in the face of hemodynamic overload. Acute administration of the endothelin-receptor antagonist, such as bosentan or tezosentan, improves hemodynamics in patients who have advanced heart failure [43,44]. Long-term clinical benefits of endothelin-receptor blockade have not been realized in several large-scale clinical trials, however [45–47], and the reasons are unclear [48]. Bosentan, when given chronically to patients who have heart failure, promotes salt and water retention with edema and weight gain. Recent evidence suggests that in patients who have heart failure, there is either increased secretion or reduced clearance of

ET-1 in the pulmonary circulation in response to congestion [49,50]. This may be why there are significant clinical benefits with endothelin-receptor antagonists in patients presenting with primary pulmonary hypertension but not in systolic heart failure per se.

The natriuretic peptide system

The discovery of the natriuretic peptide system has led to an intrinsic counterregulatory system that responds to the excessive vasopressive/volume-retaining neurohormonal systems in heart failure [51]. The most widely studied natriuretic peptides include atrial natriuretic factor (ANF or ANP) and B-type natriuretic peptide (BNP); both are released from the atria and ventricles in response to heightened ventricular wall stress. They are "counter-regulatory" because they promote vasodilation and, in some cases, a modest diuresis and natriuresis through activation of cyclic guanosine monophosphate (cGMP). They also offset excessive sympathetic nervous system and RAAS activity [52,53].

The exact mechanisms responsible for regulating synthesis, release, and clearance of the natriuretic peptides are not known [54]. The secretion patterns of ANP and BNP may vary with underlying cardiac disorders [55], and with genetic variability [56]. Several different molecular forms of ANP have been isolated, but α-ANP represents the major circulating form in humans. Synthesis of ANP occurs predominantly in the atria, where right atrial stretch seems to be an important stimulus for release. Neutral endopeptidases (NEPs), which are concentrated highly in the proximal tubule brush border of the kidney, are responsible for degradation of ANP. By contrast, BNP mRNA is synthesized in bursts in response to myocardial wall stress and then is transcribed into a 108–amino acid precursor protein, proBNP, that coexists with ANP in the same secretory granules of myocytes. ProBNP then is cleaved at the time of its secretion by corin to form BNP and its biologically inactive by-product, N-terminal proBNP (NT-proBNP). Unlike ANP, a long-term stimulus generally is required to increase plasma BNP or NT-proBNP concentration. Upon release, BNP (but not NT-proBNP) exerts its biologic effects through the A-type and B-type cGMP-mediated receptors. It is cleared by C-type receptors and NEPs, particularly along the brush border of the kidney, although some also may be degraded by NEPs.

Like many neuropeptides, ANP and BNP are released progressively into the circulation during the transition from asymptomatic left ventricular dysfunction to overt heart failure [54]. Neither ANP nor BNP genes are expressed fully until late in embryonic life and after birth, but cease in adulthood. There is heightened expression of the ANP and BNP genes in myocardium during hypertrophy and cardiomyopathy, however. Therefore, it is believed that this re-emergence of the fetal capacity to synthesize ANP in the setting of ventricular overload in hypertrophy is an adaptive response that maintains volume homeostasis in response to the progressively failing circulation (so-called "fetal gene programming").

The diagnostic usefulness of plasma BNP in patients who have symptomatic heart failure is based on observations by many investigators, and has been confirmed recently by several large multicenter clinical trials [57–59]. In the Emergency Department, plasma BNP or NT-proBNP in the normal range virtually exclude the diagnosis of heart failure as the cause of acute dyspnea. In contrast, high plasma-BNP levels are associated with the syndrome of heart failure and consistently relate to a poor prognosis, making it an important diagnostic and prognostic tool in the everyday management of heart failure [60]. Nevertheless, some patients who have advanced but stable heart failure may demonstrate normal plasma-BNP levels [61], making sequential monitoring with natriuretic peptides complex.

ANF and BNP seem to have important vasodilator, antihypertrophic, and antifibrotic properties. They can attenuate neuroendocrine activation (such as sympathetic overactivation or aldosterone secretion), reduce myocardial interstitial matrix synthesis, and promote natriuresis [52]. Based on these properties, nesiritide, a human synthetic BNP, is approved in the United States as an infusion therapy for acute heart failure [62], and a human synthetic ANP, carperitide, is being tested in clinical trials for similar indications. Although NEP inhibitors were potentially an important therapy for heart failure and hypertension, several studies using the hybrid drug omapatrilat (a NEP-ACE inhibitor) have yielded disappointing results in heart failure [63].

Other novel neurohormonal systems

The search for novel neurohormonal systems specific for heart failure continues, particularly with the help of genetic sequencing and identification. Adrenomedullin is a newly discovered vasodilating and natriuretic peptide that may have some role in the regulation of cardiorenal homeostasis [64,65]. Plasma concentrations of adrenomedullin are increased in patients who have heart failure [66], and the peptide is present in the human heart through immunoactive staining [67]. Plasma adrenomedullin levels correlate with pulmonary artery pressure and pulmonary capillary wedge pressure [65]. The precise role, if any, that adrenomedullin plays in the pathogenesis of heart failure is unknown [68]. Several other new neurohormones (eg, apelin [69], urotensin II [70], cardiotropin-1 [71], urocortin [72], and periostin [73], to name a few) have emerged in the literature, and likely will be evaluated rigorously as potential therapeutic targets.

Summary

The discovery of neurohormonal activation in chronic heart failure, like most major discoveries, was partially serendipitous. Nevertheless, by altering the natural biologic responses that are involved in the pathophysiology of heart failure, neurohormonal blockade has been an important foundation of several drugs in treating heart failure. The current approach is naïve, however. Titrating drug after drug to achieve the maximal responses fails to recognize that wide individual variations of neurohormonal upregulation exist, and, in some cases, oversuppression of neurohormonal systems may lead to adverse consequences.

The difficult and complex challenges that result are how to use these neurohormonal antagonists together more effectively, and how to embrace new and promising drugs that act on other neurohormonal systems. One way to advance the understanding is to challenge the axiom that patients who have heart failure share the same degree and sequence of neurohormonal upregulation. Clinical trials are underway to treat patients who have cardiac dysfunction with antiadrenergic blockers before ACE inhibitors (eg, CIBIS-III). Much work is in progress to look at genetic predispositions of treatment responses and the pharmacogenetic impact of neurohormonal upregulation, particularly in the area of genetic polymorphisms. It may be possible someday to develop effective strategies to individualize a patient's regimen of neurohomornal antagonists based on profiling one's neurohormonal upregulation.

References

[1] Packer M. The neurohormonal hypothesis: a theory to explain the mechanism of disease progression in heart failure. J Am Coll Cardiol 1992;20:248–54.

[2] Latini R, Masson S, Anand I, et al. The comparative prognostic value of plasma neurohormones at baseline in patients with heart failure enrolled in Val-HeFT. Eur Heart J 2004;25:292–9.

[3] Chidsey CA, Braunwald E, Morrow AG. Catecholamine excretion and cardiac stores of norepinephrine in congestive heart failure. Am J Med 1965;39:442–51.

[4] Eisenhofer G, Friberg P, Rundqvist B, et al. Cardiac sympathetic nerve function in congestive heart failure. Circulation 1996;93:1667–76.

[5] Lambert GW, Kaye DM, Lefkovits J, et al. Increased central nervous system monoamine neurotransmitter turnover and its association with sympathetic nervous activity in treated heart failure patients. Circulation 1995;92:1813–8.

[6] Meredith IT, Eisenhofer G, Lambert GW, et al. Cardiac sympathetic nervous activity in congestive heart failure. Evidence for increased neuronal norepinephrine release and preserved neuronal uptake. Circulation 1993;88:136–45.

[7] Bristow MR, Hershberger RE, Port JD, et al. Beta-adrenergic pathways in nonfailing and failing human ventricular myocardium. Circulation 1990;82:112–25.

[8] Cohn JN, Levine TB, Olivari MT, et al. Plasma norepinephrine as a guide to prognosis in patients with chronic congestive heart failure. N Engl J Med 1984;311:819–23.

[9] Kaye DM, Lefkovits J, Jennings GL, et al. Adverse consequences of high sympathetic nervous activity in the failing human heart. J Am Coll Cardiol 1995;26:1257–63.

[10] Francis GS, Benedict C, Johnstone DE, et al. Comparison of neuroendocrine activation in patients with left ventricular dysfunction with and without congestive heart failure. A substudy of the Studies of Left Ventricular Dysfunction (SOLVD). Circulation 1990;82:1724–9.

[11] Gupta R, Tang WH, Young JB. Patterns of beta-blocker utilization in patients with chronic heart failure: experience from a specialized outpatient heart failure clinic. Am Heart J 2004;147:79–83.

[12] Olivari MT, Levine TB, Cohn JN. Abnormal neurohumoral response to nitroprusside infusion in congestive heart failure. J Am Coll Cardiol 1983;2:411–7.

[13] The Cardiac Insufficiency Bisoprolol Study II (CIBIS-II): a randomised trial. Lancet 1999;353:9–13.

[14] Effect of metoprolol CR/XL in chronic heart failure: metoprolol CR/XL Randomised Intervention Trial in Congestive Heart Failure (MERIT-HF). Lancet 1999;353(9169):2001–7.

[15] Packer M, Bristow MR, Cohn JN, et al. The effect of carvedilol on morbidity and mortality in patients with chronic heart failure. US Carvedilol Heart Failure Study Group. N Engl J Med 1996;334:1349–55.

[16] Packer M, Fowler MB, Roecker EB, et al. Effect of carvedilol on the morbidity of patients with severe chronic heart failure: results of the carvedilol prospective randomized cumulative survival (COPERNICUS) study. Circulation 2002;106:2194–9.

[17] Tang WH, Militello M, Francis GS. In heart failure, all beta-blockers are not necessarily equal. Cleve Clin J Med 2003;70:1081–7.
[18] Poole-Wilson PA, Swedberg K, Cleland JG, et al. Comparison of carvedilol and metoprolol on clinical outcomes in patients with chronic heart failure in the Carvedilol Or Metoprolol European Trial (COMET): randomised controlled trial. Lancet 2003;362:7–13.
[19] Struthers AD. The clinical implications of aldosterone escape in congestive heart failure. Eur J Heart Fail 2004;6:539–45.
[20] Tang WH, Vagelos RH, Yee YG, et al. Neurohormonal and clinical responses to high- versus low-dose enalapril therapy in chronic heart failure. J Am Coll Cardiol 2002;39:70–8.
[21] Cohn JN, Tognoni G. A randomized trial of the angiotensin-receptor blocker valsartan in chronic heart failure. N Engl J Med 2001;345:1667–75.
[22] Granger CB, McMurray JJ, Yusuf S, et al. Effects of candesartan in patients with chronic heart failure and reduced left-ventricular systolic function intolerant to angiotensin-converting-enzyme inhibitors: the CHARM-Alternative trial. Lancet 2003;362:772–6.
[23] McMurray JJ, Ostergren J, Swedberg K, et al. Effects of candesartan in patients with chronic heart failure and reduced left-ventricular systolic function taking angiotensin-converting-enzyme inhibitors: the CHARM-Added trial. Lancet 2003;362:767–71.
[24] Williams JS, Williams GH. 50th anniversary of aldosterone. J Clin Endocrinol Metab 2003;88:2364–72.
[25] Farquharson CA, Struthers AD. Spironolactone increases nitric oxide bioactivity, improves endothelial vasodilator dysfunction, and suppresses vascular angiotensin I/angiotensin II conversion in patients with chronic heart failure. Circulation 2000;101:594–7.
[26] Macdonald JE, Kennedy N, Struthers AD. Effects of spironolactone on endothelial function, vascular angiotensin converting enzyme activity, and other prognostic markers in patients with mild heart failure already taking optimal treatment. Heart 2004;90:765–70.
[27] Schafer A, Fraccarollo D, Hildemann SK, et al. Addition of the selective aldosterone receptor antagonist eplerenone to ACE inhibition in heart failure: effect on endothelial dysfunction. Cardiovasc Res 2003;58:655–62.
[28] Cohn JN, Anand IS, Latini R, et al. Sustained reduction of aldosterone in response to the angiotensin receptor blocker valsartan in patients with chronic heart failure: results from the Valsartan Heart Failure Trial. Circulation 2003;108:1306–9.
[29] Pitt B, Reichek N, Willenbrock R, et al. Effects of eplerenone, enalapril, and eplerenone/enalapril in patients with essential hypertension and left ventricular hypertrophy: the 4E-left ventricular hypertrophy study. Circulation 2003;108:1831–8.
[30] Zannad F, Alla F, Dousset B, et al. Limitation of excessive extracellular matrix turnover may contribute to survival benefit of spironolactone therapy in patients with congestive heart failure: insights from the randomized aldactone evaluation study (RALES). Rales Investigators. Circulation 2000;102:2700–6.
[31] Pitt B, Remme W, Zannad F, et al. Eplerenone, a selective aldosterone blocker, in patients with left ventricular dysfunction after myocardial infarction. N Engl J Med 2003;348:1309–21.
[32] Pitt B, Zannad F, Remme WJ, et al. The effect of spironolactone on morbidity and mortality in patients with severe heart failure. Randomized Aldactone Evaluation Study Investigators. N Engl J Med 1999; 341:709–17.
[33] Goldsmith SR. Congestive heart failure: potential role of arginine vasopressin antagonists in the therapy of heart failure. Congest Heart Fail 2002;8:251–6.
[34] Lee CR, Watkins ML, Patterson JH, et al. Vasopressin: a new target for the treatment of heart failure. Am Heart J 2003;146:9–18.
[35] Benedict CR, Johnstone DE, Weiner DH, et al. Relation of neurohumoral activation to clinical variables and degree of ventricular dysfunction: a report from the Registry of Studies of Left Ventricular Dysfunction. SOLVD Investigators. J Am Coll Cardiol 1994;23:1410–20.
[36] Schrier RW, Cadnapaphornchai MA, Umenishi F. Water-losing and water-retaining states: role of water channels and vasopressin receptor antagonists. Heart Dis 2001;3:210–4.
[37] Francis GS, Tang WH. Vasopressin receptor antagonists: will the "vaptans" fulfill their promise? JAMA 2004;291:2017–8.
[38] Udelson JE, Smith WB, Hendrix GH, et al. Acute hemodynamic effects of conivaptan, a dual V(1A) and V(2) vasopressin receptor antagonist, in patients with advanced heart failure. Circulation 2001; 104:2417–23.
[39] Van Kerckhoven R, Lankhuizen I, van Veghel R, et al. Chronic vasopressin V(1A) but not V(2) receptor antagonism prevents heart failure in chronically infarcted rats. Eur J Pharmacol 2002;449:135–41.
[40] Gheorghiade M, Gattis WA, O'Connor CM, et al. Effects of tolvaptan, a vasopressin antagonist, in patients hospitalized with worsening heart failure: a randomized controlled trial. JAMA 2004;291: 1963–71.
[41] Gheorghiade M, Niazi I, Ouyang J, et al. Vasopressin V2-receptor blockade with tolvaptan in patients with chronic heart failure: results from a double-blind, randomized trial. Circulation 2003;107:2690–6.
[42] Costello-Boerrigter LC, Boerrigter G, Burnett Jr JC. Revisiting salt and water retention: new diuretics, aquaretics, and natriuretics. Med Clin North Am 2003; 87:475–91.
[43] Rich S, McLaughlin VV. Endothelin receptor blockers in cardiovascular disease. Circulation 2003;108:2184.
[44] Teerlink JR. The role of endothelin in the pathogenesis of heart failure. Curr Cardiol Rep 2002;4:206–12.
[45] Anand I, McMurray J, Cohn JN, et al. Long-term effects of darusentan on left-ventricular remodelling

and clinical outcomes in the EndothelinA Receptor Antagonist Trial in Heart Failure (EARTH): randomised, double-blind, placebo-controlled trial. Lancet 2004;364:347–54.

[46] Kalra PR, Moon JC, Coats AJ. Do results of the ENABLE (Endothelin Antagonist Bosentan for Lowering Cardiac Events in Heart Failure) study spell the end for non-selective endothelin antagonism in heart failure? Int J Cardiol 2002;85:195–7.

[47] Luscher TF, Enseleit F, Pacher R, et al. Hemodynamic and neurohumoral effects of selective endothelin A (ET(A)) receptor blockade in chronic heart failure: the Heart Failure ET(A) Receptor Blockade Trial (HEAT). Circulation 2002;106:2666–72.

[48] Spieker LE, Luscher TF. Will endothelin receptor antagonists have a role in heart failure? Med Clin North Am 2003;87:459–74.

[49] Staniloae C, Dupuis J, White M, et al. Reduced pulmonary clearance of endothelin in congestive heart failure: a marker of secondary pulmonary hypertension. J Card Fail 2004;10:427–32.

[50] von Lueder TG, Kjekshus H, Edvardsen T, et al. Mechanisms of elevated plasma endothelin-1 in CHF: congestion increases pulmonary synthesis and secretion of endothelin-1. Cardiovasc Res 2004;63:41–50.

[51] Rodeheffer RJ. Measuring plasma B-type natriuretic peptide in heart failure: good to go in 2004? J Am Coll Cardiol 2004;44:740–9.

[52] D'Souza SP, Davis M, Baxter GF. Autocrine and paracrine actions of natriuretic peptides in the heart. Pharmacol Ther 2004;101:113–29.

[53] Luchner A, Schunkert H. Interactions between the sympathetic nervous system and the cardiac natriuretic peptide system. Cardiovasc Res 2004;63:443–9.

[54] Goetze JP. Biochemistry of pro-B-type natriuretic peptide-derived peptides: the endocrine heart revisited. Clin Chem 2004;50:1503–10.

[55] Luchner A, Stevens TL, Borgeson DD, et al. Differential atrial and ventricular expression of myocardial BNP during evolution of heart failure. Am J Physiol 1998;274:H1684–9.

[56] Wang TJ, Larson MG, Levy D, et al. Heritability and genetic linkage of plasma natriuretic peptide levels. Circulation 2003;108:13–6.

[57] Maisel A, Hollander JE, Guss D, et al. Primary results of the Rapid Emergency Department Heart Failure Outpatient Trial (REDHOT): a multicenter study of B-type natriuretic peptide levels, emergency department decision making, and outcomes in patients presenting with shortness of breath. J Am Coll Cardiol 2004;44:1328–33.

[58] Maisel AS, Krishnaswamy P, Nowak RM, et al. Rapid measurement of B-type natriuretic peptide in the emergency diagnosis of heart failure. N Engl J Med 2002;347:161–7.

[59] Mueller C, Scholer A, Laule-Kilian K, et al. Use of B-type natriuretic peptide in the evaluation and management of acute dyspnea. N Engl J Med 2004;350:647–54.

[60] Young JB, Correia NG, Francis GS, et al. Testing for B-type natriuretic peptide in the diagnosis and assessment of heart failure: what are the nuances? Cleve Clin J Med 2004;71(Suppl 5):S1–17.

[61] Tang WH, Girod JP, Lee MJ, et al. Plasma B-type natriuretic peptide levels in ambulatory patients with established chronic symptomatic systolic heart failure. Circulation 2003;108:2964–6.

[62] Intravenous nesiritide vs nitroglycerin for treatment of decompensated congestive heart failure: a randomized controlled trial. JAMA 2002;287:1531–40.

[63] Packer M, Califf RM, Konstam MA, et al. Comparison of omapatrilat and enalapril in patients with chronic heart failure: the Omapatrilat Versus Enalapril Randomized Trial of Utility in Reducing Events (OVERTURE). Circulation 2002;106:920–6.

[64] Cheung BM, Li CY, Wong LY. Adrenomedullin: its role in the cardiovascular system. Semin Vasc Med 2004;4:129–34.

[65] Lainchbury JG. Novel neurohumoral factors in congestive heart failure: adrenomedullin. Curr Cardiol Rep 2001;3:208–14.

[66] Kobayashi K, Kitamura K, Etoh T, et al. Increased plasma adrenomedullin levels in chronic congestive heart failure. Am Heart J 1996;131:994–8.

[67] Baumer AT, Schumann C, Cremers B, et al. Gene expression of adrenomedullin in failing myocardium: comparison to atrial natriuretic peptide. J Appl Physiol 2002;92:1058–63.

[68] Bunton DC, Petrie MC, Hillier C, et al. The clinical relevance of adrenomedullin: a promising profile? Pharmacol Ther 2004;103:179–201.

[69] Chen MM, Ashley EA, Deng DX, et al. Novel role for the potent endogenous inotrope apelin in human cardiac dysfunction. Circulation 2003;108:1432–9.

[70] Richards AM, Nicholls MG, Lainchbury JG, et al. Plasma urotensin II in heart failure. Lancet 2002;360:545–6.

[71] Bristow MR, Long CS. Cardiotrophin-1 in heart failure. Circulation 2002;106:1430–2.

[72] Bale TL, Hoshijima M, Gu Y, et al. The cardiovascular physiologic actions of urocortin II: acute effects in murine heart failure. Proc Natl Acad Sci USA 2004;101:3697–702.

[73] Katsuragi N, Morishita R, Nakamura N, et al. Periostin as a novel factor responsible for ventricular dilation. Circulation 2004;110:1806–13.

ELSEVIER
SAUNDERS

Heart Failure Clin 1 (2005) 11 – 23

HEART
FAILURE
CLINICS

Neurohormonal Activation in Populations Susceptible to Heart Failure

Johan Ärnlöv, MD, PhD[a,b], Ramachandran S. Vasan, MD[a,c,*]

[a]*National Heart, Lung, and Blood Institute's Framingham Heart Study, Framingham, MA, USA*
[b]*Uppsala University, Uppsala, Sweden*
[c]*Boston University School of Medicine, Boston, MA, USA*

During the course of evolution, life forms moved from an aquatic to a terrestrial environment and a need for salt conservation arose. The neurohormonal defense systems that evolved to ensure salt and circulatory homeostasis have been essential for survival. For instance, the renin–angiotensin–aldosterone system (RAAS) played a fundamental role in promoting water and sodium retention, and in facilitating potassium excretion in prehistoric humans, hunter-gatherers who consumed a diet high in potassium and who were prone to death from hemorrhage or diarrhea [1]. As our living conditions have changed over millions of years, however, the need for salt conservation has diminished and the neurohormonal systems essential to survival in prehistoric times may become maladaptive under select circumstances. Consequently, the term *neurohormonal activation* often has a negative connotation, despite it being a mechanism essential for species preservation under some conditions.

This article focuses on the adverse effects of neurohormonal activation, acknowledging that it is a double-edged phenomenon. Several neurohormonal systems are activated in patients who have congestive heart failure (CHF), regardless of its etiology [2], but less is known about neurohormonal activation earlier in the cardiovascular disease continuum (ie, development of risk factors and subclinical disease). This article reviews the role of neurohormonal factors in the pathogenesis of high blood pressure, left ventricular (LV) hypertrophy, and preclinical CHF in the community (Fig. 1). The authors define neurohormonal activation, trace the contributions of relevant pathways to the development of subclinical LV dysfunction and CHF, and summarize data on the evolution of neurohormonal antagonism (or potentiation in the case of select factors such as the natriuretic peptides) as a therapeutic tool to prevent CHF.

There is no consensus on how to define "neurohormones," and the phrase "neurohormonal activation" is somewhat inaccurate. Rather than having an exclusive endocrine effect, several of the classical neurohormones (eg, angiotensin or norepinephrine) are synthesized locally in the myocardium and vascular endothelium, and exert autocrine or paracrine effects on the heart and the vasculature [3,4]. Considerable knowledge of neurohormonal activation in clinical settings is based on circulating levels of these hormones, rather than on their activity in the tissues. Accordingly, this article focuses on clinical studies that have evaluated circulating levels of neurohormones, and does not review all aspects of activation of different neurohormonal systems before the onset of CHF. The roles of the RAAS, catecholamines, endothelins, and the natriuretic peptides are

This article was supported by a Bergmarks travel grant, Viking Björks Hedersledamotstipendium, a Capio travel grant, and National Heart, Lung, and Blood Institute grants N01-HC-25195 and 2K24 HL04334.

* Corresponding author. Cardiology Section, Preventive Medicine and Epidemiology, Department of Medicine, Boston University School of Medicine, 715 Albany Street, E-113, Boston, MA 02118.

E-mail address: Vasan@bu.edu (R.S. Vasan).

1551-7136/05/$ – see front matter
doi:10.1016/j.hfc.2004.11.003

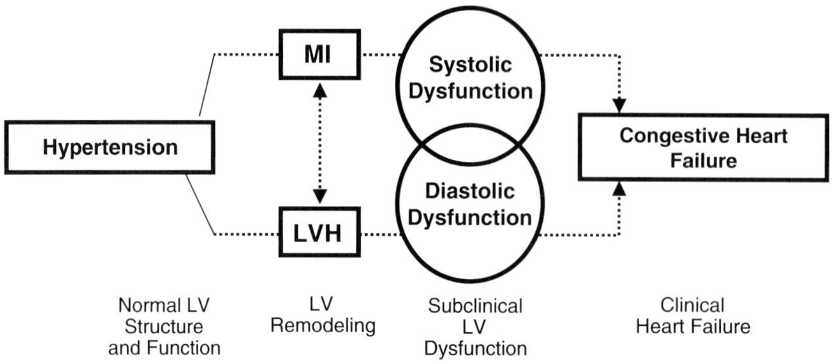

Fig. 1. Overview of the natural history of congestive heart failure. LVH, left ventricular hypertrophy; MI, myocardial infarction. (*Adapted from* Vasan RS, Levy D. The role of hypertension in the pathogenesis of heart failure. A clinical mechanistic overview. Arch Intern Med 1996;156(16):1789–96; with permission.)

discussed in populations especially susceptible to developing CHF, such as individuals who have hypertension, LV hypertrophy, and asymptomatic LV dysfunction, and post–myocardial infarction patients.

The authors' framework for evaluating evidence relating neurohormonal activation to the development of risk factors and preclinical CHF categorizes studies into the following three groups (with hierarchical increase in the level of evidence indicating a causal role):

1. Cross-sectional studies that demonstrate an association but do not establish causality;
2. Longitudinal investigations that suggest causality by establishing temporal associations; and
3. Treatment reports that support causality by demonstrating a diminution in disease risk with neurohormonal antagonism (or potentiation). (See article by Yusuf and colleagues elsewhere in this issue for treatment effects in populations at high risk for heart failure.)

Neurohormonal contributions to the development of and activation in hypertension

Broadly, four types of studies have been conducted relating neurohormones to the pathogenesis of high blood pressure. Cross-sectional studies have related plasma neurohormone levels to blood pressure levels in hypertensives and nonhypertensives. A few investigators have evaluated the longitudinal relations of plasma neurohormones to the incidence of high blood pressure and to blood pressure tracking. Other studies have related genetic variations in select candidate genes of neurohormonal pathways to the prevalence of hypertension (not discussed in this article). Finally, investigators have evaluated the effect of neurohormonal antagonism on lowering blood pressure levels in hypertensive patients and the role of such antagonism in preventing morbidity and mortality caused by CHF.

Cross-sectional studies

Renin–angiotensin–aldosterone system

Considerable experimental evidence demonstrates that the RAAS plays a major role in blood pressure homeostasis. The importance of plasma levels of RAAS hormones in the development of hypertension is less well defined, however, perhaps because circulating RAAS components may serve only partly as indicators for the activation of the RAAS in the tissues [3]. Furthermore, the pathogenesis of essential hypertension is likely multifactorial, and isolating the contributions of a specific pathway to the incidence of the condition is challenging. A clear relation of activation of select components of the RAAS to high blood pressure has been noted in patients who have renal artery stenosis and in those who have primary hyperaldosteronism. On the other hand, activation of the RAAS may occur without the development of high blood pressure, as in Bartter's and Gitelman's syndromes [5].

Plasma renin levels reportedly are correlated inversely with blood pressure levels in some studies [6,7], but not correlated to blood pressure levels at all in other reports [8].

Plasma angiotensin-converting enzyme (ACE) activity was related to blood pressure in men but not in women in a large population-based sample [9]. In another study, plasma ACE levels were significantly higher in hypertensives compared with normotensives, and a modest correlation was observed between blood pressure levels and plasma ACE activity in untreated individuals [10].

Plasma angiotensin II levels were correlated positively with blood pressure [11] and were higher in hypertensives [12]. On the other hand, plasma angiotensin II had a significant negative correlation with ambulatory blood pressure in 574 individuals [6]. Other studies showed no relation between plasma angiotensin II levels and blood pressure [13,14].

Regarding plasma/serum aldosterone and hypertension, cross-sectional studies have yielded inconsistent results: high [14,15], low [6], and normal [16,17] values have been reported in hypertensives. In another report, serum aldosterone was related positively to blood pressure in obese but not in nonobese individuals [18].

Catecholamines

A role of catecholamine overproduction in pathogenesis of high blood pressure has been well established in patients who have pheochromocytoma [19]. Plasma levels of catecholamines have been used extensively as a marker for activation of sympathetic activation, although there are several limitations of this method for assessing sympathetic activation [4]. It is difficult to measure chronic sympathetic activation, especially organ-specific sympathetic activation [20], but numerous studies show that increased plasma levels of epinephrine and norepinephrine are seen early in hypertension, as well as in patients who have established hypertension [21].

Endothelin

Endothelin-1, a hormone primarily produced in the endothelium, is an important factor in the regulation of vascular tone, vascular remodeling, and vascular injury. Endothelin has been suggested to be important in the pathophysiology of hypertension in experimental animal models [22]. Other neurohormones, such as angiotensin II and norepinephrine, stimulate endothelin synthesis.

In clinical studies of hypertensive patients, circulating levels of endothelin were reported to be elevated in most [23–26] but not all [27] cross-sectional investigations. Ethnic differences in the role of endothelin in the development of hypertension have been suggested. For example, endothelin may contribute more to hypertension in blacks [28] because blacks more often have salt-sensitive hypertension, to which endothelin may contribute more [24,29].

The vasodilatory effect of endothelin-receptor blockade in patients who have essential hypertension but not in normotensive controls [30] supports the notion that the endothelin system is activated in hypertension.

Natriuretic peptides

Although the natriuretic peptides play a fundamental role in blood pressure regulation through salt and water homeostasis [31], there are conflicting findings regarding the relations of blood pressure levels to plasma concentrations of these peptides. Cross-sectional studies have shown positive [32–35], inverse [36,37], and no correlations [38,39] between plasma natriuretic peptide levels and blood pressure. Other investigators have reported no relations of the natriuretic peptides to blood pressure levels in patients who have hypertension and a normal LV geometry [40]. Thus, the conflicting findings in cross-sectional reports may be confounded by differences in the prevalence of LV hypertrophy in different studies and by varying chronicity of hypertension in patients evaluated.

Longitudinal studies

In a recent longitudinal study from the Framingham Heart Study, normal serum levels of aldosterone predicted the development of hypertension and blood pressure progression after 4 years of follow-up [41]. The predictive capacity of aldosterone was independent of age, sex, baseline blood pressure, body mass index, and LV geometry. Although no firm conclusions could be drawn, subgroup analyses indicated that the relation between serum aldosterone and the incidence of hypertension was stronger in individuals with a high sodium intake. In another report of nonhypertensive participants from the Framingham Heart study, elevated plasma brain natriuretic peptide (BNP) levels at baseline were associated significantly with increases in blood pressure after 4 years of follow-up in men but not in women [42]. The authors concluded that further studies were needed to understand better the observed gender differences. Because both reports were performed in a predominantly white population, these findings need to be replicated in other ethnic groups.

The authors know of no prospective studies relating plasma levels of the other neurohormones (eg, renin, ACE, angiotensin II, catecholamines, or endothelin levels) to the development of essential hypertension.

Treatment studies

Several studies show that lowering blood pressure with antihypertensive agents such as ACE inhibitors and β-blockers reduces the risk for CHF in patients who have hypertension [43–46]. It is unclear whether this cardioprotective effect is related to blood pressure lowering per se, however, or whether it is a consequence of the neurohormonal antagonism seen with specific antihypertensive agents.

Several trials have compared different classes of antihypertensive agents for the development of cardiovascular morbidity and mortality, but none have used CHF as a primary endpoint. The Antihypertensive and Lipid-Lowering Treatment to Prevent Heart Attack Trial indicates potential differences between types of antihypertensive classes in their ability to prevent CHF. In that trial, the diuretic treatment was superior to treatment with α-blockers, ACE inhibitors, and calcium channel blockers [47,48] in protection against future CHF. Specifically, doxazosin (an α-blocker) increased the risk for CHF [47]. Conversely, the Second Australian National Blood Pressure study showed no differences between treatment with ACE inhibitors or with diuretics on CHF incidence [49]. In the Swedish Trial in Old Patients with Hypertension, treatment with ACE inhibitors was superior to calcium channel blockers for preventing the development of CHF in elderly hypertensives [50]. In that study, there was a nonsignificant trend toward superiority of ACE inhibitors versus β-blocker/diuretic treatment ($P = .09$) for preventing CHF. Moreover, in a post-hoc analysis of the Valsartan Antihypertensive Long-term Use Evaluation trial, treatment with valsartan lowered the incidence of hospitalization for CHF compared with amlodipine [51]. Again, these studies did not focus on CHF as a primary outcome, rendering the findings of secondary analyses hypothesis-generating, and other studies have found no difference between antihypertensive agent classes in their ability to prevent CHF [52,53].

Although some data suggest that endothelin blockers lower blood pressure in patients who have essential hypertension [54], no large clinical trials comparing endothelin-blockade to conventional treatment in hypertension patients have been published. Thus, there are no data on the effects of direct endothelin antagonism on the risk for CHF. Because ACE inhibitors lower endothelin levels in patients who have essential hypertension [55], part of the benefits of this class of agents may derive from blockade of endothelin-dependent mechanisms.

Conclusion

Cross-sectional studies have reported variable patterns of neurohormonal activation in hypertension, often without a consistent profile (summarized in Table 1). Prior studies are limited by modest referral samples and biases resulting from inclusion of patients with variable degrees and duration of blood pressure elevation and disparate extents of LV hyper-

Table 1
Cross-sectional studies of the relation between plasma levels of different neurohormones and blood pressure/hypertension and left ventricular mass

	Associations [Ref.]		
Study	Positive	None	Inverse
Blood pressure/hypertension			
Renin	—	[8]	[6,7]
ACE	[9,10]	—	—
AII	[11,12]	[13,14]	[6]
Aldosterone	[14,15]	[16,17]	[6]
Catecholamines	[21,125–127]	—	—
Endothelin	[23–26,28,29]	[27]	—
Natriuretic peptides	[32–35]	[38–40]	[36,37]
LV mass/LV hypertrophy			
Renin	[13,128,129]	[59,130,131]	[18,132]
ACE	[13,59]	[129,133]	—
AII	[13,134]	[59,130,131]	—
Aldosterone	[18,59,128,129]	[13,18,60,130–132,134,135]	—
Catecholamines	[136–138]	[129,138]	—
Endothelin	[138,139]	[140]	—
Natriuretic peptides	[61–64]	—	—

trophy. Few prospective studies relate plasma neurohormonal levels to the incidence of hypertension, partly because such studies are difficult and expensive to perform. Treatment trials show that lowering blood pressure is beneficial in hypertensives, but it is unclear whether cardioprotective effects are related to blood pressure lowering or to specific antagonism of the RAAS or sympathetic activation. Furthermore, the superiority of one antihypertension agent class over another for preventing CHF has not been established, although α-blockers increased the CHF risk in one large study [47].

Neurohormonal contributions to the development of and activation in left ventricular hypertrophy

The data on neurohormonal activation in LV hypertrophy are based mainly on cross-sectional studies and on hypertension-treatment trials (the authors identified only one small prospective study where plasma BNP levels identified hypertensive patients who were more likely to develop LV hypertrophy [56]).

Cross-sectional studies

Substantial experimental and clinical data support the role of RAAS, catecholamines, and endothelin in LV remodeling [3,57,58]. Data on the cross-sectional relations between circulating levels of these neurohormones and LV mass/hypertrophy are conflicting, however. Studies have shown positive, inverse, or no relations between various neurohormones and LV mass (summarized in Table 1).

Two large community-based investigations have evaluated the relations of neurohormones and echocardiographic indices of LV mass. In the Multinational Monitoring of Trends and Determinants in Cardiovascular Disease (MONICA) study cohort in Augsburg [59], serum ACE activity and higher serum ACE concentrations were related strongly, independently, and positively to LV mass index in men but not in women, whereas serum aldosterone was related to LV mass index in women but not in men. Serum angiotensin II and renin were not related to LV mass index in either men or women [59].

In the Framingham Heart Study, a positive relation was observed between aldosterone and an LV geometric pattern suggestive of concentric remodeling (increased LV wall thickness and relative wall thickness but decreased LV diastolic dimensions) in women but not in men [60]. The investigators reported no relation to LV mass.

In contrast, the data on the relation between the plasma levels of natriuretic peptides and LV mass are consistent. Several large population-based studies have reported that plasma natriuretic peptides are elevated in LV hypertrophy [61–63]. Plasma BNP seems to be related more closely to LV hypertrophy than N-terminal atrial natriuretic peptide (n-ANP) [64]. Natriuretic peptides have limited value for screening for LV hypertrophy in the general population, however [61–63].

Treatment studies

Numerous clinical trials [65] have evaluated the effects of antihypertensive agents in mediating regression of LV hypertrophy. In these reports, agents antagonizing the RAAS system, such as ACE inhibitors and angiotensin-II blockers, are most potent in reducing LV mass, whereas β-blockers are reported to be less potent [65]. Because different classes of antihypertensive drugs can regress LV mass differently, factors other than lowering the hemodynamic burden (ie, blood pressure) may be important in cardioprotection and consequent lowering of risk for future CHF. For instance, reduction in LV mass after treatment with angiotensin-II blockers or ACE inhibitors is related to lowering of natriuretic peptides in patients who have essential hypertension [66–68]. Although treatment with antihypertensive agents reduces the risk for CHF, the hypothesis that LV mass regression prevents the development of CHF has not been proven. In the LIFE trial [69], there was no difference between angiotensin II–blocker treatment and β-blocker treatment with regard to the development of CHF in hypertensives with LV hypertrophy, although the two classes of agents had different effects on LV mass regression.

Conclusion

There are conflicting reports on the relations of circulating neurohormones and LV hypertrophy, with the exception of the natriuretic peptides. There are no large-scale prospective studies demonstrating that the incidence of LV hypertrophy varies according to the degree and type of neurohormonal activation. Treatment trials have shown that blood pressure lowering reduces the risk for incident CHF and results in regression of elevated LV mass. It is unclear if such LV-mass regression primarily mediates the effect on lowering CHF risk, although this may be a key mechanism. For example, antihypertensive agents may influence vascular stiffness favorably, and the favorable effects of ventricular-vascular coupling may be the underlying mechanism for lowering CHF risk, rather than an effect solely on elevated LV mass.

Neurohormonal contributions to and activation in patients after a myocardial infarction or who have asymptomatic left ventricular dysfunction

Cross-sectional studies in post–myocardial infarction patients

The circulating RAAS components, catecholamines, natriuretic peptides, and endothelin increase during the acute phase of myocardial infarction. Neurohormonal activation usually begins to diminish within a few days of the acute infarction in most such patients [70–76]. Approximately 2 weeks following an uncomplicated myocardial infarction, the neurohormonal activation subsides almost completely, with plasma levels restored to normal [77,78].

Sustained neurohormonal activation in patients who have had myocardial infarction is related to multiple factors, such as the magnitude of the myocardial damage, the presence of LV systolic dysfunction or CHF symptoms, patient age, and the use of specific cardiovascular drugs [70,75,79–84]. The interactions between the different neurohormonal systems are likely intricate, however, and the data are not clear regarding the timing of elevation of a specific system and its role in evolution of preclinical CHF (see later discussion).

Renin–angiotensin–aldosterone system

Sustained activation of circulating components of RAAS such as plasma renin, aldosterone, and angiotensin II is observed up to 6 months post–myocardial infarction, principally when LV systolic dysfunction or CHF is present [75,80,85]. Although activation of RAAS also has been identified in hemodynamically compensated patients, it tends to be less sustained and of a lesser magnitude [75,86].

Catecholamines

Adrenergic activation (as measured by plasma norepinephrine and epinephrine levels) is observed during the first 5 days after an acute myocardial infarction [70]. Plasma norepinephrine levels on admission (with a myocardial infarction) correlate with LV systolic function on admission and discharge [70,82]. In patients who have acute myocardial infarction, normal plasma norepinephrine values on admission predict normal or near-normal LV ejection fraction at discharge [70]. In contrast, a small study showed no relation between serum norepinephrine and LV systolic function in asymptomatic LV dysfunction [86].

Endothelin

Within the first week of an acute myocardial infarction, plasma endothelin levels decrease and plasma atrial natriuretic peptide (ANP) levels increase [76,87]. Sustained elevation of plasma endothelin in post–myocardial infarction patients is characteristic of the presence of severe CHF, not just presence of asymptomatic LV systolic dysfunction or mild CHF [81].

Natriuretic peptides

The plasma levels of natriuretic peptides increase in the acute phase of a myocardial infarction [76,84, 88–90] and the increase is related closely to infarct size, LV systolic dysfunction, and CHF symptoms [75,76,83,84,90–93]. In patients with myocardial infarction and overall preserved LV function, plasma N-ANP and BNP were elevated within the first 14 days [88]. Plasma BNP decreased after 90 days, whereas N-ANP remained elevated.

Longitudinal studies in post–myocardial infarction patients

Renin–angiotensin–aldosterone system

Investigators have reported that patients with a sustained increase in plasma renin activity and aldosterone after a myocardial infarction had an increased mortality within 24 months [78]. In another report, plasma renin activity and aldosterone were independent predictors of the combined endpoint of cardiovascular mortality, development of severe CHF, or recurrent myocardial infarction [94] in patients who had asymptomatic LV systolic dysfunction. Other studies, however, have reported that the circulating components of the RAAS system do not predict future CHF incidence and CHF-related morbidity and mortality after accounting for clinical symptoms and other levels of plasma neurohormones, such as natriuretic peptides and norepinephrine [88,95,96]. Thus, the relative contribution of RAAS versus other neurohormones to the prognosis after myocardial infarction is unclear. It is also unclear if levels of RAAS are predictive beyond their correlation with LV systolic dysfunction or infarct size.

Catecholamines

Data on the relations of plasma catecholamines to post–myocardial infarction morbidity and mortality are not consistent. In one study, post–myocardial infarction patients who died within 2 years of the event had sustained elevations of plasma norepinephrine [78]. In another investigation, however, plasma norepinephrine levels after a myocardial infarction did not predict survival after adjustment for clinical CHF [72]. In that study, plasma ANP remained an independent predictor of survival.

Endothelin

Plasma endothelin concentrations are related to survival after a myocardial infarction [87] and some studies show that plasma endothelin provides prognostic information beyond clinical variables and ANP [97], but not independently of LV systolic function [98].

Natriuretic peptides

The prognostic value of increased natriuretic peptides after acute myocardial infarction has been studied extensively. Plasma natriuretic peptides predict mortality, clinical CHF, and myocardial infarction in patients who have acute coronary syndrome [99], post–myocardial infarction [8,72,82,94,98, 100–102], and in patients who have asymptomatic LV systolic dysfunction [95] independently of other neurohormones, LV systolic function, age, and treatment.

Studies of left ventricular dysfunction: cross-sectional and longitudinal reports

In the Studies of Left Ventricular Dysfunction (SOLVD), median values for plasma norepinephrine, plasma atrial natriuretic factor, and plasma renin activity were significantly higher in patients who had LV systolic dysfunction compared with control subjects who had normal LV systolic function [83]. Plasma neuroendocrine marker values were highest in patients who had overt CHF [83]. In this trial, plasma norepinephrine independently predicted cardiovascular morbidity (including CHF hospitalization) and mortality in patients who had asymptomatic LV systolic dysfunction [96], whereas plasma ANP and renin activity did not. Plasma norepinephrine was reported to be a useful marker for progression from asymptomatic to symptomatic LV systolic dysfunction in this report. In contrast, in the SAVE trial (which enrolled post–myocardial infarction patients), plasma renin activity, aldosterone, and ANP were independent predictors of the combined endpoints of cardiovascular mortality, development of severe CHF, or recurrent myocardial infarction [94]. Furthermore, plasma ANP and, to a lesser extent, aldosterone, measured 3 months after the infarction, predicted future cardiovascular events, but plasma norepinephrine did not [78].

Treatment studies

Treatment effects of neurohormonal levels

Short-term effects. The beneficial effects of treatment with ACE inhibitors after a myocardial infarction may not be related directly to early modulation of neurohormonal activation assessed through plasma levels. There were no differences in plasma natriuretic peptides, catecholamines, or endothelin when measured after 3 days to 3 weeks of ACE treatment in some investigations [103,104]. There are conflicting results from other studies, however. For instance, Gonzalez-Fernandez and colleagues [105] reported that 4 weeks of enalapril treatment after a myocardial infarction lowered serum norepinephrine, angiotensin II, and ANP. In another report of post–myocardial infarction patients, treatment with captopril or enalapril did not alter plasma norepinephrine, BNP, or ANP, but plasma ACE activity and angiotensin II were reduced after 5 days and after 3 months [92]. In a third report, enalapril treatment for 4 to 6 months after a myocardial infarction did not affect the plasma levels of angiotensin II, aldosterone, ANP, norepinephrine, or epinephrine, but affected LV remodeling indices favorably [106].

Long-term effects. In patients who have asymptomatic LV dysfunction, long-term treatment with enalapril lowers plasma norepinephrine after 4 and 12 months, but only in patients who had increased plasma norepinephrine at baseline [107]. In contrast, in the SAVE trial, captopril increased plasma renin activity and decreased serum aldosterone, but no changes were seen in plasma norepinephrine or ANP during 2 years of treatment [78]. In another study, ramipril treatment after a myocardial infarction lowered LV mass and plasma angiotensin II, but had no effect on plasma norepinephrine, N-ANP, or BNP [88].

There also may be differential effects of ACE inhibitors in chronic CHF compared with post–myocardial infarction regarding effect on endothelin-1 [88,108]. In CHF, ACE inhibitors lower plasma endothelin-1 [108], whereas there was no effect on endothelin levels after ramipril treatment post–myocardial infarction in one report [88].

In post–myocardial infarction patients without CHF, treatment with the calcium channel blocker diltiazem for 4 weeks lowered plasma BNP but not plasma epinephrine or norepinephrine [109].

Treatment effect on prognosis

Several studies show that antagonism of neurohormonal activation by ACE inhibitors, β-blockers, or aldosterone inhibitors is beneficial in patients who have asymptomatic LV dysfunction and in people after a myocardial infarction [110–119].

Although β-blocker treatment is beneficial after a myocardial infarction, no randomized trials have shown that β-blockers prevent the development of CHF among patients who have asymptomatic LV systolic dysfunction. The combination of ACE inhibitors and β-blockers, however, seems better than ACE inhibitors or β-blockers alone in observational studies of patients who have asymptomatic LV systolic dysfunction after a myocardial infarction [113,114,120].

Blockade of the RAAS system with a combination of ACE inhibitors and angiotension-II blockers seems to offer no benefit over treatment with either of these agents alone [121,122]. (See the article by Yusuf and colleagues elsewhere in this issue for the effect of treatment in patients who have a high risk for CHF.)

Conclusion

The plasma levels of neurohormones are increased after a myocardial infarction. Sustained neurohormonal activation is associated with poor prognosis but it is unclear if one specific marker is of greater prognostic utility than others. Treatment with neurohormonal antagonists is beneficial, but the advantageous effects are not related always to changes in circulating neurohormones.

Summary

Despite an abundance of experimental studies, there is limited information on the role of neurohormonal activation as measured by circulating neurohormonal factors during the early stages of cardiovascular disease in the general population. Because there are few prospective studies, it is not possible to distinguish whether neurohormonal activation is the cause or the consequence of subclinical LV systolic dysfunction, or both.

The interactions among the major neurohormonal systems throughout the cardiovascular disease continuum are complex. Furthermore, circulating levels of neurohormones often inadequately reflect the level of tissue activation, which explains the conflicting results, and why treatment effects often are not reflected in nor closely parallel the changes in the circulating levels of various neurohormones. It is unclear whether the blood pressure–lowering effect or the neurohormonal-antagonizing effect of the antihypertensive agents is important in lowering the risk for future CHF in hypertensives. Current data indicate, however, that it is beneficial to use antihypertensive agents at any stage of the disease progression to lower the risk for future CHF. Few trials have used CHF as the primary outcome.

Additionally, ethnicity-related variations in neurohormonal activation have not been characterized adequately. Similarly, the cardiovascular health hazards associated with neurohormonal activation may vary with age, gender, and other clinical features, such as obesity. Future studies should evaluate potential differences in adverse effects of neurohormonal activation separately in the two sexes and in larger multiethnic samples, facilitating subgroup analyses of high-risk groups such as the elderly and the obese.

There are limited data on the potential contributions of neurohormonal activation to LV diastolic dysfunction, an important precursor of diastolic CHF. Data suggest that elderly patients who have diastolic CHF have elevated vascular stiffness (at rest and upon exercise) and also demonstrate neurohormonal activation [123,124]. Such data raise the possibility that neurohormonal activation may contribute to increased vascular stiffness, exercise-induced exaggerated increases in blood pressure, subclinical LV diastolic dysfunction, and eventually diastolic CHF. There are no prospective data to establish or refute such a hypothesis.

References

[1] Harris P. Evolution and the cardiac patient. Cardiovasc Res 1983;17(8):437–45.

[2] Sigurdsson A, Swedberg K. The role of neurohormonal activation in chronic heart failure and postmyocardial infarction. Am Heart J 1996; 132(1 Pt 2 Suppl):229–34.

[3] Dzau VJ, Bernstein K, Celermajer D, et al. The relevance of tissue angiotensin-converting enzyme: manifestations in mechanistic and endpoint data. Am J Cardiol 2001;88(9A):1L–20L.

[4] Esler M. The sympathetic system and hypertension. Am J Hypertens 2000;13(6 Pt 2):99S–105S.

[5] O'Shaughnessy KM, Karet FE. Salt handling and hypertension. J Clin Invest 2004;113(8):1075–81.

[6] Walker WG, Whelton PK, Saito H, et al. Relation between blood pressure and renin, renin substrate, angiotensin II, aldosterone and urinary sodium and potassium in 574 ambulatory subjects. Hypertension 1979;1(3):287–91.

[7] Alderman MH, Sealey JE, Laragh JH. Plasma renin

activity and ischemic heart disease. N Engl J Med 1994;330(7):506–7.

[8] Richards AM, Nicholls MG, Yandle TG, et al. Plasma N-terminal pro-brain natriuretic peptide and adrenomedullin: new neurohormonal predictors of left ventricular function and prognosis after myocardial infarction. Circulation 1998;97(19):1921–9.

[9] Schunkert H, Hense HW, Muscholl M, et al. Association of angiotensin converting enzyme activity and arterial blood pressure in a population-based sample. J Hypertens 1996;14(5):571–5.

[10] Forrester T, McFarlane-Anderson N, Bennett FI, et al. The angiotensin converting enzyme and blood pressure in Jamaicans. Am J Hypertens 1997;10(5 Pt 1): 519–24.

[11] Tolagen K, Karlberg BE. Angiotensin II in primary hypertension, relationship to plasma renin activity, aldosterone and urinary electrolytes. Acta Med Scand 1979;205(7):557–62.

[12] Walker WG, Horvath JS, Moore MA, et al. Relation between plasma renin activity, angiotensin, and aldosterone and blood pressure in mild untreated hypertension. Circ Res 1976;38(6):470–6.

[13] Harrap SB, Dominiczak AF, Fraser R, et al. Plasma angiotensin II, predisposition to hypertension, and left ventricular size in healthy young adults. Circulation 1996;93(6):1148–54.

[14] Ljungman S, Aurell M, Hartford M, et al. Blood pressure in relation to the renin-angiotensin-aldosterone system. Acta Med Scand 1982;211(5): 351–60.

[15] Genest J, Nowaczynski W, Boucher R, et al. Aldosterone and renin in essential hypertension. Can Med Assoc J 1975;113(5):421–31.

[16] Wisenbaugh PE, Garst JB, Hull C, et al. Renin, aldosterone, sodium and hypertension. Am J Med 1972;52(2):175–86.

[17] Tolagen K. Aldosterone in primary hypertension relationship to plasma renin activity and urinary electrolytes and a comparison with normotensive subjects. Scand J Clin Lab Invest 1978;38(5):487–93.

[18] El Gharbawy AH, Nadig VS, Kotchen JM, et al. Arterial pressure, left ventricular mass, and aldosterone in essential hypertension. Hypertension 2001; 37(3):845–50.

[19] Vaughan Jr ED. Diseases of the adrenal gland. Med Clin North Am 2004;88(2):443–66.

[20] Lohmeier TE. The sympathetic nervous system and long-term blood pressure regulation. Am J Hypertens 2001;14(6 Pt 2):147S–54S.

[21] Goldstein DS. Plasma catecholamines and essential hypertension. An analytical review. Hypertension 1983;5(1):86–99.

[22] Touyz RM, Schiffrin EL. Role of endothelin in human hypertension. Can J Physiol Pharmacol 2003; 81(6):533–41.

[23] Saito Y, Nakao K, Mukoyama M, et al. Increased plasma endothelin level in patients with essential hypertension. N Engl J Med 1990;322(3):205.

[24] Elijovich F, Laffer CL, Amador E, et al. Regulation of plasma endothelin by salt in salt-sensitive hypertension. Circulation 2001;103(2):263–8.

[25] Kohno M, Yasunari K, Murakawa K, et al. Plasma immunoreactive endothelin in essential hypertension. Am J Med 1990;88(6):614–8.

[26] Shichiri M, Hirata Y, Ando K, et al. Plasma endothelin levels in hypertension and chronic renal failure. Hypertension 1990;15(5):493–6.

[27] Schiffrin EL, Thibault G. Plasma endothelin in human essential hypertension. Am J Hypertens 1991; 4(4 Pt 1):303–8.

[28] Ergul S, Parish DC, Puett D, et al. Racial differences in plasma endothelin-1 concentrations in individuals with essential hypertension. Hypertension 1996; 28(4):652–5.

[29] Ergul A. Hypertension in black patients: an emerging role of the endothelin system in salt-sensitive hypertension. Hypertension 2000;36(1):62–7.

[30] Cardillo C, Kilcoyne CM, Waclawiw M, et al. Role of endothelin in the increased vascular tone of patients with essential hypertension. Hypertension 1999;33(2):753–8.

[31] Levin ER, Gardner DG, Samson WK. Natriuretic peptides. N Engl J Med 1998;339(5):321–8.

[32] Buckley MG, Markandu ND, Miller MA, et al. Plasma concentrations and comparisons of brain and atrial natriuretic peptide in normal subjects and in patients with essential hypertension. J Hum Hypertens 1993;7(3):245–50.

[33] Kario K, Nishikimi T, Yoshihara F, et al. Plasma levels of natriuretic peptides and adrenomedullin in elderly hypertensive patients: relationships to 24 h blood pressure. J Hypertens 1998;16(9):1253–9.

[34] Kato J, Kitamura K, Uemura T, et al. Plasma levels of adrenomedullin and atrial and brain natriuretic peptides in the general population: their relations to age and pulse pressure. Hypertens Res 2002;25(6):887–92.

[35] Kohno M, Horio T, Yokokawa K, et al. Brain natriuretic peptide as a cardiac hormone in essential hypertension. Am J Med 1992;92(1):29–34.

[36] Talartschik J, Eisenhauer T, Schrader J, et al. Low atrial natriuretic peptide plasma concentrations in 100 patients with essential hypertension. Am J Hypertens 1990;3(1):45–7.

[37] Zachariah PK, Burnett Jr JC, Ritter SG, et al. Atrial natriuretic peptide in human essential hypertension. Mayo Clin Proc 1987;62(9):782–6.

[38] Flickinger AL, Burnett Jr JC, Turner ST. Atrial natriuretic peptide and blood pressure in a population-based sample. Mayo Clin Proc 1995;70(10):932–8.

[39] Nilsson P, Lindholm L, Schersten B, et al. Atrial natriuretic peptide and blood pressure in a geographically defined population. Lancet 1987;2(8564): 883–5.

[40] Nishikimi T, Yoshihara F, Morimoto A, et al. Relationship between left ventricular geometry and natriuretic peptide levels in essential hypertension. Hypertension 1996;28(1):22–30.

[41] Vasan RS, Evans JC, Larson MG, et al. Serum aldosterone and the incidence of hypertension in nonhypertensive persons. N Engl J Med 2004;351(1): 33–41.

[42] Freitag MH, Larson MG, Levy D, et al. Plasma brain natriuretic peptide levels and blood pressure tracking in the Framingham Heart Study. Hypertension 2003;41(4):978–83.

[43] Kostis JB, Davis BR, Cutler J, et al. Prevention of heart failure by antihypertensive drug treatment in older persons with isolated systolic hypertension. SHEP Cooperative Research Group. JAMA 1997; 278(3):212–6.

[44] Dahlof B, Lindholm LH, Hansson L, et al. Morbidity and mortality in the Swedish Trial in Old Patients with Hypertension (STOP-Hypertension). Lancet 1991;338(8778):1281–5.

[45] Staessen JA, Fagard R, Thijs L, et al. Randomised double-blind comparison of placebo and active treatment for older patients with isolated systolic hypertension. The Systolic Hypertension in Europe (Syst-Eur) Trial Investigators. Lancet 1997;350(9080): 757–64.

[46] Yusuf S, Sleight P, Pogue J, et al. Effects of an angiotensin-converting-enzyme inhibitor, ramipril, on cardiovascular events in high-risk patients. The Heart Outcomes Prevention Evaluation Study Investigators. N Engl J Med 2000;342(3):145–53.

[47] Major cardiovascular events in hypertensive patients randomized to doxazosin vs chlorthalidone: the antihypertensive and lipid-lowering treatment to prevent heart attack trial (ALLHAT). ALLHAT Collaborative Research Group. JAMA 2000; 283(15):1967–75.

[48] Major outcomes in high-risk hypertensive patients randomized to angiotensin-converting enzyme inhibitor or calcium channel blocker vs diuretic: the Antihypertensive and Lipid-Lowering Treatment to Prevent Heart Attack Trial (ALLHAT). JAMA 2002; 288(23):2981–97.

[49] Wing LM, Reid CM, Ryan P, et al. A comparison of outcomes with angiotensin-converting–enzyme inhibitors and diuretics for hypertension in the elderly. N Engl J Med 2003;348(7):583–92.

[50] Hansson L, Lindholm LH, Ekbom T, et al. Randomised trial of old and new antihypertensive drugs in elderly patients: cardiovascular mortality and morbidity the Swedish Trial in Old Patients with Hypertension-2 study. Lancet 1999;354(9192):1751–6.

[51] Weber MA, Julius S, Kjeldsen SE, et al. Blood pressure dependent and independent effects of antihypertensive treatment on clinical events in the VALUE Trial. Lancet 2004;363(9426):2049–51.

[52] Hansson L, Lindholm LH, Niskanen L, et al. Effect of angiotensin-converting-enzyme inhibition compared with conventional therapy on cardiovascular morbidity and mortality in hypertension: the Captopril Prevention Project (CAPPP) randomised trial. Lancet 1999;353(9153):611–6.

[53] Hansson L, Hedner T, Lund-Johansen P, et al. Randomised trial of effects of calcium antagonists compared with diuretics and beta-blockers on cardiovascular morbidity and mortality in hypertension: the Nordic Diltiazem (NORDIL) study. Lancet 2000; 356(9227):359–65.

[54] Krum H, Viskoper RJ, Lacourciere Y, et al. The effect of an endothelin-receptor antagonist, bosentan, on blood pressure in patients with essential hypertension. Bosentan Hypertension Investigators. N Engl J Med 1998;338(12):784–90.

[55] Uemasu J, Munemura C, Fujihara M, et al. Inhibition of plasma endothelin-1 concentration by captopril in patients with essential hypertension. Clin Nephrol 1994;41(3):150–2.

[56] Suzuki M, Yamamoto K, Watanabe S, et al. Association between elevated brain natriuretic peptide levels and the development of left ventricular hypertrophy in patients with hypertension. Am J Med 2000; 108(8):627–33.

[57] Schunkert H, Orzechowski HD, Bocker W, et al. The cardiac endothelin system in established pressure overload left ventricular hypertrophy. J Mol Med 1999;77(8):623–30.

[58] Kaddoura S, Firth JD, Boheler KR, et al. Endothelin-1 is involved in norepinephrine-induced ventricular hypertrophy in vivo Acute effects of bosentan, an orally active, mixed endothelin ETA and ETB receptor antagonist. Circulation 1996;93(11):2068–79.

[59] Schunkert H, Hense HW, Muscholl M, et al. Associations between circulating components of the renin-angiotensin-aldosterone system and left ventricular mass. Heart 1997;77(1):24–31.

[60] Vasan RS, Evans JC, Benjamin EJ, et al. Relations of serum aldosterone to cardiac structure: gender-related differences in the Framingham Heart Study. Hypertension 2004;43(5):957–62.

[61] Vasan RS, Benjamin EJ, Larson MG, et al. Plasma natriuretic peptides for community screening for left ventricular hypertrophy and systolic dysfunction—the Framingham Heart Study. JAMA 2002;288(10): 222–8.

[62] Arnlov J, Lind L, Stridsberg M, et al. N-terminal atrial natriuretic peptide and left ventricular geometry and function in a population sample of elderly males. J Intern Med 2000;247(6):699–708.

[63] Schirmer H, Omland T. Circulating N-terminal proatrial natriuretic peptide is an independent predictor of left ventricular hypertrophy in the general population. The Tromso Study. Eur Heart J 1999;20(10): 755–63.

[64] Yamamoto K, Burnett Jr JC, Jougasaki M, et al. Superiority of brain natriuretic peptide as a hormonal marker of ventricular systolic and diastolic dysfunction and ventricular hypertrophy. Hypertension 1996; 28(6):988–94.

[65] Diez J, Gonzalez A, Lopez B, et al. Effects of antihypertensive agents on the left ventricle: clinical implications. Am J Cardiovasc Drugs 2001;1(4):263–79.

[66] Anan F, Takahashi N, Ooie T, et al. Candesartan, an angiotensin II receptor blocker, improves left ventricular hypertrophy and insulin resistance. Metabolism 2004;53(6):777–81.

[67] Kohno M, Minami M, Kano H, et al. Effect of angiotensin-converting enzyme inhibitor on left ventricular parameters and circulating brain natriuretic peptide in elderly hypertensives with left venticular hypertrophy. Metabolism 2000;49(10):1356–60.

[68] Yalcin F, Aksoy FG, Muderrisoglu H, et al. Treatment of hypertension with perindopril reduces plasma atrial natriuretic peptide levels, left ventricular mass, and improves echocardiographic parameters of diastolic function. Clin Cardiol 2000;23(6):437–41.

[69] Dahlof B, Devereux RB, Kjeldsen SE, et al. Cardiovascular morbidity and mortality in the Losartan Intervention For Endpoint reduction in hypertension study (LIFE): a randomised trial against atenolol. Lancet 2002;359(9311):995–1003.

[70] Petersen CL, Nielsen JR, Petersen BL, et al. Catecholaminergic activation in acute myocardial infarction: time course and relation to left ventricular performance. Cardiology 2003;100(1):23–8.

[71] Rouleau JL, de Champlain J, Klein M, et al. Activation of neurohumoral systems in postinfarction left ventricular dysfunction. J Am Coll Cardiol 1993; 22(2):390–8.

[72] Omland T, Aarsland T, Aakvaag A, et al. Prognostic value of plasma atrial natriuretic factor, norepinephrine and epinephrine in acute myocardial infarction. Am J Cardiol 1993;72(3):255–9.

[73] McAlpine HM, Morton JJ, Leckie B, et al. Neuroendocrine activation after acute myocardial infarction. Br Heart J 1988;60(2):117–24.

[74] Remes J. Neuroendocrine activation after myocardial infarction. Br Heart J 1994;72(3 Suppl):S65–9.

[75] Sigurdsson A, Held P, Swedberg K. Short- and long-term neurohormonal activation following acute myocardial infarction. Am Heart J 1993;126(5):1068–76.

[76] Petersen CL, Munch M, Frandsen E, et al. Serial changes in atrial natriuretic peptide and endothelin-1 concentrations. Their relationships to the cardiac performance of patients hospitalized for acute myocardial infarction. Cardiology 1998;89(3):210–5.

[77] Rouleau JL, Moye LA, de Champlain J, et al. Activation of neurohumoral systems following acute myocardial infarction. Am J Cardiol 1991;68(14): 80D–6D.

[78] Vantrimpont P, Rouleau JL, Ciampi A, et al. Two-year time course and significance of neurohumoral activation in the Survival and Ventricular Enlargement (SAVE) Study. Eur Heart J 1998;19(10):1552–63.

[79] Rouleau JL, de Champlain J, Klein M, et al. Activation of neurohumoral systems in postinfarction left ventricular dysfunction. J Am Coll Cardiol 1993; 22(2):390–8.

[80] Ray SG, Morton JJ, Dargie HJ. Relationship of renin, angiotensin II and atrial natriuretic factor to clinical status in the early post-infarct period in patients with left ventricular dysfunction. Eur Heart J 1994;15(6):793–800.

[81] Wei CM, Lerman A, Rodeheffer RJ, et al. Endothelin in human congestive heart failure. Circulation 1994; 89(4):1580–6.

[82] Otterstad JE, John Sutton MG, Froeland GS, et al. Prognostic value of two-dimensional echocardiography and N-terminal proatrial natriuretic peptide following an acute myocardial infarction. Assessment of baseline values (2–7 days) and changes at 3 months in patients with a preserved systolic function. Eur Heart J 2002;23(13):1011–20.

[83] Francis GS, Benedict C, Johnstone DE, et al. Comparison of neuroendocrine activation in patients with left ventricular dysfunction with and without congestive heart failure. A substudy of the Studies of Left Ventricular Dysfunction (SOLVD). Circulation 1990;82(5):1724–9.

[84] Fontana F, Bernardi P, Spagnolo N, et al. Plasma atrial natriuretic factor in patients with acute myocardial infarction. Eur Heart J 1990;11(9):779–87.

[85] Rouleau JL, de Champlain J, Klein M, et al. Activation of neurohumoral systems in postinfarction left ventricular dysfunction. J Am Coll Cardiol 1993; 22(2):390–8.

[86] Vaughan DE, Lamas GA, Pfeffer MA. Role of left ventricular dysfunction in selective neurohumoral activation in the recovery phase of anterior wall acute myocardial infarction. Am J Cardiol 1990;66(5): 529–32.

[87] Wieczorek I, Haynes WG, Webb DJ, et al. Raised plasma endothelin in unstable angina and non-Q wave myocardial infarction: relation to cardiovascular outcome. Br Heart J 1994;72(5):436–41.

[88] White M, Rouleau JL, Hall C, et al. Changes in vasoconstrictive hormones, natriuretic peptides, and left ventricular remodeling soon after anterior myocardial infarction. Am Heart J 2001;142(6):1056–64.

[89] Rouleau JL, de Champlain J, Klein M, et al. Activation of neurohumoral systems in postinfarction left ventricular dysfunction. J Am Coll Cardiol 1993; 22(2):390–8.

[90] Bellone P, Derchi G, Tommasini G, et al. Selective activation of atrial natriuretic peptide in patients with myocardial infarction and mild left ventricular dysfunction. Int J Cardiol 1993;42(2):115–20.

[91] Svanegaard J, Angelo-Nielsen K, Pindborg T. Plasma concentration of atrial natriuretic peptide at admission and risk of cardiac death in patients with acute myocardial infarction. Br Heart J 1992;68(1): 38–42.

[92] Foy SG, Crozier IG, Richards AM, et al. Neurohormonal changes after acute myocardial infarction. Relationships with haemodynamic indices and effects of ACE inhibition. Eur Heart J 1995;16(6): 770–8.

[93] Benedict CR, Johnstone DE, Weiner DH, et al. Relation of neurohumoral activation to clinical variables and degree of ventricular dysfunction: a report

from the Registry of Studies of Left Ventricular Dysfunction. SOLVD Investigators. J Am Coll Cardiol 1994;23(6):1410–20.

[94] Rouleau JL, Packer M, Moye L, et al. Prognostic value of neurohumoral activation in patients with an acute myocardial infarction: effect of captopril. J Am Coll Cardiol 1994;24(3):583–91.

[95] Tsutamoto T, Wada A, Maeda K, et al. Plasma brain natriuretic peptide level as a biochemical marker of morbidity and mortality in patients with asymptomatic or minimally symptomatic left ventricular dysfunction. Comparison with plasma angiotensin II and endothelin-1. Eur Heart J 1999;20(24):1799–807.

[96] Benedict CR, Shelton B, Johnstone DE, et al. Prognostic significance of plasma norepinephrine in patients with asymptomatic left ventricular dysfunction. SOLVD Investigators. Circulation 1996;94(4):690–7.

[97] Omland T, Lie RT, Aakvaag A, et al. Plasma endothelin determination as a prognostic indicator of 1-year mortality after acute myocardial infarction. Circulation 1994;89(4):1573–9.

[98] Omland T, Bonarjee VV, Lie RT, et al. Neurohumoral measurements as indicators of long-term prognosis after acute myocardial infarction. Am J Cardiol 1995;76(4):230–5.

[99] de Lemos JA, Morrow DA, Bentley JH, et al. The prognostic value of B-type natriuretic peptide in patients with acute coronary syndromes. N Engl J Med 2001;345(14):1014–21.

[100] Arakawa N, Nakamura M, Aoki H, et al. Plasma brain natriuretic peptide concentrations predict survival after acute myocardial infarction. J Am Coll Cardiol 1996;27(7):1656–61.

[101] Hall C, Rouleau JL, Moye L, et al. N-terminal proatrial natriuretic factor. An independent predictor of long-term prognosis after myocardial infarction. Circulation 1994;89(5):1934–42.

[102] Richards AM, Nicholls MG, Espiner EA, et al. B-type natriuretic peptides and ejection fraction for prognosis after myocardial infarction. Circulation 2003;107(22):2786–92.

[103] Sigurdsson A, Eriksson SV, Hall C, et al. Early neurohormonal effects of trandolapril in patients with left ventricular dysfunction and a recent acute myocardial infarction: a double-blind, randomized, placebo-controlled multicentre study. Eur J Heart Fail 2001;3(1):69–78.

[104] Omland T, Aarsland T, Aakvaag A, et al. The effect of early converting enzyme inhibition on neurohumoral activation in acute myocardial infarction. Int J Cardiol 1993;42(1):37–45.

[105] Gonzalez-Fernandez RA, Altieri PI, Lugo JE, et al. Effects of enalapril on ventricular volumes and neurohumoral status after inferior wall myocardial infarction. Am J Med Sci 1993;305(4):216–21.

[106] Sigurdsson A, Held P, Swedberg K, et al. Neurohormonal effects of early treatment with enalapril after acute myocardial infarction and the impact on left ventricular remodelling. Eur Heart J 1993;14(8):1110–7.

[107] Benedict CR, Francis GS, Shelton B, et al. Effect of long-term enalapril therapy on neurohormones in patients with left ventricular dysfunction. SOLVD Investigators. Am J Cardiol 1995;75(16):1151–7.

[108] Galatius-Jensen S, Wroblewski H, Emmeluth C, et al. Plasma endothelin in congestive heart failure: effect of the ACE inhibitor, fosinopril. Cardiovasc Res 1996;32(6):1148–54.

[109] Maki N, Yoshiyama M, Omura T, et al. Effect of diltiazem on cardiac function assessed by echocardiography and neurohumoral factors after reperfused myocardial infarction without congestive heart failure. Cardiovasc Drugs Ther 2001;15(6):493–9.

[110] Effect of enalapril on mortality and the development of heart failure in asymptomatic patients with reduced left ventricular ejection fractions. The SOLVD Investigators. N Engl J Med 1992;327(10):685–91.

[111] Jong P, Yusuf S, Rousseau MF, et al. Effect of enalapril on 12-year survival and life expectancy in patients with left ventricular systolic dysfunction: a follow-up study. Lancet 2003;361(9372):1843–8.

[112] Pfeffer MA, Braunwald E, Moye LA, et al. Effect of captopril on mortality and morbidity in patients with left ventricular dysfunction after myocardial infarction. Results of the survival and ventricular enlargement trial. The SAVE Investigators. N Engl J Med 1992;327(10):669–77.

[113] Vantrimpont P, Rouleau JL, Wun CC, et al. Additive beneficial effects of beta-blockers to angiotensin-converting enzyme inhibitors in the Survival and Ventricular Enlargement (SAVE) Study. SAVE Investigators. J Am Coll Cardiol 1997;29(2):229–36.

[114] Exner DV, Dries DL, Waclawiw MA, et al. Beta-adrenergic blocking agent use and mortality in patients with asymptomatic and symptomatic left ventricular systolic dysfunction: a post hoc analysis of the Studies of Left Ventricular Dysfunction. J Am Coll Cardiol 1999;33(4):916–23.

[115] Pitt B, Remme W, Zannad F, et al. Eplerenone, a selective aldosterone blocker, in patients with left ventricular dysfunction after myocardial infarction. N Engl J Med 2003;348(14):1309–21.

[116] Fox KM. Efficacy of perindopril in reduction of cardiovascular events among patients with stable coronary artery disease: randomised, double-blind, placebo-controlled, multicentre trial (the EUROPA study). Lancet 2003;362(9386):782–8.

[117] Ambrosioni E, Borghi C, Magnani B. The effect of the angiotensin-converting-enzyme inhibitor zofenopril on mortality and morbidity after anterior myocardial infarction. The Survival of Myocardial Infarction Long-Term Evaluation (SMILE) Study Investigators. N Engl J Med 1995;332(2):80–5.

[118] Kober L, Torp-Pedersen C, Carlsen JE, et al. A clinical trial of the angiotensin-converting-enzyme inhibitor trandolapril in patients with left ventricular dysfunction after myocardial infarction. Trandolapril

Cardiac Evaluation (TRACE) Study Group. N Engl J Med 1995;333(25):1670–6.

[119] Indications for ACE inhibitors in the early treatment of acute myocardial infarction: systematic overview of individual data from 100,000 patients in randomized trials. ACE Inhibitor Myocardial Infarction Collaborative Group. Circulation 1998;97(22): 2202–12.

[120] Aronow WS, Ahn C, Kronzon I. Effect of beta blockers alone, of angiotensin-converting enzyme inhibitors alone, and of beta blockers plus angiotensin-converting enzyme inhibitors on new coronary events and on congestive heart failure in older persons with healed myocardial infarcts and asymptomatic left ventricular systolic dysfunction. Am J Cardiol 2001; 88(11):1298–300.

[121] Pfeffer MA, McMurray JJ, Velazquez EJ, et al. Valsartan, captopril, or both in myocardial infarction complicated by heart failure, left ventricular dysfunction, or both. N Engl J Med 2003;349(20):1893–906.

[122] Dickstein K, Kjekshus J. Effects of losartan and captopril on mortality and morbidity in high-risk patients after acute myocardial infarction: the OPTIMAAL randomised trial. Optimal Trial in Myocardial Infarction with Angiotensin II Antagonist Losartan. Lancet 2002;360(9335):752–60.

[123] Kitzman DW, Little WC, Brubaker PH, et al. Pathophysiological characterization of isolated diastolic heart failure in comparison to systolic heart failure. JAMA 2002;288(17):2144–50.

[124] Hundley WG, Kitzman DW, Morgan TM, et al. Cardiac cycle-dependent changes in aortic area and distensibility are reduced in older patients with isolated diastolic heart failure and correlate with exercise intolerance. J Am Coll Cardiol 2001;38(3):796–802.

[125] Carstensen E, Ramaiya K, Denver E, et al. The contribution of the sympathoadrenomedullary system to the etiology of essential hypertension: a study using plasma and platelet catecholamine concentrations. J Clin Endocrinol Metab 1995;80(2):455–60.

[126] Jacobs MC, Lenders JW, Willemsen JJ, et al. Adrenomedullary secretion of epinephrine is increased in mild essential hypertension. Hypertension 1997;29(6):1303–8.

[127] Beilin LJ, Vandongen R, Arkwright PD, et al. Adrenal and sympathetic nervous activity in subjects with "low" and "high" normal blood pressure. J Hypertens 1983;1(1):13–8.

[128] Muscholl MW, Schunkert H, Muders F, et al. Neurohormonal activity and left ventricular geometry in patients with essential arterial hypertension. Am Heart J 1998;135(1):58–66.

[129] Malmqvist K, Ohman KP, Lind L, et al. Relationships between left ventricular mass and the renin-angiotensin system, catecholamines, insulin and leptin. J Intern Med 2002;252(5):430–9.

[130] Schlaich MP, Klingbeil A, Hilgers K, et al. Relation between the renin-angiotensin-aldosterone system and left ventricular structure and function in young normotensive and mildly hypertensive subjects. Am Heart J 1999;138(5 Pt 1):810–7.

[131] Schlaich MP, Schobel HP, Hilgers K, et al. Impact of aldosterone on left ventricular structure and function in young normotensive and mildly hypertensive subjects. Am J Cardiol 2000;85(10):1199–206.

[132] du Cailar G, Pasquie JL, Ribstein J, et al. Left ventricular adaptation to hypertension and plasma renin activity. J Hum Hypertens 2000;14(3):181–8.

[133] Reneland R, Andren B, Lind L, et al. Circulating angiotensin converting enzyme levels are increased in concentric, but not eccentric, left ventricular hypertrophy in elderly men. J Hypertens 1997;15(8): 885–90.

[134] Schmieder RE, Messerli FH, Garavaglia GE, et al. Does the renin-angiotensin-aldosterone system modify cardiac structure and function in essential hypertension? Am J Med 1988;84(3A):136–9.

[135] Schroeder AP, Sihm I, Morn B, et al. Influence of humoral and neurohormonal factors on cardiovascular hypertrophy in untreated essential hypertensives. Am J Hypertens 1996;9(3):207–15.

[136] Corea L, Bentivoglio M, Verdecchia P, et al. Plasma norepinephrine and left ventricular hypertrophy in systemic hypertension. Am J Cardiol 1984;53(9): 1299–303.

[137] Corea L, Bentivoglio M, Verdecchia P. Echocardiographic left ventricular hypertrophy as related to arterial pressure and plasma norepinephrine concentration in arterial hypertension. Reversal by atenolol treatment. Hypertension 1983;5(6):837–43.

[138] Olsen MH, Wachtell K, Hermann KL, et al. Is cardiovascular remodeling in patients with essential hypertension related to more than high blood pressure? A LIFE substudy. Losartan Intervention For Endpoint-Reduction in Hypertension. Am Heart J 2002;144(3):530–7.

[139] Hua L, Li C, Xia D, et al. Relationship between hypertensive left ventricular hypertrophy and levels of endothelin and nitric oxide. Hypertens Res 2000; 23(4):377–80.

[140] Sayama H, Nakamura Y, Saito N, et al. Relationship between left ventricular geometry and brain natriuretic peptide levels in elderly subjects. Gerontology 2000;46(2):71–7.

ELSEVIER
SAUNDERS

Heart Failure Clin 1 (2005) 25 – 37

HEART
FAILURE
CLINICS

Role and Optimal Dosing of Angiotensin-Converting Enzyme Inhibitor Therapy

Dhruv Kazi, MD[a], Anita Deswal, MD, MPH[b,*]

[a]Baylor College of Medicine, Houston, TX, USA
[b]Michael E. DeBakey Veterans Affairs Medical Center and Baylor College of Medicine, Houston, TX, USA

An understanding of the important role of neurohormonal upregulation in disease progression in heart failure has been translated into therapeutic strategies using neurohormonal antagonists to improve cardiac function, alter disease progression, and improve survival. Angiotensin-converting enzyme (ACE) inhibitors, which were the first of this class of drugs proved to alter the natural history of heart failure and lead to long-term benefit, remain a cornerstone of therapy in all stages of heart failure. This article reviews the rationale for their use, key clinical trial data supporting the major role of ACE inhibitors in heart failure, and the recommended dosing in this patient population.

Rationale for the use of angiotensin-converting enzyme inhibitors in heart failure

Activation of the renin-angiotensin system plays a critical role in the pathogenesis of heart failure [1]. The deleterious effects of renin-angiotensin system activation in heart failure are mediated primarily through increased circulating and tissue levels of the neurohormone angiotensin II. Angiotensin II is an extremely potent vasoconstrictor, acting directly on vascular smooth muscles and indirectly by increasing sympathetic tone [2,3]. In addition, it produces sodium retention (through aldosterone and renal vasoconstriction), as well as fluid retention (through antidiuretic hormone) [4,5]. At the cellular level, angiotensin II promotes migration, proliferation, and hypertrophy, thus producing numerous adverse effects, including remodeling of the left ventricle, alterations in the morphology and mechanical properties of the vasculature, and the development of endothelial dysfunction [6,7].

Angiotensin II promotes cardiac remodeling in several ways. By increasing arterial smooth muscle tone and causing salt and water retention, it increases cardiac preload and afterload, and increased wall stress is a potent stimulus for remodeling. In addition, angiotensin II has direct effects on the myocardium, causes hypertrophy of cardiac myocytes and hyperplasia of cardiac fibroblasts associated with an increase in extracellular matrix deposition [8], and stimulates the release of other growth factors, including norepinephrine and endothelin, which in turn stimulate cardiac remodeling [9]. These actions of angiotensin II are mediated largely through the angiotensin type 1 (AT_1) receptor.

The renin-angiotensin system may be inhibited at various levels, as shown in Fig. 1. ACE inhibitors block the action of ACE, the enzyme responsible for the conversion of angiotensin I to angiotensin II, thereby reducing the angiotensin II available to stimu-

Dr. Deswal is a recipient of the Advanced Clinical Research Career Development Award (CRCD 712A) from the Veterans Affairs (VA) Cooperative Studies Program.

This article is supported in part by grants from the VA Health Services Research and Development Service (IIR 02-082-1) and the VA Clinical Science Research and Development Service.

* Corresponding author. Winters Center for Heart Failure Research and Houston Center of Quality of Care and Utilization Services, Michael E. DeBakey Veterans Affairs Medical Center (152) and Baylor College of Medicine, 2002 Holcombe Boulevard, Houston, TX 77030.

E-mail address: adeswal@bcm.tmc.edu (A. Deswal).

1551-7136/05/$ – see front matter. Published by Elsevier Inc.
doi:10.1016/j.hfc.2004.10.002

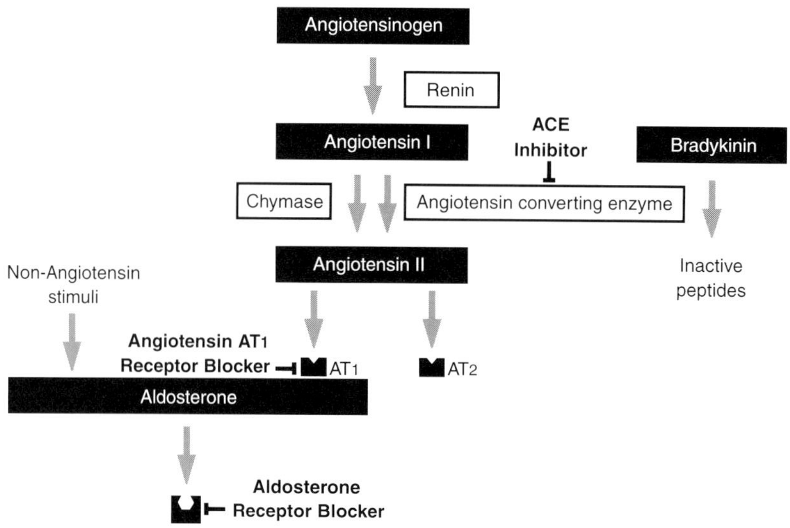

Fig. 1. Activation of the renin-angiotensin-aldosterone system. Angiotensin (AT) is converted to angiotensin I (ATI) by renin. ATI can be converted to angiotensin II (ATII) through ACE and chymase-dependent pathways. ATII exerts its biological effects by binding to AT receptors. Aldosterone production is stimulated by ATII as well as by AT-independent mechanisms. ACE inhibitors block ACE-dependent conversion of ATI to ATII. ACE inhibitors also prevent the catabolism of bradykinin, which can lead to an increase in the local generation of nitric oxide and prostaglandins.

late the angiotensin receptors. Thus, ACE inhibition attenuates many of the key hemodynamic, mechanical, and functional disturbances crucial to the pathophysiology of heart failure. In addition to its ACE blocking effects, ACE also catalyzes the degradation of bradykinin (see Fig. 1). Bradykinin has direct and indirect vasodilator activity mediated by release of nitric oxide and prostaglandin, as well as antimitotic and antithrombotic actions that could be of benefit in heart failure [10]. It also causes natriuresis by a direct tubular effect in the kidney [11]. ACE inhibition results in an accumulation of kinins and accentuation of kinin-mediated prostaglandin synthesis, and experimental data have shown that the hemodynamic and remodeling modification response to ACE inhibition is attenuated significantly by the simultaneous administration of a bradykinin antagonist [12,13]. Thus, in addition to blocking the production of angiotensin II, the therapeutic effects of ACE inhibition in patients who have heart failure may be caused in part by its effect on the kallikrein-kinin system and the attendant increase in endogenous kinin levels.

Although first developed as antihypertensive agents, ACE inhibitors occupy a central role in the management of heart failure [7,14]. Initially, the hemodynamic effects of ACE inhibitors were believed to be central to their role in heart failure. They were expected to optimize loading conditions imposed on the failing heart by reducing peripheral vascular resistance, thus enhancing cardiac output. Studies with the ACE inhibitor captopril demonstrated an increase in cardiac output, lowering of left ventricular (LV) filling pressures, and modest reductions in systolic blood pressure and heart rate in patients who had heart failure and LV systolic dysfunction. These effects were sustained with long-term ACE inhibition [15–17]. It has since been recognized that the effect of ACE inhibitors on LV remodeling may be one of the most important mechanisms for their efficacy in patients who have heart failure [18]. Recently, it has been recognized increasingly that the antiatherogenic, anti-inflammatory, antiproliferative, and antithrombotic properties of ACE inhibitors likely contribute to the vascular protective effects noted in patients with and without heart failure [19,20].

Angiotensin-converting enzyme inhibitors in symptomatic heart failure: evidence from clinical trials

A large body of evidence supports the use of ACE inhibitors in heart failure: ACE inhibitors have been evaluated in clinical trials of more than 7000 patients who have symptomatic heart failure. A meta-analysis based on 7105 patients from 32 published and unpublished trials investigated the efficacy of ACE inhibition in patients who have heart failure [21]. All patients in the analysis had symptomatic heart failure (New York Heart Association [NYHA] functional class II–IV), LV systolic dysfunction, or limitation of exercise duration. In most trials, patients were on background therapy with either digoxin and diuretics or only diuretics. Of these 32 trials, 28 trials with 6726 patients used captopril, enalapril, ramipril, quinapril, or lisinopril. The remaining agents, benazepril hydrochloride, cilazapril, and perindopril, were used in 379 patients. ACE inhibitors significantly reduced mortality (odds ratio [OR] 0.77; 95% confidence interval [CI] 0.67–0.88), which was caused chiefly by a substantial reduction in deaths attributable to progressive heart failure (OR 0.69; 95% CI 0.58–0.83; $P < .001$); point estimates for effects on sudden or presumed arrhythmic deaths and fatal myocardial infarction were not significant. The odds of developing the combined endpoint of death or hospitalization for heart failure were 0.65 (95% CI 0.57–0.74), and there was no evidence of heterogeneity across the different agents. In addition, there were significant reductions in myocardial infarction and nonsignificant reductions in strokes and other thromboembolic events.

Although most of the effect was noted in the first 90 days of treatment, additional benefit continued to accrue with longer use. Most trials were short with duration of 3 months; 12 trials had patient follow-up beyond 90 days. The reductions in total mortality and the combined endpoint of total mortality or hospitalization for heart failure were consistent in the various subgroups based on age, sex, NYHA class, and etiology, although the patients with greater LV systolic dysfunction (LV ejection fraction [LVEF] ≤ 25%) benefited the most. The largest amount of data was from the trials using enalapril, in which there was a significant reduction in mortality (Table 1). Although the reductions in mortality were not statistically significant in the trials using captopril, ramipril, quinapril, and lisinopril, the point estimates were consistent with the overall effect of enalapril (see Table 1). Thus these trials have established the role of ACE inhibitors in reducing mortality and heart failure hospitalization in patients who have heart failure.

Salient features of the three landmark trials with ACE inhibitors in symptomatic heart failure—the Studies of Left Ventricular Dysfunction (SOLVD) treatment trial, the Cooperative North Scandinavian Enalapril Survival Study (CONSENSUS), and the Veterans Administration Cooperative Vasodilator-Heart Failure Trial II (V-HeFT II)—are detailed in

Table 1
Total mortality or hospitalization for heart failure by duration of follow-up and agent for randomized trials of angiotensin-converting enzyme inhibitors

Agent	No. of trials	ACE inhibitors (no. of events/no. randomized)	Controls (no. of events/no. randomized)	OR (95% CI)
90 days or less of follow-up				
Captopril	4	27/292	42/288	0.60 (0.36–1.00)
Enalapril	7	157/1690	259/1691	0.52 (0.42–0.65)
Lisinopril	4	10/351	10/195	0.50 (0.19–1.27)
Quinapril	5	3/548	3/327	0.68 (0.13–3.66)
Ramipril	6	33/714	44/513	0.52 (0.32–0.83)
All other trials	4	9/215	14/164	0.51 (0.21–1.24)
Total	**30**	**239/3810**	**372/3178**	**0.53 (0.44–0.63)**
More than 90 days of follow-up				
Captopril	3	52/214	66/206	0.68 (0.44–1.04)
Enalapril	3	559/1282	592/1187	0.78 (0.66–0.91)
Lisinopril	0	—	—	—
Quinapril	2	2/218	2/210	0.96 (0.14–6.87)
Ramipril	2	2/120	3/83	0.58 (0.10–3.48)
Total	**10**	**615/1834**	**663/1686**	**0.76 (0.66–0.88)**

Data from Garg R, Yusuf S. Overview of randomized trials of angiotensin-converting enzyme inhibitors on mortality and morbidity in patients with heart failure. Collaborative Group on ACE Inhibitor Trials. JAMA 1995;273(18):1450–6.

Table 2
Selected clinical trials establishing the benefit of angiotensin-converting enzyme inhibitors in symptomatic and asymptomatic left ventricular systolic dysfunction

Trial [Ref.] (no. of patients; average follow-up)	Study population	ACE inhibitor and dose	Key results
CONSENSUS I [22] (n = 253; 6 mo)	NYHA IV	Enalapril vs. placebo 2.5 mg twice daily titrated to 20 mg twice daily	6-mo mortality decreased 40% 1-y mortality decreased 31% Improvement in NYHA class Decrease in cardiac size
V-HeFT II [24] (n = 804; 2.5 y)	NYHA II–IV LVEF <45%	Target enalapril 10 mg twice daily vs. hydralazine 75 mg four times daily + isosorbide dinitrate 40 mg four times daily	2-y mortality decreased 28% No difference in HF hospitalization Lesser improvement in exercise capacity and ventricular function with enalapril
SOLVD Treatment Trial [65] (n = 2569; 41 mo)	NYHA II–IV (90% II-III) LVEF ≤35%	Enalapril vs. placebo 2.5 mg twice daily titrated to 10 mg twice daily	16% decrease in mortality 22% decrease in progressive HF mortality 26% decrease in either death or HF hospitalization 8.6-mo increase in median life expectancy [76]
SOLVD Prevention Trial [29] (n = 4228; 37.4 mo)	NYHA I LVEF ≤35%	Enalapril vs. placebo 2.5 mg twice daily titrated to 10 mg twice daily	20% decrease in either death or HF hospitalization 29% decrease in either death or development of HF

Table 2. These trials were included in the meta-analysis discussed above and individually established the role of the ACE inhibitor enalapril in prolonging survival in patients with the complete range of symptomatic heart failure (NYHA class II–IV) secondary to LV systolic dysfunction [22–24].

In addition to their benefit on mortality, several trials have shown that ACE inhibitors improve symptoms and exercise capacity in patients who have heart failure. Narang and colleagues [25] reviewed 35 published, double-blind, randomized placebo-controlled trials involving 3411 patients that compared the effect of ACE inhibitors and placebo on exercise capacity in patients who had symptomatic chronic heart failure. Exercise duration improved in 23 of the studies, whereas symptoms improved in 25 of the 33 studies that evaluated this. In most trials (27 of 33), there was concordance between the effect on symptoms and on exercise capacity, but six trials showed discrepant results. All nine trials with sample size more than 50, follow-up of 3 to 6 months, and use of treadmill exercise tests showed improved exercise capacity as well as symptoms.

Thus far, no trials have established the role of ACE inhibitors specifically in patients who have heart failure and preserved ejection fraction. Continuing trials such as the Perindopril for Elderly People with Chronic Heart Failure (PEP-CHF) study should clarify the benefit of ACE inhibition in this patient population.

Angiotensin-converting enzyme inhibitors in asymptomatic left ventricular systolic dysfunction

Patients who have asymptomatic LV dysfunction are at high risk for developing heart failure and for death [26]. Studies have shown some degree of neurohormonal activation in patients who have asymptomatic LV dysfunction and mild heart failure, and that this activation may be more marked during exercise [27,28]. These factors led to the evaluation of the effect of ACE inhibitors on morbidity, mortality, and development of heart failure in patients who have asymptomatic LV systolic dysfunction in the SOLVD Prevention Trial [29]. In this trial of asymptomatic patients with depressed LVEF who were not receiving any therapy for heart failure, enalapril significantly reduced the rate of the combined endpoint of death or hospitalization for heart failure and significantly delayed the development of heart failure (see Table 2). Enalapril produced an 8%, nonsignificant reduction in mortality (P = .30), however. Notably, 41% of all patients in the placebo group and 51% of patients in the placebo group who were hospitalized for heart failure were prescribed an open-label ACE inhibitor, suggesting an underestimation of the effect of ACE inhibition in patients who have asymptomatic LV systolic dysfunction. Thus, in a patient population with asymptomatic LV dysfunction, ACE inhibitors were associated with a significant benefit on morbidity but not on mortality. A substudy demonstrated that chronic ACE inhibition resulted in slowing or reversal of LV dilatation in patients who had asymptomatic LV dysfunction, suggesting that as in systolic heart failure, the clinical benefits of ACE inhibition may have been caused in part by its impact on ventricular remodeling [30].

Angiotensin-converting enzyme inhibition in patients who have heart failure or left ventricular systolic dysfunction post–myocardial infarction

There is a marked increase in fatal and nonfatal cardiovascular events among survivors of acute myocardial infarction [31], with the degree of LV dysfunction being the most important determinant of the increased risk [32,33]. After the initial insult, residual viable myocardium undergoes progressive remodeling and dilatation, leading to deterioration in LV performance [34–36]. The degree of LV dysfunction is proportionate to the size and age of the scar. Animal experiments as well as clinical studies with surrogate endpoints (ventricular size and function) have demonstrated the efficacy of ACE inhibition in the attenuation of LV dilatation and progressive LV dysfunction [18,37,38]. In addition, ACE inhibitors may have antiatherogenic, anti-inflammatory, antiproliferative, and antithrombotic effects that may reduce recurrent myocardial infarction in these patients [19,20].

The three long-term trials that demonstrated benefit of the ACE inhibitors captopril, ramipril, and trandolapril in patients who had LV systolic dysfunction or heart failure after an acute myocardial infarction are detailed in Table 3 [31,39,40]. An overview of these three trials established that the use of ACE-inhibitor therapy, begun within 3 to 16 days after an acute myocardial infarction and continued long-term, was associated with an overall reduction in mortality (OR 0.74; 95% CI 0.66–0.83), recurrent myocardial infarction (OR 0.80; 95% CI 0.69–0.94), hospitalization for heart failure (OR 0.73; 95% CI 0.63–0.85), and development of heart failure [41]. The results indicated that 15 patients would need to be treated for 2.5 years to prevent one death. Long-term follow-up of patients in two of these trials also demonstrated a sustained benefit on survival [42,43].

Angiotensin-converting enzyme inhibition and prevention of heart failure in patients without left ventricular systolic dysfunction

Having demonstrated the efficacy of ACE inhibitors in patients who have LV systolic dysfunction, irrespective of clinical symptoms of heart failure, the next logical step was to investigate their role in the

Table 3
Selected clinical trials establishing the benefit of angiotensin-converting enzyme inhibitors after an acute myocardial infarction

Trial [Ref.] (no. of patients; average follow-up)	Study population	ACE inhibitor and dose	Key results
SAVE [31] (n = 2231; 42 mo)	3–16 d post-MI LVEF<40% No overt HF	Captopril 12.5 mg three times daily titrated to 50 mg three times daily	19% decrease in all-cause mortality 21% decrease in CV mortality 37% decrease in severe HF 25% decrease in recurrent MI
AIRE [40,43] (n = 2006; 15 mo)	3–10 d post-MI Clinical HF irrespective of LVEF	Ramipril 2.5 mg twice daily titrated 5 mg twice daily	27% decrease in all cause mortality 19% decrease in death, reinfarction, severe HF, or stroke 23% decrease in severe HF 30% decrease in sudden death No effect on recurrent MI
TRACE [39] (n = 2606; 36 mo)	3–7 d post-MI Wall motion index ≤1.2 LVEF ≤35%	Trandolapril 1 mg once daily titrated up to 4 mg once daily	22% decrease in all-cause mortality 25% decrease in CV mortality 29% decrease in severe HF 24% decrease in sudden death

Abbreviations: CV, cardiovascular; HF, heart failure; MI, myocardial infarction.

prevention of heart failure in patients without LV systolic dysfunction, in patients who have hypertension, for example, or in patients at high risk for cardiovascular events. In patients who have hypertension, ACE inhibitors may prevent or delay the progression of myocardial fibrosis and structural disarray in the hypertensive heart by blunting the renin-angiotensin system over a prolonged period, and thus may prevent or delay the onset of heart failure [44,45].

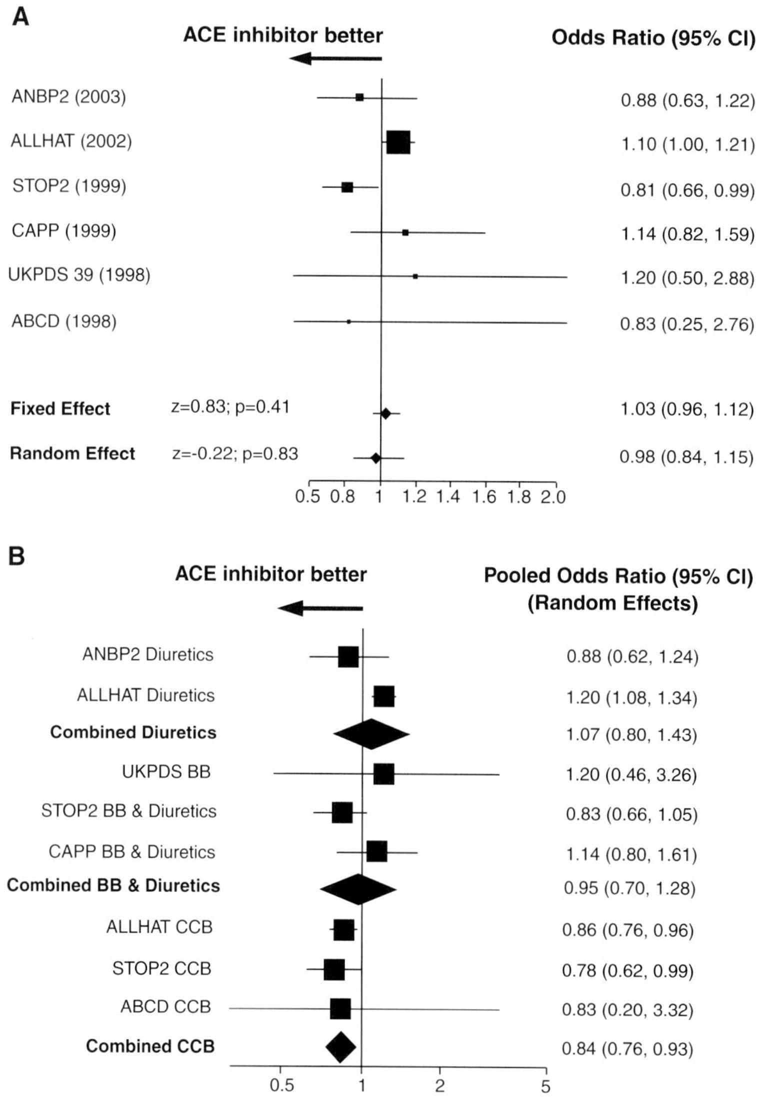

Fig. 2. (*A*) Meta-analysis of effectiveness of ACE inhibitors in the prevention of heart failure in patients who have hypertension: comparison of ACE inhibitors to all other drugs. ABCD, Appropriate Blood Pressure Control in Diabetes; ANBP2, Second Australian National Blood Pressure Project; ALLHAT, Antihypertensive and Lipid-Lowering Treatment to Prevent Heart Attack Trial; CAPP, Captopril Prevention Project; STOP-2, Swedish Trial in Old Patients with Hypertension-2; UKPDS, UK Prospective Diabetes Study Group. (*From* Angeli F, Verdecchia P, Reboldi GP, et al. Meta-analysis of effectiveness or lack thereof of angiotensin-converting enzyme inhibitors for prevention of heart failure in patients with systemic hypertension. Am J Cardiol 2004;93(2):240–3; with permission.) (*B*) Meta-analysis of effectiveness of ACE inhibitors in the prevention of heart failure in patients who have hypertension: comparison of ACE inhibitors to other drug classes. (*From* Mills E, Montori VM, Thabane L. Angiotensin-converting enzyme inhibitor meta-analysis provides misleading conclusion. Am J Cardiol 2004; 94(1):149; with permission.)

A recent meta-analysis of six trials of antihypertensive therapy evaluated the benefits of ACE inhibitors versus all other antihypertensive agents (including diuretics, beta blockers, calcium channel blockers, and alpha blockers) [46]. The main finding of this analysis was that the risk for heart failure did not differ between patients randomized to receive ACE inhibitors and those randomized to receive other classes of antihypertensives (Fig. 2). This analysis assumed, however, that all other antihypertensive agents evaluated were equal in their effects on the development of heart failure. Using the same trials, but evaluating ACE inhibitors against individual drug classes (diuretics, beta blockers, calcium channel blockers, and beta blocker and diuretic combination) yielded slightly different results [47]. As shown in Fig. 2, although diuretics seemed superior to or no different than ACE inhibitors (OR for ACE inhibitors versus other drugs 1.07; 95% CI 0.80–1.43) in the prevention of heart failure, ACE inhibitors seemed superior to calcium channel blockers in preventing heart failure (OR 0.84; 95% CI 0.76–0.93). Based on these data, one may conclude that in a general population with hypertension, ACE inhibitors may not have a consistent benefit in preventing heart failure, but may be superior to calcium channel blockers.

Results were different, however, in patients who were at high risk for the development of cardiovascular events. The Heart Outcome Evaluation Project (HOPE) examined benefit of the ACE inhibitor ramipril in reducing mortality and morbidity in high-risk patients without heart failure or known depressed LVEF [48]. A total of 9297 elderly patients (>55 years of age) with a history of coronary artery disease, stroke, peripheral vascular disease, or diabetes mellitus plus at least one other cardiovascular risk factor (hypertension, elevated total cholesterol levels, low high-density lipoprotein cholesterol levels, cigarette smoking, or documented microalbuminuria) were randomized to receive either ramipril at a target dose of 10 mg/d or placebo for an average of 5 years. Overall, patients in the ramipril group had a 22% reduction in the primary composite outcome of myocardial infarctions, stroke, or death from cardiovascular causes. In addition, the allocation to treatment with ramipril significantly reduced the rate of all heart failure (composite of heart failure death, heart failure requiring hospitalization, heart failure requiring ACE inhibitor, or any reported heart failure) by 23% and the rate of combined cardiovascular death and all heart failure by 24% [49]. When analyzed separately, each component of the composite endpoint of heart failure showed benefit with ramipril. Documentation of LVEF was not required for entry into the study, but of 5193 patients who had known LVEF at baseline, 92% had a normal LVEF and a subgroup analysis of patients who had documented normal LVEF at baseline (n = 4775) found similar benefits to those seen in the overall group. The benefits of ramipril on heart failure development were consistent across most subgroups. There was a significant interaction between baseline blood pressure and treatment group. Ramipril was associated with a 9% reduction in heart failure in patients who had baseline systolic blood pressure below the median (139 mm Hg) compared with a larger 33% reduction in patients who had blood pressure above the median. Thus, mechanisms for prevention of heart failure in patients at high risk could include better control of blood pressure in addition to prevention of myocardial infarction, as well as beneficial effects in diabetics with ACE inhibition [49].

Choice of angiotensin-converting enzyme inhibitors and optimal dosing

Although most evidence supporting an effect of ACE inhibitors on the survival of patients who have symptomatic heart failure is derived from experience with enalapril, the available data suggest that there are no differences among available ACE inhibitors in their effects on symptoms or survival (see Table 1) [21]. It has been suggested that drugs in this class may differ in their ability to inhibit tissue ACE, but no trial has shown that tissue ACE-inhibiting agents are superior to other ACE inhibitors in any clinical aspect of heart failure. In selecting among ACE inhibitors, however, it is recommended that preference be given to ACE inhibitors that reduced morbidity and mortality in clinical trials (eg captopril, enalapril, lisinopril, and ramipril), because such studies have defined a dose that effectively modifies the natural history of the disease. Such information generally is lacking for ACE inhibitors that were not evaluated in large-scale studies [50].

Despite overwhelming evidence of the benefits of ACE inhibitors on morbidity and mortality in heart failure, initial surveys reflected significant underuse as well as use of doses much lower than those used in clinical trials. This may be based on the perception that the degree of benefit accrued depends on the use of ACE inhibitors (irrespective of their dose), whereas the adverse events are dose-dependent, although these assumptions have not been validated [51]. Additionally, there is a marked reluctance to initiate or advance therapy in patients who have baseline hypotension or renal insufficiency or in elderly patients, despite evidence that these patients receive as much benefit from the ACE inhibitor therapy as other patients [52–54]. Because many patients are treated at doses below the target doses used in clinical trials, there remains significant interest in whether lower doses of ACE inhibitors confer similar reductions in morbidity and mortality.

Earlier clinical studies showed that higher doses of ACE inhibitors offered greater hemodynamic [16,55,56] and symptomatic [57] benefit compared with lower doses, and experimental data indicated reduction in mortality with higher doses of ACE inhibition in animal models [58]. Therefore, clinical studies were performed to evaluate the use of ACE inhibitors at low dose, at target doses used in large clinical trials, and at higher than target doses.

Tang and colleagues [59] compared the neurohormonal responses and clinical effects of high-dose (40 mg/d) versus low-dose (5 mg/d) enalapril over 6 months in 75 patients who had chronic heart failure and LV systolic dysfunction. In the 48 patients who remained in the study at the end of 6 months, high-dose enalapril was associated with a greater reduction in serum ACE activity compared with the low-dose group. High-dose enalapril was not associated with greater suppression of angiotensin II, aldosterone, or norepinephrine levels, however. There were nearly twice the number of predetermined clinical events including emergency room visits, hospital admissions, deaths, and sustained increases in diuretic doses in the low-dose group compared with the high-dose group (53% versus 30%), but this finding did not reach statistical significance ($P = .06$). Similarly, a trend toward a greater reduction in LV diastolic dimensions was noted in the high-dose arm ($P = .08$). Enalapril was well tolerated even at the high doses. More adverse events were reported in the low-dose group than in the high-dose group.

Conversely, the NETWORK study of 1532 patients, which compared low-dose (2.5 mg twice daily), intermediate (5 mg twice daily), or high-dose (10 mg twice daily) enalapril for 6 months, found no significant differences in mortality or hospitalization among the three groups. It should be noted, however, that this study was of short duration and overall only had 53 deaths and 90 hospitalizations for heart failure in the randomized patients, thus allowing suboptimal power for detection of smaller differences between groups [60]. Nanas and colleagues [61] took a different approach. They compared differences in survival, clinical, and hemodynamic variables between patients treated with either standard dose (target 20 mg/d; mean dose achieved 17.9 ± 4.3 mg/d) or higher than standard dose (target 60 mg/d; mean dose achieved 42 ± 19.3 mg/d) enalapril in 248 patients. At the end of 1 year of follow-up, they found no significant differences in survival or in clinical or hemodynamic variables between the two groups. Thus, these smaller studies did not define clearly the importance of ACE-inhibitor dosing in patients who have heart failure on mortality, morbidity, or exercise tolerance [62].

The Assessment of Treatment with Lisinopril and Survival (ATLAS) Trial was performed with the objective of definitively comparing the efficacy and safety of low- versus high-dose ACE inhibition on mortality and morbidity in chronic heart failure [63]. The ATLAS trial randomized 3164 patients with LVEF $\leq$ 30% and chronic heart failure (NYHA II–IV) to either low-dose (target 2.5–5.0 mg/d) or high-dose (target 32.5–35.0 mg/d) of the ACE inhibitor lisinopril. This dose selection was based on previous studies that showed the lower dose of 2.5 to 5 mg of lisinopril to have favorable hemodynamic effects [56], whereas doses of lisinopril, 20 to 40 mg/d, were comparable to the doses of ACE inhibitors that had demonstrated beneficial effects on morbidity and mortality in prior clinical trials [63,64]. The trial had an initial open-label phase for at least 4 weeks in which an attempt was made to up-titrate to and maintain patients at lisinopril, 12.5 mg/d to 15 mg/d. Almost 5% of patients were excluded from participation in the trial because they could not tolerate the intermediate doses of lisinopril during this open-label period. Of the 3164 patients that were randomized, 93% achieved target dose in the low-dose group and 91% achieved target dose in the high-dose group. During the course of the study, 31% of patients in the low-dose and 27% patients in the high-dose group discontinued therapy. In addition, 22% of patients in the low-dose and 18% of the high-dose group were started on open label therapy, potentially decreasing the magnitude of differences in benefit between the two groups.

After a median follow-up of 46 months, compared with the low-dose group, patients receiving the higher dose of lisinopril had a nonsignificant 8% reduction in all-cause mortality ($P = .128$), a 10% reduction in cardiovascular mortality ($P = .073$) and a 12% reduction in the combined endpoint of all-cause mortality or hospitalization for any reason ($P = .002$). Patients on high-dose lisinopril, however, had 24% fewer hospitalizations for heart failure ($P = .002$), 13% reduction in all-cause hospitalizations ($P = .021$), and 16% reduction in cardiovascular hospitalizations ($P = .05$). This study also demonstrated the relative safety of high-dose ACE inhibition. Although high-dose lisinopril was associated with more frequent dizziness, hypotension, mild decrease in renal function, and hyperkalemia, these side effects did not lead patients to stop the study medication more frequently in the high-dose group than in the low-dose group (17% versus 18%). Compared with the low-dose group, fewer patients in the high-dose group experienced cough or reported worsening heart failure as an adverse event [63].

Thus the ATLAS trial demonstrated that when compared with low doses of ACE inhibitors, the use of high doses reduces the risk for major clinical events, especially cardiovascular and heart failure hospitalizations. This can translate into significant cost savings as well as improvement in quality of life. There was no significant reduction in all-cause mortality with the use of high-dose ACE inhibitors, however. The benefit achieved with low-dose ACE inhibition compared with high-dose inhibition was approximately half that noted when comparable high-dose ACE inhibitors were compared with placebo in the SOLVD studies [65], suggesting that low-dose ACE inhibitors may provide about half the benefits associated with the high dose of these agents. Also, the study results do not clarify whether there is any incremental benefit from intermediate to high-dose ACE inhibition [63].

Therefore, available data support trying to up-titrate ACE inhibitor doses beyond the low doses, if tolerated. Until further data are available, it may be prudent to attempt up-titration to the target doses shown beneficial in clinical trials of ACE inhibitors in patients who have heart failure [50]. If target doses of an ACE inhibitor cannot be tolerated, lower doses should be used with the expectation that the lower doses exert benefit, albeit less than higher doses. Table 4 lists the initial and target doses of ACE inhibitors that are recommended in the treatment of patients who have heart failure.

Patient characteristics as a determinant of benefit from angiotensin-converting enzyme inhibition

Although the numerous clinical trials of ACE inhibition in patients who have heart failure provide incontrovertible evidence in its favor, it is unclear whether this benefit extends equally across all subgroups. This section discusses various patient characteristics that may influence the degree of benefit achieved from ACE inhibitors.

Disease severity

In most clinical trials of ACE inhibition in heart failure, patients who had greater severity of clinical heart failure and lower LVEF obtained the greatest benefit. The CONSENSUS trial demonstrated a 31% reduction in mortality in patients who had NYHA class-IV heart failure after treatment with enalapril for 6 months, whereas the SOLVD treatment trial, which predominantly included patients in NYHA class II and III, demonstrated a 16% reduction in mortality at 41 months [22,65]. On a similar note, the SOLVD prevention trial, which looked at patients with asymptomatic LV dysfunction, produced only an 8% nonsignificant trend toward reduced mortality with enalapril [29].

Patients who have hyponatremia (serum sodium $<$135 mEq/L) tend to be more sensitive to ACE inhibition, likely because of higher plasma renin levels [66]. Hyponatremia identifies patients more likely to develop hypotension and worsening azotemia after the initiation of ACE inhibitors.

Baseline azotemia identifies a group of patients at increased risk for all-cause mortality in patients who have heart failure [67,68]. On the other hand, some patients are at a higher risk for deterioration of renal function after initiation of an ACE inhibitor, particu-

Table 4
Recommended doses of angiotensin-converting enzyme inhibitors in heart failure

Drug	Initial dose	Target/maximum dose
Captopril	6.25 mg three times daily	50 mg three times daily
Enalapril	2.5 mg twice daily	10 to 20 mg twice daily
Fosinopril	5 to 10 mg once daily	40 mg once daily
Lisinopril	2.5 to 5.0 mg once daily	20 to 40 mg once daily
Quinapril	10 mg twice daily	40 mg twice daily
Ramipril	1.25 to 2.5 mg once daily	10 mg once daily

Data from Hunt SA, Baker DW, Chin MH, et al. ACC/AHA Guidelines for the evaluation and management of chronic heart failure in the adult. Circulation 2001;104(24):2996–3007.

larly those who are older or on diuretics [69]. It is therefore imperative to start at a low dose and up-titrate the dose cautiously in patients who have pre-existing renal disease with close monitoring of renal function and serum potassium during the initiation and up-titration phase. Worsening renal function or hypotension usually can be improved after reduction in the dose of concomitantly administered diuretics, if possible. If renal function continues to deteriorate, however, lower doses of ACE inhibitors may need to be tried, or, in some cases, the ACE inhibitors may need to be discontinued. Patients who are unable to tolerate ACE inhibitors because of progressive renal dysfunction or other circulatory-renal limitations while on ACE inhibitors have a higher risk for mortality [70].

Gender and race

Most patients enrolled in the large randomized clinical trials that established the benefit of ACE inhibitors in patients who have LV systolic dysfunction were white men. Whether an equal effect is achieved in women and blacks has been controversial. There are several reasons to believe that certain subpopulations may not experience the same benefits as white men. There is evidence that ACE inhibitors exert a lesser effect on blood pressure in black compared with non-black hypertensive patients [71], and retrospective analyses have suggested that ACE inhibitors may not be as effective in black patients who have heart failure [72,73]. Similarly, men and women may respond differently to cardiac therapies. A preliminary analysis of one ACE inhibitor study suggested a trend toward lower mortality reduction in women compared with men [74]. A recent gender- and race-specific analysis of pooled data from seven large clinical trials, however, suggested that ACE inhibitors have survival benefit in women who have symptomatic heart failure and LV dysfunction, as well in black patients. Because of smaller numbers of these subgroups in the trials, definitive conclusions regarding the magnitude of the benefits compared with those seen in white males are not possible [75]. Pending the availability of more definitive data, however, current guidelines continue to recommend the use of ACE inhibition in women and black patients who have heart failure. Although clinical trials designed to address the issue of ACE inhibition in racial minorities may be desirable, a placebo-controlled trial would be unethical at this juncture. Finally, ethnic minorities such as blacks are genetically inhomogeneous populations, and data from subgroup analyses of large trials should not be used to withhold this life-saving treatment.

Summary

Based on overwhelming data demonstrating reduced morbidity and mortality, ACE inhibitors are a mainstay of therapy in patients with symptomatic and asymptomatic LV systolic dysfunction. Furthermore, ACE inhibitors may be beneficial in the prevention of heart failure in patients with high-risk cardiovascular profiles. Data are not available to recommend their use in patients who have heart failure and preserved LVEF. Although ACE inhibitors likely exert a class effect, it is recommended that ACE inhibitors that reduced morbidity and mortality in clinical trials (eg, captopril, enalapril, lisinopril, and ramipril) be used preferentially because studies have defined clearly a dose for these agents that is effective in modifying the natural history of the disease. Attempts should be made to up-titrate patients to target doses of ACE inhibitors that have been used in clinical trials, if tolerated.

References

[1] Schrier RW, Abraham WT. Hormones and hemodynamics in heart failure. N Engl J Med 1999;341(8): 577–85.

[2] Folkow B, Johansson B, Mellander S. The comparative effects of angiotensin and noradrenaline on consecutive vascular sections. Acta Physiol Scand 1961; 53:99–104.

[3] Zimmerman BG, Sybertz EJ, Wong PC. Interaction between sympathetic and renin-angiotensin system. J Hypertens 1984;2(6):581–7.

[4] Weber KT. Aldosterone in congestive heart failure. N Engl J Med 2001;345(23):1689–97.

[5] Padfield PL, Morton JJ. Effects of angiotensin II on arginine-vasopressin in physiological and pathological situations in man. J Endocrinol 1977;74(2):251–9.

[6] Williams B. Angiotensin II and the pathophysiology of cardiovascular remodeling. Am J Cardiol 2001; 87(8A):10C–7C.

[7] Brown NJ, Vaughan DE. Angiotensin-converting enzyme inhibitors. Circulation 1998;97(14):1411–20.

[8] Sadoshima J, Izumo S. Molecular characterization of angiotensin II–induced hypertrophy of cardiac myocytes and hyperplasia of cardiac fibroblasts. Critical role of the AT1 receptor subtype. Circ Res 1993;73:413–23.

[9] Greenberg BH. Effects of angiotensin converting enzyme inhibitors on remodeling in clinical trials. J Card Fail 2002;8(6 Suppl):S486–90.

[10] Gavras I. Bradykinin-mediated effects of ACE inhibition. Kidney Int 1992;42(4):1020–9.

[11] Stein JH, Congbalay RC, Karsh DL, et al. The effect of bradykinin on proximal tubular sodium reabsorption in the dog: evidence for functional nephron heterogeneity. J Clin Invest 1972;51(7):1709–21.

[12] Gainer JV, Morrow JD, Loveland A, et al. Effect of bradykinin-receptor blockade on the response to angiotensin-converting-enzyme inhibitor in normotensive and hypertensive subjects. N Engl J Med 1998; 339(18):1285–92.

[13] McDonald KM, Mock J, d'Aloia A, et al. Bradykinin antagonism inhibits the antigrowth effect of converting enzyme inhibition in the dog myocardium after discrete transmural myocardial necrosis. Circulation 1995;91(7):2043–8.

[14] Antonaccio MJ. Development and pharmacology of angiotensin converting enzyme inhibitors. J Pharmacol 1983;14(Suppl 3):29–45.

[15] Ader R, Chatterjee K, Ports T, et al. Immediate and sustained hemodynamic and clinical improvement in chronic heart failure by an oral angiotensin-converting enzyme inhibitor. Circulation 1980;61(5): 931–7.

[16] DiCarlo L, Chatterjee K, Parmley WW, et al. Enalapril: a new angiotensin-converting enzyme inhibitor in chronic heart failure: acute and chronic hemodynamic evaluations. J Am Coll Cardiol 1983;2(5):865–71.

[17] Chatterjee K, Parmley WW, Cohn JN, et al. A cooperative multicenter study of captopril in congestive heart failure: hemodynamic effects and long-term response. Am Heart J 1985;110(2):439–47.

[18] Pfeffer JM, Pfeffer MA, Braunwald E. Influence of chronic captopril therapy on the infarcted left ventricle of the rat. Circ Res 1985;57:84–95.

[19] O'Keefe JH, Wetzel M, Moe RR, et al. Should an angiotensin-converting enzyme inhibitor be standard therapy for patients with atherosclerotic disease? J Am Coll Cardiol 2001;37(1):1–8.

[20] Banerjee A, Talreja A, Sonnenblick EH, et al. Evolving rationale for angiotensin-converting enzyme inhibition in chronic heart failure. Mt Sinai J Med 2003;70(4): 225–31.

[21] Garg R, Yusuf S. Overview of randomized trials of angiotensin-converting enzyme inhibitors on mortality and morbidity in patients with heart failure. JAMA 1995;273:1450–6.

[22] CONSENSUS Trial Study Group. Effects of enalapril on mortality in severe congestive heart failure: results of the Cooperative North Scandanavian Enalapril Survival Study. N Engl J Med 1987;316:1429–35.

[23] SOLVD Investigators. Effect of enalapril on survival in patients with reduced left ventricular ejection fractions and congestive heart failure. N Engl J Med 1991;325:293–302.

[24] Cohn JN, Johnson G, Ziesche S, et al. A comparison of enalapril with hydralazine-isosorbide dinitrate in the treatment of chronic congestive heart failure. N Engl J Med 1991;325:303–10.

[25] Narang R, Swedberg K, Cleland JG. What is the ideal study design for evaluation of treatment for heart failure? Insights from trials assessing the effect of ACE inhibitors on exercise capacity. Eur Heart J 1996; 17(1):120–34.

[26] Wang TJ, Evans JC, Benjamin EJ, et al. Natural history of asymptomatic left ventricular systolic dysfunction in the community. Circulation 2003;108(8): 977–82.

[27] Francis GS, Benedict C, Johnstone DE, et al. Comparison of neuroendocrine activation in patients with left ventricular dysfunction with and without congestive heart failure A substudy of the Studies of Left Ventricular Dysfunction (SOLVD). Circulation 1990; 82(5):1724–9.

[28] Kirlin PC, Grekin R, Das S, et al. Neurohumoral activation during exercise in congestive heart failure. Am J Med 1986;81(4):623–9.

[29] The SOLVD Investigators. Effect of enalapril on mortality and the development of heart failure in asymptomatic patients with reduced left ventricular ejection fractions. N Engl J Med 1992;327(10):685–91.

[30] Konstam MA, Kronenberg MW, Rousseau MF, et al. Effects of the angiotensin converting enzyme inhibitor enalapril on the long-term progression of left ventricular dilatation in patients with asymptomatic systolic dysfunction. SOLVD (Studies of Left Ventricular Dysfunction) Investigators. Circulation 1993; 88(5 Pt 1):2277–83.

[31] Pfeffer MA, Braunwald E, Moye LA, et al. Effect of captopril on mortality and morbidity in patients with left ventricular dysfunction after myocardial infarction. Results of the Survival and Ventricular Enlargement trial. The SAVE Investigators. N Engl J Med 1992; 327(10):669–77.

[32] Stadius ML, Davis K, Maynard C, et al. Risk stratification for 1 year survival based on characteristics identified in the early hours of acute myocardial infarction. The Western Washington Intracoronary Streptokinase Trial. Circulation 1986;74(4):703–11.

[33] White HD, Norris RM, Brown MA, et al. Left ventricular end-systolic volume as the major determinant of survival after recovery from myocardial infarction. Circulation 1987;76(1):44–51.

[34] McKay RG, Pfeffer MA, Pasternak RC, et al. Left ventricular remodeling after myocardial infarction: a corollary to infarct expansion. Circulation 1986;74(4): 693–702.

[35] Gaudron P, Eilles C, Ertl G, et al. Early remodelling of the left ventricle in patients with myocardial infarction. Eur Heart J 1990;11(Suppl B):139–46.

[36] Pfeffer MA, Braunwald E. Ventricular remodeling after myocardial infarction. Experimental observations and clinical implications. Circulation 1990;81(4): 1161–72.

[37] Pfeffer MA, Lamas GA, Vaughan DE, et al. Effect of captopril on progressive ventricular dilatation after anterior myocardial infarction. N Engl J Med 1988; 319:80–6.

[38] Sharpe N, Murphy J, Smith H, et al. Treatment of patients with symptomless left ventricular dysfunction after myocardial infarction. Lancet 1988;1(8580): 255–9.

[39] Kober L, Torp-Pedersen C, Carlsen JE, et al. A clinical trial of the angiotensin-converting-enzyme inhibitor trandolapril in patients with left ventricular dysfunction after myocardial infarction. Trandolapril Cardiac Evaluation (TRACE) Study Group. N Engl J Med 1995;333(25):1670–6.

[40] AIRE Study. Effect of ramipril on mortality and morbidity of survivors of acute myocardial infarction with clinical evidence of heart failure. Lancet 1993; 342:821–8.

[41] Flather MD, Yusuf S, Kober L, et al. Long-term ACE-inhibitor therapy in patients with heart failure or left- ventricular dysfunction: a systematic overview of data from individual patients. ACE-Inhibitor Myocardial Infarction Collaborative Group. Lancet 2000; 355(9215):1575–81.

[42] Torp-Pedersen C, Kober L. Effect of ACE inhibitor trandolapril on life expectancy of patients with reduced left-ventricular function after acute myocardial infarction. TRACE Study Group. Trandolapril Cardiac Evaluation. Lancet 1999;354(9172):9–12.

[43] Hall AS, Murray GD, Ball SG. Follow-up study of patients randomly allocated ramipril or placebo for heart failure after acute myocardial infarction: AIRE Extension (AIREX) Study Acute Infarction Ramipril Efficacy. Lancet 1997;349(9064):1493–7.

[44] Brilla CG, Funck RC, Rupp H. Lisinopril-mediated regression of myocardial fibrosis in patients with hypertensive heart disease. Circulation 2000;102(12): 1388–93.

[45] Weber KT, Brilla CG. Pathological hypertrophy and cardiac interstitium. Fibrosis and renin-angiotensin-aldosterone system. Circulation 1991;83(6):1849–65.

[46] Angeli F, Verdecchia P, Reboldi GP, et al. Meta-analysis of effectiveness or lack thereof of angiotensin-converting enzyme inhibitors for prevention of heart failure in patients with systemic hypertension. Am J Cardiol 2004;93(2):240–3.

[47] Mills E, Montori VM, Thabane L. Angiotensin-converting enzyme inhibitor meta-analysis provides misleading conclusion. Am J Cardiol 2004; 94(1):149.

[48] Yusuf S, Sleight P, Pogue J, et al. Effects of an angiotensin-converting-enzyme inhibitor, ramipril, on cardiovascular events in high-risk patients. The Heart Outcomes Prevention Evaluation Study Investigators. N Engl J Med 2000;342(3):145–53.

[49] Arnold JM, Yusuf S, Young J, et al. Prevention of heart failure in patients in the Heart Outcomes Prevention Evaluation (HOPE) study. Circulation 2003;107(9): 1284–90.

[50] Hunt SA, Baker DW, Chin MH, et al. ACC/AHA guidelines for the evaluation and management of chronic heart failure in the adult: executive summary. A report of the American College of Cardiology/American Heart Association Task Force on Practice Guidelines. Circulation 2001;104(24):2996–3007.

[51] Packer M. Do angiotensin-converting enzyme inhibitors prolong life in patients with heart failure treated in clinical practice. J Am Coll Cardiol 1996;28: 1323–7.

[52] Ljungman S, Kjekshus J, Swedberg K. Renal function in severe congestive heart failure during treatment with enalapril (the Cooperative North Scandinavian Enalapril Survival Study [CONSENSUS] Trial). Am J Cardiol 1992;70(4):479–87.

[53] Massie BM, Kramer BL, Topic N. Lack of relationship between the short-term hemodynamic effects of captopril and subsequent clinical responses. Circulation 1984;69(6):1135–41.

[54] Chen YT, Wang Y, Radford MJ, et al. Angiotensin-converting enzyme inhibitor dosages in elderly patients with heart failure. Am Heart J 2001;141(3): 410–7.

[55] Pacher R, Stanek B, Globits S, et al. Effects of two different enalapril dosages on clinical, haemodynamic, and neurohumoral response of patients with severe congestive heart failure. Eur Heart J 1996;17(8): 1223–32.

[56] Uretsky BF, Shaver JA, Liang CS, et al. Modulation of hemodynamic effects with a converting enzyme inhibitor: acute hemodynamic dose-response relationship of a new angiotensin converting enzyme inhibitor, lisinopril, with observations on long-term clinical, functional, and biochemical responses. Am Heart J 1988;116(2 Pt 1):480–8.

[57] Riegger GA. Effects of quinapril on exercise tolerance in patients with mild to moderate heart failure. Eur Heart J 1991;12(6):705–11.

[58] Wollert KC, Studer R, von Bulow B, et al. Survival after myocardial infarction in the rat. Role of tissue angiotensin-converting enzyme inhibition. Circulation 1994;90:2457–67.

[59] Tang WH, Vagelos RH, Yee YG, et al. Neurohormonal and clinical responses to high- versus low-dose enalapril therapy in chronic heart failure. J Am Coll Cardiol 2002;39(1):70–8.

[60] Clinical outcome with enalapril in symptomatic chronic heart failure; a dose comparison. The NETWORK Investigators. Eur Heart J 1998;19(3): 481–9.

[61] Nanas JN, Alexopoulos G, Anastasiou-Nana MI, et al. Outcome of patients with congestive heart failure treated with standard versus high doses of enalapril: a multicenter study. High Enalapril Dose Study Group. J Am Coll Cardiol 2000;36(7):2090–5.

[62] Williams SG, Cooke GA, Wright DJ, et al. Disparate results of ACE inhibitor dosage on exercise capacity in heart failure: a reappraisal of vasodilator therapy and study design. Int J Cardiol 2001; 77(2–3):239–45.

[63] Packer M, Poole-Wilson PA, Armstrong PW, et al. Comparative effects of low and high doses of the angiotensin-converting enzyme inhibitor, lisinopril,

on morbidity and mortality in chronic heart failure. ATLAS Study Group. Circulation 1999;100(23): 2312–8.

[64] Zannad F, van den Broek SA, Bory M. Comparison of treatment with lisinopril versus enalapril for congestive heart failure. Am J Cardiol 1992;70(10): 78C–83C.

[65] The SOLVD Investigators. Effect of enalapril on survival in patients with reduced left ventricular ejection fractions and congestive heart failure. N Engl J Med 1991;325:293–302.

[66] Packer M, Medina N, Yushak M. Relation between serum sodium concentration and the hemodynamic and clinical responses to converting enzyme inhibition with captopril in severe heart failure. J Am Coll Cardiol 1984;3(4):1035–43.

[67] Dries DL, Exner DV, Domanski MJ, et al. The prognostic implications of renal insufficiency in asymptomatic and symptomatic patients with left ventricular systolic dysfunction. J Am Coll Cardiol 2000; 35(3):681–9.

[68] McAlister FA, Ezekowitz J, Tonelli M, et al. Renal insufficiency and heart failure: prognostic and therapeutic implications from a prospective cohort study. Circulation 2004;109(8):1004–9.

[69] Knight EL, Glynn RJ, McIntyre KM, et al. Predictors of decreased renal function in patients with heart failure during angiotensin-converting enzyme inhibitor therapy: results from the studies of left ventricular dysfunction (SOLVD). Am Heart J 1999;138(5 Pt 1): 849–55.

[70] Kittleson M, Hurwitz S, Shah MR, et al. Development of circulatory-renal limitations to angiotensin-converting enzyme inhibitors identifies patients with severe heart failure and early mortality. J Am Coll Cardiol 2003;41(11):2029–35.

[71] Materson BJ, Reda DJ, Cushman WC, et al. Single-drug therapy for hypertension in men. A comparison of six antihypertensive agents with placebo. The Department of Veterans Affairs Cooperative Study Group on Antihypertensive Agents. N Engl J Med 1993;328(13):914–21.

[72] Vasan RS, Benjamin EJ, Levy D. Congestive heart failure with normal left ventricular systolic function. Clinical approaches to the diagnosis and treatment of diastolic heart failure. Arch Intern Med 1996;156(2): 146–57.

[73] Carson P, Ziesche S, Johnson G, et al. Racial differences in response to therapy for heart failure: analysis of the vasodilator-heart failure trials. Vasodilator-Heart Failure Trial Study Group. J Card Fail 1999; 5(3):178–87.

[74] Limacher MC, Yusuf S, for the SOLVD Investigators. Gender differences in the Studies of Left Ventricular Dysfunction (SOLVD): a preliminary report. In: Wenger NK, Sperof L, Packard B, editors. Cardiovascular health and disease and women. Greenwich (CT): Le Jaq Communications; 1993. p. 345–8.

[75] Shekelle PG, Rich MW, Morton SC, et al. Efficacy of angiotensin-converting enzyme inhibitors and beta-blockers in the management of left ventricular systolic dysfunction according to race, gender, and diabetic status: a meta-analysis of major clinical trials. J Am Coll Cardiol 2003;41(9):1529–38.

[76] Jong P, Yusuf S, Rousseau MF, et al. Effect of enalapril on 12-year survival and life expectancy in patients with left ventricular systolic dysfunction: a follow-up study. Lancet 2003;361(9372):1843–8.

ELSEVIER
SAUNDERS

Heart Failure Clin 1 (2005) 39 – 47

HEART
FAILURE
CLINICS

Angiotensin-Converting Enzyme Inhibitors, Angiotensin-Receptor Blockers, or Both in Chronic Heart Failure

James B. Young, MD*

Case Western University, Cleveland, OH, USA

Heart failure remains a substantial worldwide public health problem [1–4]. In the United States alone, approximately 5 million residents are affected, representing 2.2% of the population, with over 500,000 new cases diagnosed annually [1]. Irrespective of index age, the lifetime risk for developing congestive heart failure for men and women is approximately 20% [3]. More important, heart failure causes over 300,000 deaths annually and 1 million hospitalizations, primarily for decompensation. There are an estimated 3 million office visits for heart failure, which is the number-one cause of hospitalization in the elderly. The estimated direct and indirect costs for this problem are $30 billion annually. Although progress in treatments has been made, the 5-year survival rate for men has improved from approximately 35% to 55% in the "modern" heart failure treatment era (the last decade of the 20th century) [4]. Clearly, new therapeutic approaches must be developed.

Angiotensin-converting enzyme inhibitors and angiotensin-receptor blockers in chronic heart failure

As the pathophysiology of heart failure was studied more intently, it became apparent that the malady is a continuation of difficulties rooted primarily in ventricular remodeling manifested by cardiac muscle hypertrophy and heart chamber dilation. This results in varying degrees of diastolic and systolic ventricular dysfunction that can lead to the symptomatic syndrome of heart failure and, subsequently, death. Hypertension and ischemic heart disease are prime drivers of the difficulty, and prevention and treatment of these problems are important [5].

Pharmacotherapeutic strategies focus on interdicting the progression of remodeling and its adverse consequences. Particular attention has been placed on the nuances of the renin-angiotensin-aldosterone system by using agents that can attenuate ill pathophysiologic effects precipitated by stimulating the angiotensin-II receptor (specifically, the angiotensin-II type-1 receptor [AT_1]). By inhibiting formation of angiotensin II with angiotensin-converting-enzyme (ACE) inhibitors, angiotensin-II levels decrease and seemingly beneficial bradykinin-breakdown molecules increase, stimulating nitric oxide release (which stabilizes cardiovascular endothelial function) [6]. ACE inhibitors, however, do not inhibit completely conversion of angiotensin I to angiotensin II because nonspecific tissue chymase enzymes facilitate this conversion as well. Angiotensin-receptor blockers (ARBs), with their further downstream effects, could be more effective because of this pharmacologic action in attenuating the adverse effects of angiotensin II. Of particular interest, a combination of an ARB and an ACE inhibitor may produce optimal outcomes in heart failure. Important questions regarding ARBs, ACE inhibitors, or their combination in

* Department of Medicine, Lerner College of Medicine, Case Western Reserve University, Cleveland Clinic Foundation, 9500 Euclid Avenue/T13, Cleveland, OH 44195.

E-mail address: youngj@ccf.org

doi:10.1016/j.hfc.2004.11.004

chronic heart failure (CHF) patients are summarized in Box 1.

ACE inhibitors have been studied well in patients who have heart failure. Their benefits are incontrovertible [7]. Several guidelines recommend that ACE inhibitors (usually in combination with beta-blockers) are the core of CHF treatment programs [5,7–9]. Nonetheless, despite the morbidity attenuation of ACE inhibitors in heart failure, 50% of treated patients will die within 5 years and another 30% may be rehospitalized for heart failure within 3 months of an index hospital admission [2]. Perhaps 10% to 20% of patients have difficulties with these agents and are ACE-inhibitor "intolerant" (see Box 1) [10].

When considering new tactics in managing patients who have insipient or manifest heart failure, one should remember that the treatment goals are to increase patient survival, reduce morbidity (particularly heart failure hospitalizations), and improve symptoms and clinical functional status when patients are symptomatic. Clinical trials help determine if treatment strategies achieve these important endpoints safely.

Traditionally, drug therapy of CHF, particularly congestive heart failure, has focused on diuretics and digitalis glycosides [5]. Today, ACE inhibitors, beta-blockers, and aldosterone antagonists are important additions in specific populations. Because of the limitations of current drug therapy, including that patients remain at high risk for cardiovascular death, recurrent heart failure hospitalizations, and functional limitation despite optimal therapy, newer approaches including use of ARBs in heart failure have been pursued.

As Box 1 shows, combining an ACE inhibitor and an ARB is logical because one likely would preserve the ACE inhibitor–induced bradykinin-potentiating activity while allowing preferential AT_2-receptor stimulation by angiotensin II. A combination of an ACE inhibitor and an ARB also has lowered blood pressure incrementally [11]. A few trials provide insight into the strategy of using ACE inhibitors, ARBs, or a combination thereof in patients who have CHF [12–19]. ACE inhibitors are the standard agent to which ARBs and a combination of an ACE inhibitor and an ARB should be compared [5]. The relevant questions include: (1) are ARBs equally effective as ACE inhibitors in treating patients who have CHF, (2) are ARBs better than or inferior to ACE inhibitors in treating CHF, and (3) is the combination of an ACE inhibitor and an ARB superior to either agent alone in treating CHF? Most data available to answer these questions are from clinical trials studying patients who had depressed left ventricular ejection fraction (LVEF, or left ventricular systolic dysfunction).

Box 1. Theoretical issues in chronic heart failure: angiotensin-receptor blockers, angiotensin-converting enzyme inhibitors, or both

Angiotensin-converting enzyme inhibitors

- Reduce morbidity–mortality in CHF
- Attenuate detriment of CHF remodeling
- Are core CHF medications
- Incompletely block angiotensin I conversion to angiotensin II
- Are bradykinin-potentiating agents (activate nitric oxide)
- Cannot be taken in 10% to 20% of population (ACE-inhibitor intolerance)

Angiotensin-receptor blockers

- Can be used safely in ACE inhibitor–intolerant patients
- Are generally well tolerated
- Effectively lower blood pressure
- Block AT_1 receptor, allowing angiotensin-II type-2 receptor (AT_2) activity
- Lack bradykinin-potentiating activity

Angiotensin-converting enzyme inhibitor/angiotensin-receptor blocker combination

- Preserves ACE inhibitors' bradykinin-potentiating activity
- Allows preferential AT_2-receptor stimulation by angiotensin
- Lowers blood pressure incrementally

Morbidity–mortality endpoint clinical trials of angiotensin-receptor blockers in heart failure

The first randomized clinical trial of an ARB in CHF powered to determine effects on morbidity and mortality was the second Losartan Heart Failure Survival Study II (ELITE) [18]. The first ELITE trial was a small, 48-week, randomized, controlled clinical trial in 722 elderly patients who had symptomatic heart failure and who had not been treated previously with an ACE inhibitor [17]. ELITE originally was designed to test the hypothesis that the ARB losartan would be better tolerated (with respect to renal function) than the ACE inhibitor captopril. In that study, which was not powered primarily to detect a significant difference in morbidity and mortality, an unexpected 46% mortality decrease (a secondary safety endpoint) was observed with losartan compared with captopril. Although the primary endpoint of the study was not different (ie, a similar rate of persistent rise in serum creatinine concentration was noted in the ARB and ACE-inhibitor groups), losartan generally was tolerated more than captopril (there were significantly fewer discontinuations of the ARB because of adverse events). Furthermore, losartan reduced the rate of all-cause hospital admissions. The survival benefit with losartan in the first ELITE study seemed directly related to a reduction in sudden cardiac death.

Because of this unexpected morbidity and mortality benefit with losartan in ELITE, a larger, double-blind, randomized controlled trial of 3152 patients 60 or more years of age who had New York Heart Association (NYHA) Class II to IV heart failure and an ejection fraction of 40% or less was undertaken [18]. ELITE II randomized patients to either losartan, 50 mg/d, or captopril, 50 mg three times daily. Endpoints were all-cause mortality and sudden death or resuscitated cardiac arrest. Median follow-up was 555 days. There was no significant difference in all-cause mortality or sudden cardiac death/resuscitated arrest events between losartan and captopril groups. All-cause mortality was 11.7% in the captopril group and 10.4% in the losartan group. Significantly fewer patients in the losartan group discontinued study treatment because of adverse effects (9.7% versus 14.7%, $P < .001$). (The Valsartan in Heart Failure [ValHeFT] trial [19] provided a retrospective subset observation that patients on a beta-blocker in ELITE II [approximately 22% of the overall population] had a significantly better outcome when randomized to captopril rather than losartan [hazard ratio 1.77; 95% confidence interval [CI] approximately 1.10–2.90].) Although losartan did not prove to be superior to captopril in symptomatic patients who were elderly and had CHF, the trial suggested that this ARB was well tolerated. Some have speculated that the dose of the ARB was too low. Others believe that the lack of bradykinin-potentiating effects of losartan accounted for the observation. Regardless, the ELITE II trial set the stage for further study of ARBs in CHF [20].

The next large morbidity–mortality powered randomized clinical trial of an ARB in patients who had CHF was ValHeFT [19]. Unlike ELITE II, which was an active drug-controlled trial (losartan versus captopril), ValHeFT was a placebo-controlled trial with 5010 patients who had NYHA Class II to IV heart failure. Valsartan was given in higher doses than usually used for hypertension (160 mg twice daily). The coprimary endpoints of ValHeFT were total mortality and the combined endpoint of mortality and morbidity, which was defined as the incidence of resuscitated cardiac arrest, hospitalization for heart failure, or the need to receive intravenous inotropic or vasodilator therapy in any setting for at least 4 hours.

Total mortality was not significantly different between the valsartan and placebo groups. The combined endpoint was 13.2% lower in the valsartan arm than placebo, however (relative risk [RR] = 0.87; 97.5% CI 0.77–0.97; $P = .009$). Driving this reduction in combined endpoint risk was a decrease in the number of patients hospitalized for heart failure in the valsartan group (18.2% placebo versus 13.8% valsartan; $P < .001$). Other important observations in ValHeFT included that valsartan improved NYHA functional class, increased ejection fraction, and diminished signs and symptoms of congestive heart failure. Quality of life also improved in the valsartan arm compared with placebo.

In a retrospectively defined subgroup analysis, however, mortality and the combined endpoint were affected unfavorably when the combination of an ACE inhibitor, a beta-blocker, and valsartan occurred [19]. This finding prompted the investigators to raise a caution regarding this combination, and when regulatory authorities subsequently approved this ARB for clinical use in heart failure, the safety of this combination was questioned. Another important ValHeFT outcome observation was that most of the benefit with valsartan was noted in the group of patients not on an ACE inhibitor. With only 5% of patients receiving spironolactone, the safety and efficacy of valsartan when an aldosterone-receptor antagonist also is used is unclear.

More recently, the ARB candesartan has been studied in a series of clinical trials culminating in the Candesartan in Heart Failure Assessment of Reduction in Mortality and Morbidity (CHARM) program [13–16,21]. Leading up to this large-scale mortality-morbidity clinical effort was the Study of Patients Intolerant to Converting Enzyme Inhibitors (SPICE) registry and study, which demonstrated that approximately 10% of CHF patients were ACE-inhibitor intolerant, primarily because of cough [10]. In a subset of patients in SPICE, a randomized, double-blind clinical trial was performed with candesartan and placebo. No difference in tolerability was noted in these ACE-inhibitor intolerant patients. Approximately 80% of the placebo and candesartan groups continued medication therapy without difficulties.

The Randomized Evaluation of Strategies for Left Ventricular Dysfunction (RESOLVD) pilot study tested the feasibility of an intense neurohormonal blocking approach to heart failure by assessing the impact of adding candesartan to an ACE inhibitor (enalapril) and a beta-blocker (metoprolol) [12]. Not only was the triple-therapy approach feasible and safe, the combination of candesartan, enalapril, and metoprolol produced the most significant benefit on neurohormones and cardiac remodeling during a short follow-up period.

CHARM was a program of three clinical trials designed to address a broad spectrum of heart failure, including patients who had symptomatic congestive heart failure but relatively preserved left ventricular systolic function [13–16]. Three double-blind, placebo-controlled, randomized clinical trials of candesartan ran in parallel [14–16]. Each had the combined morbidity–mortality primary endpoint of risk reduction for cardiovascular death or heart failure hospital admission. The CHARM-Added trial included 2548 patients who had an ejection fraction less than 40% already treated with an ACE inhibitor [15]. The CHARM-Alternative trial randomized 2028 patients who could not tolerate an ACE inhibitor [14]. The third trial, CHARM-Preserved, studied 3025 patients who had LVEF greater than 40% [16]. An overall CHARM program analysis included all 7601 patients in the program with the overarching endpoint of total mortality, irrespective of background therapy or baseline LVEF [13]. An additional aspect of the CHARM program was a prespecified analysis of the combined CHARM-Low LVEF trials that included all patients having an ejection fraction less than 40% (the pooled CHARM-Added and CHARM-Alternative trials) [21]. This design feature was a carefully considered and important component of CHARM because earlier studies with ACE inhibitors, beta-blockers, and aldosterone antagonists, particularly ELITE II and ValHeFT, were conducted specifically in this population [18,19].

There were 4576 patients in the CHARM-Low LVEF analysis [21]. The primary outcome (time to first event by intention to treat) was cardiovascular death or hospitalization for heart failure, with all-cause mortality a secondary endpoint. Of the patients in the candesartan group, 35.7% experienced cardiovascular death or a heart failure hospitalization compared with 41.3% in the placebo group (hazard ratio [HR] 0.82; 95% CI 0.74–0.90; $P < .001$). Both endpoints in this combined analysis were impacted beneficially. There was a reduced risk for cardiovascular death of 22.8% versus 26.2% (HR 0.84; 95% CI 0.75–0.95; $P = .005$) and heart failure hospitalization (22.5% versus 28.1%; HR 0.76; 95% CI 0.68–0.85; $P < .001$). This trial's analysis was the first to note a statistically significant decrease in all-cause mortality with an ARB in heart failure. Total mortality in the candesartan group was 28% versus 31% in the placebo group (HR 0.88; 95% CI 0.79–0.98; $P = .018$) (Fig. 1). No significant heterogeneity for the beneficial effects of candesartan was found across prespecified and subsequently identified subgroups, including treatment with ACE inhibitors, beta-blockers, and aldosterone antagonists, or various combinations thereof.

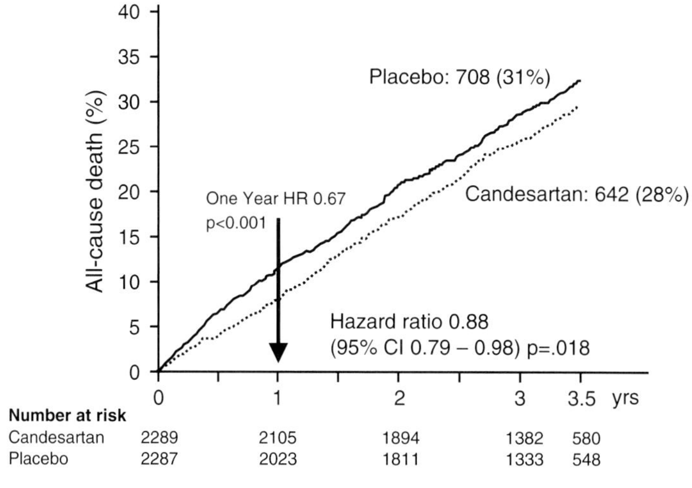

Fig. 1. Total mortality in the CHARM Low LVEF trials analysis.

Specifically addressing the question of combination ARB and ACE-inhibitor therapy was the CHARM-Added trial. In this study the combined endpoint of cardiovascular mortality and heart failure hospitalizations was reduced by 15% with candesartan and an ACE inhibitor compared with placebo (HR 0.85; 95% CI 0.75–0.96; $P = .011$). There was only a trend toward decrement in all-cause mortality (HR 0.86; 95% CI 0.77–1.02; $P = .086$).

CHARM showed that candesartan reduces mortality and morbidity in patients in patients who have CHF with left ventricular systolic dysfunction. Furthermore, there seems to be an incremental benefit to an ACE inhibitor when used in combination with candesartan [15]. Importantly, benefits were evident in major subgroups analyzed in CHARM, including individuals with other medical conditions, such as diabetes mellitus, and across a wide age range. Males and females seem to benefit similarly and, unlike the ValHeFT trial, patients seemed to benefit when a combination of beta-blocker, ACE inhibitor, and candesartan was used [21]. Even with the addition of spironolactone to this protocol, benefits seemed apparent, although these latter subgroups had wide CIs because of small patient numbers. Obviously, care needs to be used when interpreting retrospective subset analyses of large clinical trials such as CHARM and ValHeFT.

The differences in outcomes between ELITE II [18], ValHeFT [19], and the CHARM-Low LVEF trials analyses [21] should be considered in the context of several observations. Table 1 compares some baseline characteristics of patients in ELITE II, ValHeFT, and the CHARM-Low LVEF trials analysis. ELITE II patients were older with a mean age of 71.4 years, compared with 62.4 years in ValHeFT and 65.2 years in CHARM-Low LVEF. None of the trials were well populated with women. In ELITE II, 30% of the participants were female, with 20% of participants female in ValHeFT, and 26% female in CHARM-Low LVEF. Likewise, minorities were underrepresented in these clinical trials. Black enroll-

Table 1
Angiotensin-receptor blocker morbidity–mortality endpoint clinical trials

	Study and year [Ref.]		
Characteristics	ELITE-II 2000 [18]	ValHeFT 2001 [19]	CHARM-Low EF 2004 [21]
Mean age (± SD)	71.4 y (± 6.7)	62.4 y (± 11.1)	65.2 y (± 10.9)
% male	70	80	74
Ethnicity			
% white	82	90	89
% black	2	7	4
NYHA class in %			
Class II	52	62	34
Class III	43	36	62
Class IV	5	2	3
Diagnosis: % with			
Myocardial infarction/ischemia	58	57	58
Hypertension	48	6	49
Atrial fibrillation	31	12	26
Fiabetes	24	25	28
Taking medications in %			
Angiotensin-converting enzyme inhibitor	N/A	93	56
Beta-blocker	23	35	55
Diuretic	77	86	88
Cardiac glycoside	50	67	53
Spironolactone	N/A	N/A	20
Ca^{++} blocker	23	N/A	13
Aspririn	22	N/A	54
Mean % ejection fraction (± SD)	31 (± 7)	27 (± 7)	29 (± 8)
Mean % with heart failure (± SD)	75 (± 12)	N/A	74 (± 14)
Mean systolic blood pressure (± SD)	134 (± 19)	123 (± 19)	127 (± 19)
Mean diastolic blood pressure (± SD)	78 (± 10)	76 (± 11)	76 (± 11)
Control for study	Captopril	Placebo	Placebo

Abbreviations: EF, ejection fraction; N/A, not applicable/available.

ees made up 2% of ELITE II, 7% of ValHeFT, and 4% of CHARM-Low LVEF participants. Perhaps the most striking difference among the three trials is the severity of heart failure, with only 34% of CHARM-Low LVEF patients being NYHA Class II at randomization, whereas ValHeFT contained 62% and ELITE II 52% in this category. Similar rates of ischemic heart disease and diabetes were seen in the trials. ValHeFT had a much lower reported incidence of "hypertension," but this likely resulted from definition. Also, ValHeFT had only 12% of patients with atrial fibrillation compared with 31% of ELITE II patients and 26% of CHARM-Low LVEF patients. Mean ejection fraction was approximately 30% in all three trials, but blood pressure was higher in ELITE II (mean systolic blood pressure 134 mm Hg in ELITE II compared with 123 mm Hg in ValHeFT and 127 mm Hg in CHARM-Low LVEF). The trial with the most NYHA Class II patients and lowest mean systolic blood pressure, ValHeFT, did not demonstrate a reduction in overall mortality when compared with CHARM-Low LVEF. An additional difference between the three studies was that ELITE II was an actively controlled trial using captopril as the comparator.

Whenever benefit is considered for a therapeutic maneuver, side effects and risk of therapy must be taken into account. Perhaps it is best to look at differences between active drug therapy and placebo groups. In the ValHeFT trial, valsartan was reasonably well tolerated but more patients stopped valsartan than placebo for dizziness (1.6% versus 0.4%; $P<.001$), hypotension (1.3% versus 0.8%; $P=.124$), and renal impairment (1.1% versus 0.2%; $P<.001$) [19]. The mean change in serum potassium concentration was 0.12 mmol/L with valsartan compared with 0.07 mmol/L with placebo ($P<.001$). In the CHARM-Low LVEF analysis group, concerns regarding creatinine increase caused study-drug discontinuation in 7.1% of candesartan versus 3.5% of placebo patients ($P<.001$), hypotension in 4.2% versus 2.1% ($P<.001$), and hyperkalemia in 2.8% versus 0.5% ($P<.001$), respectively [21].

This analysis also gives insight into the important question of the safety of multidrug therapy for heart failure, particularly the risk for hypotension, hyperkalemia, and renal insufficiency when spironolactone was used in addition to an ACE inhibitor, beta-blocker, and candesartan. Although a small subset, study drug was stopped in 26.6% of patients taking this combination versus 18% taking an ACE inhibitor, spironolactone, beta-blocker, and placebo ($P=.110$). This suggests that only a small increase in adverse events is noted with this particular polypharmaceutical approach.

Meta-analysis: angiotensin-receptor blockers in chronic heart failure

A meta-analysis published by Jong and colleagues [22] in 2002 suggested that ARBs had no statistically significant impact on mortality or heart failure hospitalizations compared with placebo. This analy-

Table 2
Meta-analysis of angiotension-receptor blockers in chronic heart failure

	All cause mortality			Chronic heart failure hospitalizations		
	ARB vs.			ARB vs.		
Characteristics	Placebo	ACEI	ACEI/ARB vs. ACEI	Placebo	ACE	ARB/ACEI vs. ACEI
Sample size	4623	5201	8260	2590	4310	8101
Total events	618	426	1804	544	654	1507
Test for heterogeneity						
x^2 statistic	9.28	11.47	5.85	0.88	4.29	4.21
P	0.32	0.12	0.21	0.64	0.12	0.24
Test for overall effect						
z statistic	1.98	0.71	0.52	4.50	0.55	4.44
P	0.05	0.48	0.60	< 0.001	0.58	< 0.001
OR	0.83	1.06	0.97	0.64	0.95	0.77
95% CI	0.69–1.00	0.90–1.26	0.87–1.08	0.53–0.78	0.80–1.13	0.69–0.87

Abbreviations: ACEI, angiotensin converting enzyme inhibitor; CI, confidence interval; OR, odds ratio.
Data from Lee VC, Rhew DC, Dylan M, et al. Meta-analysis: angiotensin-receptor blockers in chronic heart failure and high-risk acute myocardial infarction. Ann Intern Med 2004;141:693–704.

sis, which included randomized controlled clinical trials published through May 2001, focused on patients who had CHF and low LVEF.

With the subsequent publication of the 7601-patient CHARM program (4576 with low LVEF), Lee and colleagues [23] performed an updated meta-analysis. This compulsive and elegant overview identified 24 relevant clinical trials using exacting, predefined meta-analysis criteria. Table 2 summarizes the statistical analysis focusing on all-cause mortality and prevention of heart failure hospitalizations. Lee and colleagues suggested that in 24 trials involving 38,080 patients, ARBs were associated with reduced all-cause mortality (HR 0.83; 95% CI 0.69–1.00) and heart failure hospitalizations (HR 0.64; 95% CI 0.53–0.78) compared with placebo (see Table 2). When data comparing ARBs to ACE inhibitors were analyzed, all-cause mortality (HR 1.06; 95% CI 0.90–1.26) and heart failure hospitalization (HR 0.95; 95% CI 0.80–1.13) did not differ significantly. For the combination of an ARB plus an ACE inhibitor versus an ACE inhibitor alone, all-cause mortality was not reduced significantly (HR 0.97; 95% CI 0.87–1.08), but hospitalization for heart failure was (HR 0.77; 95% CI 0.69–0.87).

These data suggest that ARBs are comparable to ACE inhibitors in reducing mortality and morbidity in patients who have CHF and, in addition, heart failure hospitalizations are reduced significantly when ARBs and ACE inhibitors are combined. These authors therefore suggest that ARBs should be regarded as suitable alternatives to ACE inhibitors. The Heart Failure Society of America in a recent Physicians' Statement recommended that quality indicators for heart failure treatment recognize ARBs as an acceptable alternative to ACE inhibitors [24]. This was in response to Joint Commission on Accreditation of Hospitals Organization and Centers for Medicare Services statements indicating that quality indicators should not recognize ARBs as alternatives to ACE inhibitors for treating CHF [9,23].

Are angiotensin-receptor blocker benefits in chronic heart failure a class effect?

Unless direct drug-to-drug comparisons are done in CHF populations using noninferiority trial designs, a perplexing question will remain: are all ARBs alike? Perhaps the variability in outcomes noted in ValHeFT and CHARM simply are related to differences in patient populations studied. Baseline characteristics were dissimilar in many respects (see Table 1). Dosing may have played a role in the ELITE II trial observations. Finally, ARB effects may not be class-specific because candesartan has a different pharmacologic profile than valsartan and losartan. It is reasonable, therefore, to recommend that when treating patients in general, clinicians use the drugs studied in the clinical trials demonstrating efficacy. Also important is that clinicians treat the same type of patients entered into the clinical trials, use the same dosing strategies, and monitor the patients as was done in trials for metabolic and physiologic changes.

The "class effect" question of agents in treating cardiovascular disease is difficult. It recently has been suggested that survival benefits the first year after an acute myocardial infarction differ according to the specific ACE inhibitor used. Pilote and colleagues [25] suggested in a retrospective cohort study using linked hospital discharge and prescription databases that ramapril was associated with lower mortality post–myocardial infarction compared with most other ACE inhibitors. This controversy extends into mega-trials with cardiovascular endpoints in hypertension patients. Kjeldsen and Julius [26] recently overviewed six trials of ACE inhibitors and five trials of ARBs in hypertension designed to detect beneficial impact on cardiovascular endpoints.

It has been suggested that ACE inhibitors and ARBs have a "vasculo-protective property" that goes beyond the benefits of lowering blood pressure and that these agents are not all alike. In the recently completed Comparison of Amlodipine Versus Enalapril to Limit Occurrences of Thrombosis study, the calcium channel blocker amlodipine proved more effective than enalapril in normotensive patients who had coronary artery disease with respect to time to first occurrence of an adverse cardiovascular event [27]. These observations and conclusions are, however, controversial. Properly designed and more powerful clinical trials are necessary to answer these questions.

Summary

The compendium of evidence suggests that ACE inhibitors should remain drugs of first choice for treating patients who have CHF but that ARBs are suitable and equally effective alternatives. In symptomatic CHF patients, the addition of an ARB to an ACE inhibitor likely diminishes morbidity further, particularly the morbidity of multiple heart failure hospitalizations.

References

[1] American Heart Association. Heart disease and stroke statistics: 2003 update. Dallas (TX): American Heart Association; 2004.

[2] Young JB. The prognosis of heart failure. In: Mann DL, et al, editors. Heart failure: a companion to Braunwald's heart disease. Philadelphia: W.B. Saunders; 2004. p. 489–505.

[3] Lloyd-Jones DM, Larson MG, Leip EP, et al. Framingham Heart Study. Lifetime risk for developing heart failure. The Framingham Heart Study. Circulation 2002;106:3068–72.

[4] Levy D, Kenchaiah S, Larson MG, et al. Long-term trends in the incidence of and survival with heart failure. New Engl J Med 2002;347:1397–402.

[5] Hunt SA, Baker DW, Chin MH, et al. ACC/AHA guidelines for the evaluation and management of chronic heart failure in the adult: executive summary. A report of the American College of Cardiology/American Heart Association Task Force on Practice Guidelines (Committee to Revise the 1995 Guidelines for the Evaluation and Management of Heart Failure): developed in collaboration with the International Society for Heart and Lung Transplantation; endorsed by the Heart Failure Society of America. Circulation 2001;104:2996–3007.

[6] Goodfriend TL, Elliott ME, Carr KJ. Angiotensin receptors and their antagonists. N Engl J Med 1996; 334:1649–54.

[7] Flather MD, Yusuf S, Kober L, et al. Long-term ACE-inhibitor therapy in patients with heart failure or left ventricular dysfunction: a systematic overview of data from individual patients. ACE-Inhibitor Myocardial Infarction Collaborative Group. Lancet 2000; 355:1575–81.

[8] Heart Failure Society of America (HFSA) practice guidelines. HFSA guidelines for management of patients with heart failure caused by left ventricular systolic dysfunction—pharmacological approaches. J Card Fail 1999;5:357–82.

[9] Joint Commission on Accreditation of Healthcare Organizations. Overview of the Heart Failure (HF) Core Measure Set. Oakbrook Terrace (IL): Joint Commission on Accreditation of Healthcare Organizations. Available at: http://www.jcaho.org/dscc/dsc/performance+measures/heart+failure+measure+set.htm. Accessed on December 8, 2004.

[10] Granger CB, Erd G, Kuch J, et al. Randomized trial of candesartan cilexetil in the treatment of patients with congestive heart failure and a history of intolerance to angiotensin-converting enzyme inhibitors. Am Heart J 2000;139:609–17.

[11] Hamroff G, Katz SD, Mancini D, et al. Addition of angiotensin II receptor blockade to maximal angiotensin-converting enzyme inhibition improves exercise capacity in patients with severe congestive heart failure. Circulation 1999;99:990–2.

[12] McKelvie RS, Yusuf S, Pericak D, et al. Comparison of candesartan, enalapril, and their combination in congestive heart failure: randomized evaluation of strategies for left ventricular dysfunction (RESOLVD) pilot study. The RESOLVD Pilot Study Investigators. Circulation 1999;100:1056–64.

[13] Pfeffer MA, Swedberg K, Granger CB, et al. Effects of candesartan on mortality and morbidity in patients with chronic heart failure: the CHARM-Overall programme. Lancet 2003;362:759–66.

[14] Granger CB, McMurray JJ, Yusuf S, et al. Effects of candesartan in patients with chronic heart failure and reduced left ventricular systolic function intolerant to angiotensin-converting enzyme inhibitors: the CHARM-Alternative trial. Lancet 2003;362: 772–6.

[15] McMurray JJ, Ostergren J, Swedberg K, et al. Effects of candesartan in patients with chronic heart failure and reduced left ventricular systolic function taking angiotensin-converting enzyme inhibitors: the CHARM-Added trial. Lancet 2003;362:767–71.

[16] Yusuf S, Pfeffer MA, Swedberg K, et al. Effects of candesartan in patients with chronic heart failure and preserved left ventricular ejection fraction: the CHARM-Preserved Trial. Lancet 2003;362:777–81.

[17] Pitt B, Segal R, Martinez FA, et al. Randomised trial of losartan versus captopril in patients over 65 with heart failure (Evaluation of Losartan in the Elderly Study, ELITE). Lancet 1997;349:747–52.

[18] Pitt B, Poole-Wilson PA, Segal R, et al. Effect of losartan compared with captopril on mortality in patients with symptomatic heart failure: randomized trial—the Losartan Heart Failure Survival Study ELITE II. Lancet 2000;355:1582–7.

[19] Cohn JN, Tognoni G. A randomized trial of the angiotensin-receptor blocker valsartan in chronic heart failure. N Engl J Med 2001;345:1667–75.

[20] Gring CN, Francis GS. A hard look at angiotensin-receptor blockers in heart failure. J Am Coll Cardiol 2004;44:1841–6.

[21] Young JB, Dunlap ME, Pfeffer MA, et al. Mortality and moribity reduction with candesartan in patients with chronic heart failure and left ventricular systolic dysfunction: results of the CHARM Low Left Ventricular Ejection Fraction Trials. Circulation 2004;110: 1618–26.

[22] Jong P, Demers C, McKelvie RS, et al. Angiotensin receptor blockers in heart failure: meta-analysis of randomized controlled trials. J Am Coll Cardiol 2002; 39:463–70.

[23] Lee VC, Rhew DC, Dylan M, et al. Meta-analysis: angiotensin-receptor blockers in chronic heart failure and high-risk acute myocardial infarction. Ann Intern Med 2004;141:693–704.

[24] Executive Council of the Heart Failure Society of America. Implications of recent clinical trials for heart failure performance measures. J Card Fail 2004;10:4–5.

[25] Pilote L, Abrahamowicz M, Rodriguez E, et al. Mortality rates in elderly patients who take different angiotensin-converting enzyme inhibitors after acute

myocardial infarction: a class effect? Ann Intern Med 2004;141:102–12.

[26] Kjedsen SE, Julius S. Hypertension mega-trials with cardiovascular end points: effect of angiotensin-converting enzyme inhibitors and angiotensin receptor blockers. Am Heart J 2004;148:747–54.

[27] Nissen SE, Tuzcu EM, Libber P, et al. Effect of antihypertensive agents on cardiovascular events in patients with coronary disease and normal blood pressure. The CAMELOT study: a randomized controlled trial. JAMA 2004;292:2217–26.

ELSEVIER
SAUNDERS

Heart Failure Clin 1 (2005) 49 – 56

HEART
FAILURE
CLINICS

Role of Aldosterone Blockade in Heart Failure

Bertram Pitt, MD*

University of Michigan School of Medicine, Ann Arbor, MI, USA

Angiotensin-converting enzyme inhibitors (ACE-Is) [1,2] and β-adrenergic receptor–blocking agents (BBs) [3–5] reduce cardiovascular mortality and hospitalization for heart failure (HF) in patients who have chronic HF caused by systolic left ventricular dysfunction (SLVD). ACE-Is and BBs are indicated in patients who have HF unless specifically contraindicated or not tolerated. There is increasing evidence that aldosterone blockade (AB) also reduces cardiovascular mortality and hospitalization for HF when added to an ACE-I or an angiotensin receptor–blocking agent (ARB) and a BB in patients who have chronic HF and those who have HF post–myocardial infarction with SLVD [6,7].

The evidence for the effectiveness of AB in patients who have HF caused by SLVD, however, is emerging, and currently AB is recommended in patients who have severe chronic HF and in those who have HF early post–myocardial infarction with SLVD. Before discussing the role of AB in patients with HF caused by SLVD, this article reviews the potential mechanisms by which AB is believed to be effective.

The role of aldosterone and activation of mineralocorticoid receptors in heart failure

By activating mineralocorticoid receptors (MR) in the renal tubule, aldosterone causes sodium retention and loss of potassium and magnesium. AB causes naturesis in patients who have chronic HF and is effective in patients who become resistant to loop diuretics [8,9]. Low dosages of an AB, which have no effect on blood pressure or naturesis, are effective in causing naturesis when combined with subthreshold dosages of a loop diuretic [10]. Thus, AB, even at relatively low dosages, can result in naturesis when used in conjunction with a loop diuretic. MRs, however, are present not only in the renal tubular but in endothelial cells, the myocardium, kidney, and brain [11,12]. Thus, activation of MRs has several pathophysiologic effects in the vascular wall, myocardium, kidney, and brain. MR activation in the vascular wall and myocardium is associated with an increase in reduced NAD(P) vascular oxidase, reactive oxygen species (ROS), epidermal growth factor, activation of the nuclear factor κ-B and activator protein-1 signaling pathways, as well as destruction of nitric oxide (NO) [13,14].

In part, aldosterone-induced ROS production may be caused by a reduction in glucose-6-phosphate dehydrogenase activity with a resultant decrease in glutathione, and therefore a decrease in antioxidant reserve and an increase in ROS [15].

The increase in NADPH oxidase activity and a decrease in tetrahydrobiopterin [16], an important cofactor for the production of NO, result in uncoupling of endothelial nitric oxide synthase and the production of ROS. Aldosterone and angiotensin II (ATII) share a common signaling pathway and work through the epidermal growth factor receptor (EGFR) with stimulation of mitogen-activated protein kinases (extracellular-regulated protein kinase and c-Jun amino terminal kinase) [17]. Specific EGFR blockade inhibits aldosterone- and ATII-induced ROS signal-

* Division of Cardiology, Department of Internal Medicine, University of Michigan School of Medicine, 1500 East Medical Center Drive, Taubman Center, Ann Arbor, MI 48109-0366.

E-mail address: bpitt@med.umich.edu

1551-7136/05/$ – see front matter
doi:10.1016/j.hfc.2004.12.003

heartfailure.theclinics.com

ing. Not all effects of ATII on ROS signaling can be attributed to EGFR activation, however [17]. Although ACE-Is or ARBs decrease ATII-induced aldosterone production from the adrenal gland and local production in the myocardium, ATII is not the only stimulus for aldosterone production; other factors such as potassium are important [18]. In fact, ATII is not required for aldosterone production from the adrenal gland, as evidenced by the ability to stimulate aldosterone production in the angiotensinogen knockout mouse, in which ATII is not present [19]. Thus, aldosterone may be produced (aldosterone escape) [20] under circumstances in which ATII is inhibited maximally or blocked by an ACE-I or ARB. Increasing evidence suggests that there is added benefit of blocking ATII and aldosterone to prevent many pathophysiologic mechanisms contributing to myocardial damage in patients who have HF.

The full consequences of MR-induced ROS are not understood. In brief, aldosterone increases various adhesion molecules, including cyclooxygenase-2, intercellular adhesion molecule, vascular cell adhesion molecule, and osteopontin [21]. Activation of these adhesion molecules results in perivascular and myocardial inflammation with subsequent perivascular and myocardial fibrosis [22]. Aldosterone and increased sodium intake result in perivascular infiltration and fibrosis in the kidney, brain, and myocardium [22].

Evidence of increased collagen formation associated with MR activation has been seen in several models of HF and in patients who have HF and SLVD [23–27]. Continuing myocardial collagen formation, as evidenced by an increase in circulating procollagen I and III, has been seen in patients who have chronic HF and is an independent risk factor for mortality [24]. An increase in myocardial and perivascular fibrosis has important effects on ventricular function, vascular stiffness, and coronary flow reserve [28–30]. Myocardial fibrosis also correlates with diastolic ventricular function. Conversely, AB decreases myocardial and perivascular fibrosis and vascular stiffness, prevents ventricular remodeling, decreases metalloproteinases 2 and 9, and improves coronary flow reserve. Aldosterone also causes ventricular hypertrophy and AB reverses ventricular hypertrophy [31,32].

AB, by decreasing ROS, improves the availability of NO and endothelial function. The improvement in endothelial function in animals and in patients who have HF has been shown on top of ACE-I [33,34]. This is of importance because endothelial dysfunction is an independent predictor of cardiovascular events in patients who have HF and SLVD [35]. An increase in availability of NO also has implications for platelet activation, monocyte adhesion, and infiltration into the vascular wall.

AB improves platelet activation, the ratio of plasminogen activator inhibitor – 1 to tissue plasminogen activator, and fibrinogen levels, suggesting an important role in thrombosis and fibrinolysis [36,37]. AB also improves norepinephrine uptake into the myocardium, decreases circulating norepinephrine levels, and increases heart rate variability and baroreceptor function, suggesting an improvement in parasympathetic nervous activity [38,39]. AB decreases central MR-induced sympathetic nervous activation [40].

The effect of AB on norepinephrine uptake, heart rate variability, and baroreceptor function can be explained by its effects on ROS and NO availability. An increase in NO availability tends to decrease sympathetic discharge and improve heart rate variability and baroreceptor function [41,42]. The effects of AB on the parameters discussed above seem to be similar in magnitude to those seen with an ACE-I or an ARB and are additive when an ACE-I or an ARB are combined with AB.

Aldosterone increases tissue angiotensin-converting enzyme (ACE) activity [43] and prevents ATII-induced down-regulation of the AT_1 receptor [44], resulting in an increase in ATII-mediated aldosterone production and a vicious cycle. Aldosterone also decreases AT_2-receptor levels during experimental ischemia [44] and reduces ACE_2 activity [45], both of which would tend to decrease NO availability. Other vicious cycles involve endothelin, vasopressin, and norepinephrine. Continued activation of these neurohumeral factors results in increased ROS with its consequences, including continuing myocardial, renal, and vascular damage.

Aldosterone also stimulates the low-density lipoprotein receptor 1 [46], which is responsible for oxidation of low-density lipoprotein-cholesterol (LDL-C) to oxidized LDL-C (OX-LDL-C), another important cause of ROS production, suggesting an important role of MR activation in the atherosclerotic process. Evidence suggesting a role of MR activation in atherosclerosis comes from studies showing that aldosterone increases the OX-LDL-C content of macrophages in the aorta and atherosclerotic lesion area [47]. In the Apolipoprotein-E knockout mouse, ATII causes an increase in atherosclerotic lesion area that can be blocked by an ARB or AB [47,48], suggesting that the effects of ATII on atherosclerosis are mediated, at least in part, by activation by the MR.

Although aldosterone has several deleterious effects associated with progressive myocardial and vascular damage, the effectiveness of AB cannot be predicted from serum aldosterone levels. In patients who have severe HF, serum aldosterone levels correlate with cardiovascular events [49]. In the Randomized Aldactone Evaluation Study (RALES), however, there was a poor correlation between circulating aldosterone levels and the effectiveness of spironolactone.

The role of aidosterone blockade in patients who have chronic heart failure caused by systolic left ventricular dysfunction

AB with spironolactone is effective in improving total mortality in patients who have New York Heart Association (NYHA) Class-III to -IV HF caused by SLVD [2]. The reduction in total mortality by spironolactone was caused by a reduction in death from progressive HF and sudden cardiac death. This reduction in mortality was accompanied by a 35% reduction in the incidence of hospitalization for HF. These effects of spironolactone were seen at a mean dosage of 26 mg/d and were shown across several subsets, including age, gender, ischemic/nonischemic etiology, left ventricular ejection fraction (LVEF), whether or not ACE-Is were used, and whether or not BBs or digoxin were used. Only 10% to 11% of patients in RALES were on a BB because when the trial was begun, the effects of BB on mortality in patients who had HF caused by SLVD were unknown. Subsequent experience in patients who have mild to moderate HF and in patients who have SLVD and HF post–myocardial infarction, however, shows that AB reduces ventricular remodeling and mortality when added to an ACE-I, ARB, or BB [7,50–52].

The combination of an AB and digoxin on mortality is of particular interest. In the Digitalis Investigator Group trial digoxin had no significant effect in reducing overall mortality [53]. Digoxin did, however, reduce death from progressive HF, but increased sudden cardiac death and death from ischemic events such that total mortality was not reduced. The effectiveness of digoxin and an AB in reducing total mortality more than when an AB is used alone can be attributed to AB's effectiveness in preventing sudden cardiac death while preserving the effectiveness of digoxin on death from progressive HF. This hypothesis will require prospective confirmation, however.

In RALES [6], patients with a baseline serum potassium level $\geq$ 5 mEq/L or a serum creatinine level of 2.5 or more mg/dL were excluded. Serum potassium was measured at baseline before beginning spironolactone at 1 week, 1 month, and every 3 to 6 months thereafter. If serum potassium increased to 5.5 mEq/L or greater, the dosage of study medication was reduced by half, and if serum potassium was 6 mEq/L or greater at any time without a clear reason (eg, the use of a nonsteroidal anti-inflammatory agent or potassium supplement), study medication was discontinued but could be restarted if serum potassium decreased to 5.0 mEq/L or less. If there was no evidence of hyperkalemia (potassium $\geq$ 5.5 mEq/L) after 1 month but evidence of progressive HF, the dosage of study medication could be increased to 50 mg/d.

With this strategy, there was no clinically significant increase in the incidence of serious hyperkalemia (potassium $\geq$ 6 mEq/L). There was one death attributable to hyperkalemia in the RALES study: a placebo patient. After publication of RALES, however, several papers pointed out that the incidence of hyperkalemia when spironolactone was used under clinical conditions was much greater than reported in RALES, and was associated with an increase in renal failure, occasionally requiring dialysis, and death [54–58].

A review of these reports reveals that the increased incidence of hyperkalemia could be attributed largely to the use of higher dosages of spironolactone than those used in RALES, failure to exclude patients with a baseline serum potassium level of 5 or more meq/L or a serum creatinine level of 2.5 mg/dL or greater, or failure to monitor serum potassium and adjust the dosage of spironolactone if potassium was 5.5 mEq/L or greater or to discontinue spironolactone if potassium was 6 mEq/L or greater. There were, however, instances of hyperkalemia in patients treated according to the recommendations in RALES. This happened largely because serum creatinine does not always reflect the degree of renal insufficiency (eg, in patients with low body weight, the elderly, or those with diabetes mellitus). Calculation of renal clearance by the Cockcroft and Gault or other formula would have avoided this risk [59]. Regardless, it is clear from experience in randomizing over 4000 patients to an AB that if the recommendations for dosing and monitoring of serum potassium outlined in RALES are followed, and patients with severe renal dysfunction (creatinine clearance $\leq$ 30 mL/min) are avoided, that the risks for hyperkalemia associated with AB are relatively low and the net effect on mortality highly favorable.

In RALES there was a significant increase in sexually related side effects, including gynecomastia, breast pain, and impotence in males. Spironolactone also causes menstrual irregularities and libido changes in premenstrual females. Although most of the women in RALES were postmenopausal, these sexual changes are a detriment to the extrapolation of AB to other less symptomatic populations, including those with asymptomatic SLVD and hypertension. The increased incidence of sexual side effects associated with spironolactone has been attributed to the fact that spironolactone, although an effective blocker of the MR, downregulates androgen receptors and upregulates progesterone receptors.

As a result of the RALES study, AB is recommended in the American College of Cardiology/American Heart Association and European guidelines for use in patients who have severe HF caused by SLVD. The effectiveness of AB on mortality and morbidity in patients who have mild to moderate HF caused by SLVD has not been evaluated prospectively, however. Several studies in patients who had mild to moderate HF caused by SLVD treated with an ACE-I and a BB showed that AB improves ventricular remodeling, decreases collagen formation, and improves endothelial function, norepinephrine uptake, heart rate variability, baroreceptor function, and fibrinolysis, however. Thus, it can be postulated that AB is effective in reducing mortality and morbidity in these patients. A prospective, randomized, double-blind study of the aldosterone-blocking agent eplerenone in patients with mild to moderate HF (NYHA Class II) is under consideration. Until the results of further trials are available, the effectiveness of AB in patients who have mild to moderate HF is uncertain.

Further support for the effectiveness of AB in patients who have HF comes from the use of the AB eplerenone in the Eplerenone Post-AMI Heart Failure Efficacy and Survival Study (EPHESUS) [7]. Eplerenone is a relatively selective blocker of the MR with relatively little effect on androgen and progesterone receptors. In EPHESUS, eplerenone at a dosage of 25 mg uptitrated to 50 mg at 1 month, if there was no evidence of hyperkalemia (potassium $\geq$ 5.5 mEq/L), was tested in a prospective double-blind protocol in patients with evidence of an acute myocardial infarction, SLVD (LVEF $\leq$ 40%), and clinical evidence of HF. Clinical evidence of HF was not required if a patient had diabetes mellitus, however, because its presence was believed sufficient to increase the risk for mortality similar to that of clinical HF.

When the EPHESUS study was undertaken there was relatively little experience with AB in patients post–myocardial infarction, and it was believed prudent to begin randomization 3 to 14 days post–myocardial infarction to avoid the potential of hypotension immediately postinfarction while ACE-Is, ARBs, and BBs were initiated. Over 6600 patients were randomized to eplerenone or placebo with a planned termination of the trial after 1032 deaths. There were two coprimary endpoints: total mortality and cardiovascular mortality/cardiovascular hospitalization.

Mean LVEF was 33%, and patients were randomized at a mean of 7.3 days from onset of infarction. LVEF could be determined at anytime from onset of infarction to randomization, however, and at randomization the LVEF likely was higher than 33% because of recovery from ventricular stunning, hibernation, and the effect of myocardial reperfusion. Also, although clinical signs of chronic HF were required to be present at baseline, except in those with diabetes mellitus, they were often transient as a result of a change in myocardial compliance or the use of nitroglycerine and diuretics. Approximately one third of patients had evidence of diabetes mellitus, 25% had a prior history of myocardial infarction, but only 15% had a prior history of chronic HF. Background medication included an ACE-I or ARB in approximately 87% and a BB in 75% of patients. Slightly less than 50% of the patients underwent reperfusion and less than 50% received a statin.

At a mean follow-up of 16 months, eplerenone at a mean dosage of 42 mg/d resulted in a significant 15% reduction in total mortality and a 13% reduction in the coprimary combined endpoint of cardiovascular mortality/cardiovascular hospitalization. The benefit of eplerenone in reducing total mortality was seen in patients on an ACE-I or ARB and a BB and in patients on "optimal therapy" including an ACE-I or ARB, BB, aspirin, statin, and undergoing reperfusion. Thus, eplerenone provides additional benefit to current standard therapy in reducing total mortality.

The major cardiovascular cause of mortality in EPHESUS was sudden cardiac death, which was reduced by 21%. In a retrospective analysis of patients with a baseline LVEF of 30% or less, eplerenone reduced sudden death by 33%. This retrospective analysis was undertaken in view of the current focus on the use of electrical and mechanical devises in patients with an ejection fraction of 30% to 35% or less post–myocardial infarction. The use of an automatic implanted cardiac defibrillator (AICD) in patients with severe systolic dysfunction post–myocardial infarction is attractive because these patients have a relatively high incidence of sudden cardiac death.

In the recent Defibrillator in Acute Myocardial Infarction Trial [60], patients who had had an acute myocardial infarction and had an LVEF of 35% or less were randomized to contemporary therapy or contemporary therapy with an AICD between day 6 and 40 post–myocardial infarction. Patients randomized to the AICD strategy had a reduction in sudden cardiac death [60], but there was an increase in nonarrhythmic death such that total mortality was increased at 1 year.

In the Multicenter Automatic Defibrillator Implantation Trial–II, implantation of an AICD more than 30 days postinfarction was associated with a significant reduction in sudden cardiac death and total mortality [61]. There was no apparent benefit of AICD implantation on total mortality for the first year postimplantation. Thus, eplerenone may provide an important bridge in the strategy to reduce sudden cardiac death and total mortality early after myocardial infarction.

Of potentially greater importance is that AB can prevent ventricular remodeling early post–myocardial infarction. For example, Hyashi and colleagues [50] randomized patients with their first anterior myocardial infarction on day 1 postinfarction immediately after undergoing primary percutaneous transluminal coronary angioplasty. Patients randomized to the AB strategy for 1 month had a significant increase in LVEF and decrease in myocardial collagen formation. The mean LVEF at baseline was approximately 47%. It is therefore likely that patients with a lower baseline LVEF (30%–35%) also would improve, fewer patients would reach 1 month postinfarction with a LVEF of 30% to 35% or less, and fewer would require electrical or mechanical intervention. This hypothesis will require prospective evaluation in patients with a baseline LVEF of 30% to 35% or less, however.

The major cause of cardiovascular hospitalization in EPHESUS was HF, which was reduced by 15%; episodes of HF were reduced by 23%. In the retrospective study of patients with a baseline LVEF of 30% or less the combined endpoint of HF mortality/HF hospitalization was reduced by 25%.

There was no increase in the risk for sexually related side effects in patients randomized to eplerenone, attesting to the selectivity of eplerenone for the MR. There was an increase in the incidence of serious hyperkalemia (potassium $\geq$ 6 mEq/L), but there were no deaths attributable to hyperkalemia in patients randomized to eplerenone. Although there was an increase in the risk for hyperkalemia with eplerenone, the risk for hypokalemia (potassium $<$ 3.5 mEq/L) post–myocardial infarction was greater than that for hyperkalemia and eplerenone significantly reduced this incidence. Hypokalemia may be a more serious risk factor than hyperkalemia postinfarction and predisposes to sudden cardiac death and death from progressive HF.

Although eplerenone reduces mortality in patients who have SLVD and HF postinfarction, several clinicians have suggested that spironolactone be used for this indication because of its lower cost and that eplerenone be considered only if the patient fails to tolerate spironolactone because of gynecomastia, breast pain, impotence, or menstrual irregularities. Given the increasing emphases on cost-effectiveness, this strategy seems reasonable.

Although less expensive, spironolactone may not be as cost-effective as eplerenone in the long run, however. Experience shows that many patients do not tolerate spironolactone because of its sexually related side effects. If patients could be switched immediately to eplerenone after they experience a sexually related side effect, the strategy of using eplerenone only for patients who do not tolerate spironolactone might be cost-effective. In clinical practice, however, many patients will discontinue spironolactone and it may be several months before they are seen by their physician and switched to eplerenone. If during this interval a few patients developed manifest HF or die, the strategy of beginning therapy with spironolactone would not be as cost-effective as eplerenone. Only a prospective comparative study will give definitive insight into which of these AB agents is most cost-effective in reducing mortality and morbidity post–myocardial infarction.

Use of aldosterone blockade in patients who have heart failure caused by preserved systolic function

AB effectively reduces myocardial hypertrophy and fibrosis. There is a good correlation between the extent of myocardial fibrosis and diastolic myocardial function, as measured by the echocardiographic E-A ratio. AB improves the echocardiographic E-A ratio, reduces vascular stiffness, improves coronary flow reserve [29,30], and improves diastolic function associated with a reduction in myocardial fibrosis [62].

In view of the failure of ARBs to decrease significantly cardiovascular mortality/hospitalization for HF in the Candesartan in Heart Failure Assessment of Reduction in Mortality and Morbidity Preserved Trial [63] and the lack of clinical evidence for the effectiveness of any other strategy in reducing mortality/morbidity in patients who have diastolic HF, the National Heart, Lung, and Blood Institute is planning a large-scale study of AB in patients who have HF associated with preserved systolic function.

Given the effectiveness of AB on ventricular hypertrophy, fibrosis, coronary flow reserve, and autonomic function, a beneficial effect of AB can be predicted. It is prudent to await the results of this and other studies before applying this strategy clinically, however. Similarly, one should not extrapolate the results of AB in patients who have severe HF and SLVD to those who have asymptomatic SLVD without further prospective, large-scale, randomized studies. Although AB improves several surrogate endpoints including LVEF, collagen formation, exercise tolerance, endothelial function, norepinephrine uptake, heart rate variability, baroreceptor function, and fibrinolysis in patients who have mild to moderate HF caused by SLVD, it is prudent to await further data before recommending AB in these patients.

Thus, AB with either spironolactone or eplerenone is effective in reducing total mortality in patients who have SLVD and signs of HF. The evidence from preclinical and clinical studies suggests that many effects of ATII on the myocardium and the vascular wall are mediated through aldosterone, and that the combination of an ACE-I or ARB and AB is more effective in correcting the pathophysiology of HF than either alone. Although further data are needed on the effectiveness of AB in patients who have mild to moderate HF caused by SLVD, asymptomatic SLVD, and HF caused by preserved left ventricular dysfunction, AB likely will reduce further mortality/morbidity and hence reduce health care costs in many patients who have HF.

References

[1] The CONSENSUS Trial Study Group. Effects of enalapril on mortality in severe congestive heart failure. Results of the Cooperative North Scandinavian Enalapril Survival Study (CONSENSUS). The CONSENSUS Trial Study Group. N Engl J Med 1987;316:1429–35.

[2] The SOLVD INVESTIGATORS. Effect of enalapril on survival in patients with reduced left ventricular ejection fractions and congestive heart failure. N Engl J Med 1991;325:293–302.

[3] CIBS-II Investigators and Committees. The Cardiac Insufficiency Bisoprolol Study II (CIBIS-II): a randomized trial. Lancet 1999;353:9–13.

[4] MERIT-HF Study Group. Effect of metoprolol CR/XL in chronic heart failure: Metoprolol CR/XL Randomized Intervention Trial in Congestive Heart Failure (MERIT-HF). Lancet 1999;353:2001–7.

[5] Packer M, Coats AJ, Fowler MB, et al. Effect of carvedilol on survival in severe chronic heart failure. N Engl J Med 2001;344:1651–8.

[6] Pitt B, Zannad F, Remme WJ, et al. The effect of spironolactone on morbidity and mortality in patients with severe heart failure. N Engl J Med 1999;341: 709–17.

[7] Pitt B, Remme W, Zannad F, et al. of the Eplerenone Post-Acute Myocardial Infarction Heart Failure Efficacy and Survival Study Investigators. Eplerenone, a selective aldosterone blocker, in patients with left ventricular dysfunction after myocardial infarction. N Engl J Med 2003;348(14):1309–21.

[8] van Vliet AA, Donker AJ, Nauta JJ, et al. Spironolactone in congestive heart failure refractory to high-dose loop diuretic and low-dose angiotensin-converting enzyme inhibitor. Am J Cardiol 1993;71: 21A–8A.

[9] MacFadyen RJ, Gorski JC, Brater DC, et al. Furosemide responsiveness non-adherence and resistance during the chronic treatment of heart failure: a longitudinal study. Br J Clin Pharmacol 2004;57:622–31.

[10] Muller J. Spironolactone in the management of congestive cardiac failure: a review. Clin Ther 1986;9: 63–76.

[11] Funder JW, Pearce PT, Smith R, et al. Vascular type I aldosterone binding sites are physiological mineralocorticoid receptors. Endocrinology 1989;125:2224–6.

[12] Lombes M, Oblin ME, Gasc JM, et al. Immunohistochemical and biochemical evidence for a cardiovascular mineralocorticoid receptor. Circ Res 1992;71: 503–10.

[13] Rajagopalan S, Duquaine D, King S, et al. Mineralocorticoid receptor antagonism in experimental atherosclerosis. Circulation 2002;105:2212–6.

[14] Luft FC. Mechanisms and cardiovascular damage in hypertension. Hypertension 2001;37:594–8.

[15] Leopold JA, Scribner AE, Dam A, et al. Aldosterone impairs vascular reactivity by decreasing glucose 6-phosphate dehydrogenase activity [abstract]. Circulation 2004;110:III–154.

[16] Mitchell BM, Smith AD, Webb RC, et al. Aldosterone decreases endothelium-dependent relaxation by down-regulating GTP cyclohydrolase [abstract]. Hypertension 2003;42(435):161.

[17] Mazak I, Fiebler A, Dominik N, et al. Aldosterone potentiates angiotensin II-induced signaling in vascular smooth muscle cells. Circulation 2004;109:2792–800.

[18] Quinn S, Williams G. Regulation of aldosterone secretion. Annu Rev Physiol 1988;50:409–26.

[19] Okubo S, Niimura F, Nishimura H, et al. Angiotensin-independent mechanism for aldosterone synthesis during chronic extracellular fluid volume depletion. J Clin Invest 1997;99(5):855–60.

[20] Pitt B. "Escape" of aldosterone production in patients with left ventricular dysfunction treated with an angiotensin-converting enzyme inhibitors: implications for therapy. Cardiovasc Drugs Ther 1995;99:145–9.

[21] Blasi ER, Frierdrich GE, De Ciechi PA, et al. Aldosterone/salt-induced myocardial injury: a vascular inflammatory disease. Amer J Hypertens 2001;14: 8A–9A.

[22] Weber KT. Fibrosis and hypertensive heart disease. Curr Opin Cardiol 2000;25:264–72.

[23] MacFadyen RJ, Barr CS, Struthers AD. Aldosterone blockade reduces vascular collagen turnover, improves heart rate variability and reduces early morning rise in heart rate in heart failure patients. Cadiovasc Res 1997; 35:30–4.

[24] Zannad F, Alla F, Dousset B, et al. Limitation of excessive extracellular matrix turnover may contribute to survival benefit of spironolactone therapy in patients with congestive heart failure: insights from the Randomized Aldactone Evaluation Study (RALES). Circulation 2000;102:2700–6.

[25] Benetos A, Lacolley P, Safar ME. Prevention of aortic fibrosis by spironolactone in spontaneously hypertensive rats. Arterioscler Thromb Vasc Biol 1997;17: 1152–6.

[26] Brilla CG, Pick R, Tan LB, et al. Remodeling of the rat right and left ventricles in experimental hypertension. Circ Res 1990;67:1355–64.

[27] Iglarz M, Touyz RM, Viel EC, et al. Involvement of oxidative stress in the profibrotic action of aldosteone. Interaction with the renin-angiotension system. Am J Hypertens 2004;17:597–603.

[28] Suzuki G, Morita H, Mishima T, et al. Effects of long-term monotherapy with eplerenone, a novel aldosterone blocker, on progression of left ventricular dysfunction and remodeling in dogs with heart failure. Circulation 2002;106:2967–72.

[29] Susic D, Varagic J, Ahn I, et al. Eplerenone improves coronary hemodynamics and reduces cardiac fibrosis in aging spontaneously hypertensive rats [abstract]. J Am Coll Cardiol 2004;43:482A.

[30] LaColley P, Labat C, Pujol A, et al. Increased carotid wall elastic modulus and fibronectin in aldosterone-salt-treated rats effects of eplerenone. Circulation 2002; 106:2848–53.

[31] Pitt B, Reichek N, Willenbrock R, et al. Effect of eplerenone, enalapril, and eplerenone/enalapril in patients with essential hypertension and left ventricular hypertrophy study. Circulation 2003;108:1831–8.

[32] Qin W, Rudolph AE, Bond BR, et al. Transgenic model of aldosterone-driven cardiac hypertrophy and heart failure. Circ Res 2003;93:69–76.

[33] Lim PO, Donnan PT, Struthers AD. Exercise capacity and brain natruiretic peptide in hypertensin. J Cardiovasc Pharmacol 2002;40:519–27.

[34] Bauersachs J, Heck M, Fraccarollo D, et al. Addition of spironolactone to angiotensin-converting enzyme inhibition in heart failure improves endothelial vasomotor dysfunction: role of vascular superoxide anion formation and endothelial nitric oxide synthase expression. J Am Coll Cardiol 2002;39:351–8.

[35] Meyer B, Huelsmann M, Strecker K, et al. Flow-mediated vasodilation predicts outcome in patients with chronic heart failure. J Am Coll Cardiol 2004; 43:198A.

[36] Brown NJ, Kim KS, Chen YQ, et al. Synergistic effect of adrenal steroids and angiotensin II on plasminogen activator inhibitor-1 production. J Clin Endocrinol Metab 2000;85:336–44.

[37] Schaefer A, Fraccarollo D, Hildemann S, et al. Inhibition of platelet activation in congestive heart failure by selective aldosterone receptor antagonism and angiotensin-converting enzyme inhibition [abstract]. Eur Heart J 2002;23(Suppl):401.

[38] Barr CS, Lang CC, Hanson J, et al. Effects of adding spironolactone to an angiotensin-converting enzyme inhibitor in chronic congestive heart failure secondary to coronary artery disease. Am J Cardiol 1995;76(17): 1259–65.

[39] Kasama S, Toyama T, Kumakura H, et al. Effect of spironolactone on cardiac sympathetic nerve activity and left ventricular remodeling in patients with dilated cardiomyopathy. J Am Coll Cardiol 2003;41(4): 574–81.

[40] Zhang ZH, Francis J, Weiss RM, et al. The rennin-angiotensin-aldosterone system excites hypothalmic paraventricular nucleus neurons in heart failure. Am J Physiol Heart Circ Physiol 2002;283:H423–33.

[41] Chowdhary S, Vaile JC, Fletcher J, et al. Nitric oxide and cardiac autonomic control in humans. Hypertension 2000;36:264–9.

[42] Schwarz P, Diem R, Dun NJ, et al. Endogenous and exogenous nitric oxide inhibits norepinephrine release from rat heart sympathetic nerves. Circ Res 1995;77: 841–8.

[43] Harada E, Yoshimura M, Yasue H, et al. Aldosterone induces angiotensin-converting-enzyme gene expression in cultured neonatal rat cardiocytes. Circulation 2001;104:137–9.

[44] Michel F, Ambroisine ML, Duriez M, et al. Aldosterone enhances ischemia-induced neovascularization through angiotensin II-dependent pathway. Circulation 2004;109:1933–7.

[45] Yamamuro M, Yoshimura M, Nakayama M. Aldosterone reduces gene expression of angiotensin-converting enzyme 2 in rat neonatal cardiomyocytes. Circulation 2004;110:III–635.

[46] Kobayashi N, Honda T, Hara K, et al. Eplerenone shows renoprotective effects by reducing LOX-1 mediated adhesion molecule expression and PK cepsilon-MAP kinase –p90 RSK pathway activation. [abstract] Hypertension 2003;42(446):216.

[47] Keridar S, Kaplan M, Pavlotsky E, et al. Aldosterone administration to mice stimulates macrophage NADPH oxidase and increases atherosclerosis development: a possible role for angiotensin-converting enzymes and the receptors for angiotensin II and aldosterone. Circulation 2004;109:2213–20.

[48] Zhou Y, Chen R, Hu L. Angiotensin II and aldosterone are both required to stimulate atheosclerosis in Apo-E deficient mice [abstract]. Hypertension 2003; 42:403A.

[49] Swedberg K, Eneroth P, Kjekshus J, et al. Hormones regulating cardiovascular function in patients with severe congestive heart failure and their relation to mortality. Circulation 1990;82:1730–60.

[50] Hayashi M, Tsutamoto T, Wada A, et al. Immediate administration of mineralocorticoid receptor antagonist spironolactone prevents post-infarct left ventricular remodeling associated with suppression of a marker of myocardial collagen synthesis in patients with first anterior acute myocardial infarction. Circulation 2003; 107:2259–65.

[51] Tsutamoto T, Wada A, Maeda K, et al. Effect of spironolactone on plasma brain natriuretic peptide and left ventricular remodeling in patients with congestive heart failure. J Am Coll Cardiol 2001;37:1228–33.

[52] Cicoira M, Zanolla L, Rossi A, et al. Long-term, dose dependent effects of spironolactone on left ventricular function and exercise tolerance in patients with chronic heart failure. J Am Coll Cardiol 2002;40:304–10.

[53] The Digitalis Investigation Group. The effect of digoxin on mortality and morbidity in patients with heart failure. N Engl J Med 1997;336:525–33.

[54] Berry C, McMurray JJ. Serious adverse events experienced by patients with chronic heart failure taking spironolactone. Heart 2001;85(4):E8.

[55] Schepkens H, Vanholder R, Billiouw JM, et al. Life-threatening hyperkalemia during combined therapy with angiotensin-converting enzyme inhibitors and spironolactone: an analysis of 25 cases. Am J Med 2001;110:438–41.

[56] Sveensson M, Gustafsson F, Galatius S, et al. Hyperkalaemia and impaired renal function in patients taking spironolactone for congestive heart failure. Retrospective study. Br Med J 2003;327:1141–2.

[57] Wrenger E, Muller R, Moesenthin M, et al. Interaction of spironolactone with ACE inhibitors or angiotensin receptor blockers; analysis of 44 cases. Br Med J 2003; 327:147–9.

[58] Juurlink DN, Mamdani MM, Lee DS, et al. Rates of hyperkalemia after publication of the Randomized Aldactone Evaluation Study. N Engl J Med 2004; 351:543–51.

[59] Cockcroft DW, Gault MH. Prediction of creatinine clearance from serum creatinine. Nephron 1976;16: 31–41.

[60] Hohnloser SH, Kuck KH, Dorian P, et al. Prophylactic use of an implantable cardioverter-defibrillator after acute myocardial infarction. N Engl J Med 2004;351: 2481–8.

[61] Moss AJ, Vyas A, Greenberg H, et al. Temporal aspects of improved survival with the implanted defibrillator (MADIT-II). Am J Cardiol 2004;109: 2792–800.

[62] Izawa H, Murase Y, Xu JL, et al. Spironolactone improves left ventricular chamber stiffness and diastolic function associated with regression of myocardial fibrosis in asymptomatic patients with dilated cardiomyopathy [abstract]. Circulation 2004;110: III–479.

[63] Pfeffer MA, McMurray JJ, Velazquez EJ, et al. for the Valsartan in Acute Myocardial Infarction Trial Investigators. Valsartan, captopril, or both in myocardial infarction complicated by heart failure, left ventricular dysfunction or both. N Engl J Med 2003;349:1893–906.

ELSEVIER
SAUNDERS

Heart Failure Clin 1 (2005) 57 – 66

HEART
FAILURE
CLINICS

Are There Clinically Important Differences Between Beta-Blockers in Heart Failure?

John G.F. Cleland, MD*, Huan Loh, MBChB, B Med Sci, Jonathan Windram, MBChB, BSc

University of Hull, Castle Hill Hospital, Kingston-upon-Hull, UK

Three beta-blockers (bisoprolol, carvedilol, and metoprolol succinate) are known to reduce the mortality of patients with heart failure due to left ventricular systolic dysfunction [1–4]. Recently, a fourth agent (nebivolol) was shown to reduce the composite outcome of death or cardiovascular hospitalization [5]. Other beta-blockers have failed to show benefit [6,7]. Overall, including only trials that have reported more than 40 deaths, beta-blockers have reduced all-cause mortality by 28% (Fig. 1) [5]. Three of the agents used in the successful landmark trials were beta-1-selective agents (bisoprolol, metoprolol succinate and nebivolol) and one was a nonselective agent (carvedilol) (Fig. 2).

These studies suggest that metoprolol succinate and bisoprolol are rather similar in their effect. The SENIORS trial failed to show a reduction in all-cause mortality with nebivolol, suggesting that it might be somewhat less effective than other beta-1-selective agents. This difference may be apparent rather than real and explained by the fact that SENIORS recruited only elderly patients and was under-powered. Less benefit was observed in patients aged > 75 years, a group not well represented in previous studies [5]. Bucindolol, a nonselective beta-blocker that also partially stimulates beta-receptors (partial agonism), in one of the most highly powered trial programs amongst beta-blockers for heart failure, also failed to show a reduction in mortality. Xamoterol, an agent that blocks the beta-1 receptor and has even more powerful partial agonist properties than bucindolol, was associated with an increase in mortality when introduced abruptly, without dose-titration, in patients with severe heart failure. Carvedilol, a nonselective beta-blocker that also blocks alpha-1-receptors and has antioxidant properties, has shown a reduction in all-cause mortality in three separate trials [1,4,8] and one trial of postinfarction left ventricular dysfunction [9,10]. The benefits appear somewhat greater than with most other agents. Interestingly, propranolol also appeared to exert a greater reduction in mortality than did beta-1-selective blockers in the one small study that has assessed this agent [11]. Finally, no large long-term study of a beta-1-selective blocker has ever shown a reduction in mortality after myocardial infarction [12,13]. The positive, large, long-term studies of beta-blockers after myocardial infarction were reported with timolol, propranolol, and carvedilol.

The above studies strongly suggest that all beta-blockers are not equally effective in patients with heart failure. However, it is difficult to compare the benefits of effective agents using information from different trials because differences may be due to the type of patient recruited or their background management. Head-to-head trials are required. Fortunately, there is one large, adequately powered study comparing a beta-1-selective and a nonselective beta-blocker in patients with heart failure. The COMET [14] trial

* Corresponding author. Department of Cardiology, University of Hull, Castle Hill Hospital, Kingston-upon-Hull, UK.

E-mail address: g.m.porter@hull.ac.uk (J.G.F. Cleland).

1551-7136/05/$ – see front matter
doi:10.1016/j.hfc.2004.12.004

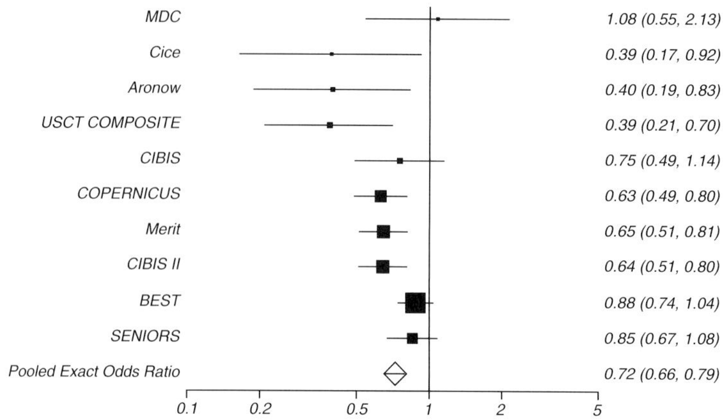

Fig. 1. Pooled exact odds ratio and 95% confidence intervals for all-cause mortality. Meta-analysis of trials comparing beta-blocker versus placebo or inactive control in which 40 or more deaths occurred. Hazard ratio with 95% confidence intervals are shown. For references, see text. MDC and MERIT were conducted with metoprolol. Cice, USCT Composite, and COPERNICUS were conducted with carvedilol. Aronow was conducted with propranolol and included only patients with LV ejection fraction > 40%. CIBIS and CIBIS-II were conducted with bisoprolol. BEST was conducted with bucindolol. SENIORS was conducted with nebivolol. (*From* Cleland JGF, Loh PH, Freemantle N, et al. Clinical trials update from the European Society of Cardiology. Eur J Heart Failure 2004;6:787–91; with permission.)

showed that, compared with metoprolol tartrate (target dose 50 mg twice daily), carvedilol (target dose 25 mg twice daily) reduced all-cause mortality. The reduction in mortality with carvedilol compared with metoprolol, both relative and absolute, was similar in size to that of other accepted therapies for heart failure (Table 1). Patients randomized to carvedilol not only lived longer but also reported improved symptoms and well-being [15]. Despite living longer and therefore having a greater period of risk, there was no increase in the number or duration of hospitalizations. As carvedilol, compared with metoprolol, improves both the quality and quantity of life for patients with heart failure, there is a strong argument for making it the beta-blocker of choice for patients with heart failure.

There is no dispute that a difference between metoprolol and carvedilol was observed in COMET. However, there is debate about why the difference occurred [16]. The original hypothesis of the trial was that the myocardial and peripheral effects of comprehensive adrenergic receptor blockade with carvedilol would be superior to those of beta-1-selective blockade with metoprolol [14,17]. However, most scientific evidence has weaknesses and limitations that can be exploited by those who do not wish to believe the obvious conclusions. Convoluted and speculative lines of reasoning can lead to distorted alternative interpretations of seemingly secure data. Obvious, simple, straightforward interpretation of data is not always correct but it often is. In this article, simple and complex interpretations of the data are juxtaposed so that the reader can decide on the best interpretation of the data.

The History of COMET

Planning of the COMET study began in 1995, after the US Carvedilol Trials data had been presented but before it had even been published. The first patients were randomized in 1996. The MERIT study started recruitment 1 year later. Patient recruitment to COMET was complete before the results of MERIT were known.

Information from randomized, placebo-controlled trials available during planning

By 1996, there were 29 published trials of beta-blockers and meta-analysis of these suggested that beta-blockers reduced mortality and morbidity and that metoprolol and carvedilol were both effective [18]. The largest bodies of data at the time were with carvedilol (n = 1658), metoprolol (n = 620), bisoprolol (n = 641), and bucindolol (n = 222), of which only metoprolol was generically available and licensed for use in patients with heart failure due to dilated cardiomyopathy in some European countries. Publications with each of these agents had suggested benefit, but only one study, using carvedilol, had shown a reduction in all-cause mortality [1]; other individual studies had been inconclusive. The benefit with carvedilol in the US Carvedilol Trials Program appeared greater than with other beta-blockers and various explanations were put forward including chance, the fact that the trial was stopped early (which tends to over-estimate benefit), and differences in the pharmacological properties of carvedilol. The uncertainty about whether the effects of carvedilol were a class effect of beta-blockers or whether some agents in this class were more effective than others was the prime rationale for the COMET study.

Supportive evidence that beta-blockers might not all be similarly effective in patients with heart failure was provided by long-term trials of beta-blockers post–myocardial infarction, although these were

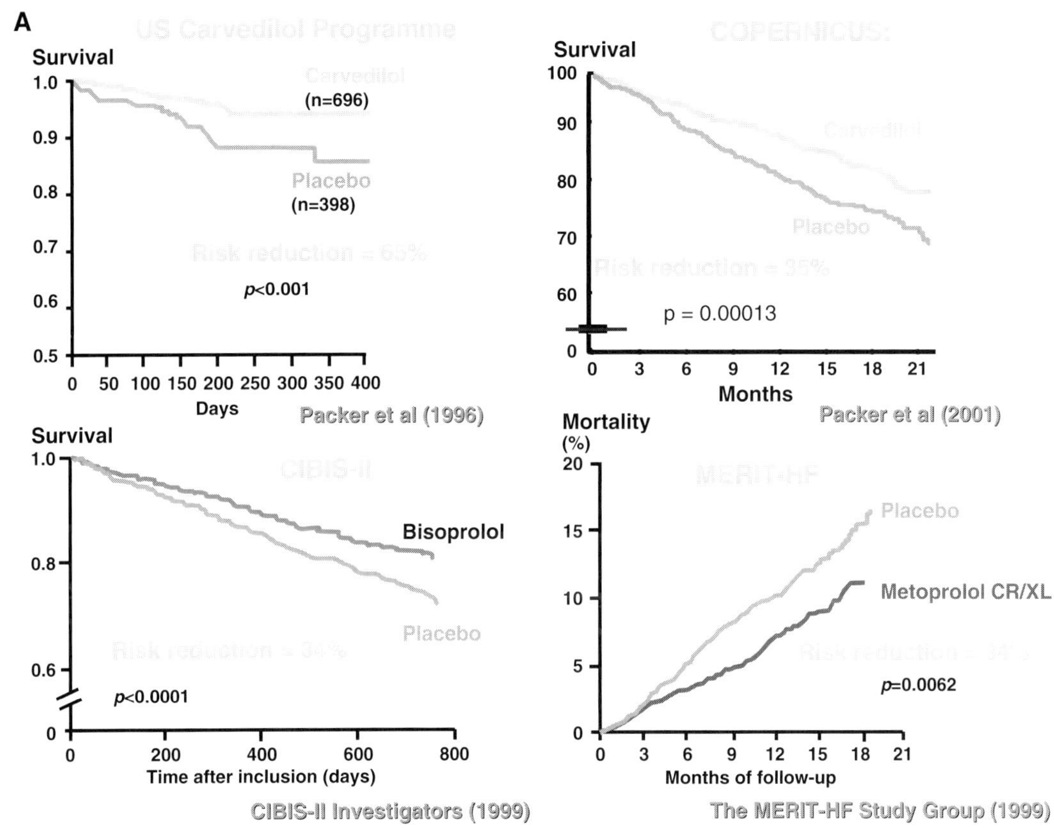

Fig. 2. (*A*) Effects of beta-blockers on mortality compared with placebo in the four positive landmark studies. US Carvedilol program [1], COPERNICUS [4], CIBIS-II [2], and MERIT-HF [3]. (*B*) Subgroup analysis of the MERIT-HF study suggesting that, compared to the placebo group, the effects of metoprolol were similar amongst patients who received ≤ 100 and > 100 mg once daily of metoprolol succinate [28]. Metoprolol succinate 100 mg once daily is equivalent to 30 to 35 mg twice daily of metoprolol tartrate and the actual mean dose received of metoprolol succinate was 76 mg once daily, which is equivalent to about 25 mg twice daily of metoprolol tartrate. (*From* Wikstrand J, Hjalmarson A, Waagstein F, et al for the MERIT-HF study group. Dose of metoprolol CR/XL and clinical outcomes in patients with heart failure: analysis of the experience in metoprolol CR/XL randomised intervention trial in chronic heart failure (MERIT-HF). J Am Coll Cardiol 2002;40(3):491–8; with permission.) (*C*) Comparison of mortality on metoprolol tartrate (target dose of 50 mg twice daily, 78% of patients achieved target and mean achieved dose was 40 to 45 mg twice daily) and carvedilol (target dose 25 mg twice daily, 75% achieved target and mean achieved dose was about 21 mg twice daily) [14]. Note that there is little separation of the mortality curves until after 1 year. (*From* Poole-Wilson PA, Swedberg K, Cleland JGF, et al for the COMET investigators. Comparison of carvedilol and metoprolol on clinical outcomes in patients with chronic heart failure in the Carvedilol Or Metoprolol European Trial (COMET): randomised controlled trial. Lancet 2003;362:7–13; with permission.)

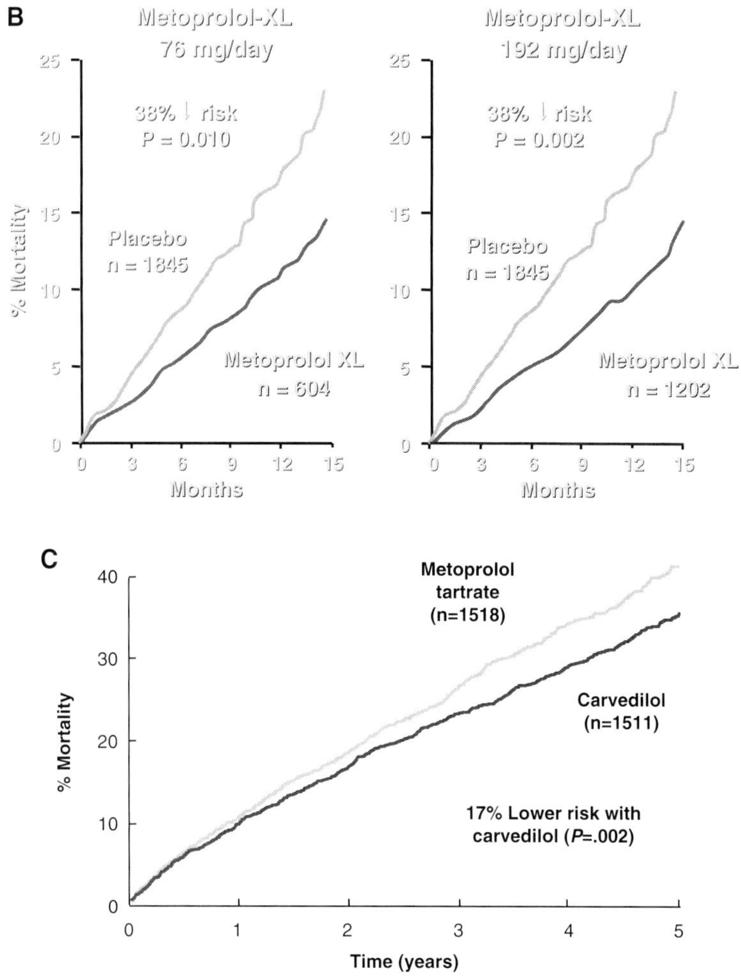

Fig. 2 (*continued*).

conducted in the era before thrombolysis and ACE inhibitors became widely available [13]. Overall, metoprolol tartrate reduced mortality after myocardial infarction by about 20%, propranolol by 29%, and timolol by 41%. Subsequently, one large and several smaller trials of carvedilol were published in patients who were receiving contemporary management [10], showing that carvedilol also reduced mortality after myocardial infarction in the modern era of post-infarction therapy.

There was a lengthy and careful debate during the planning phase of COMET over the formulation and dose of metoprolol to be used. Metoprolol XL/CR, a product that had been launched only 4 years earlier in 1992, was considered as a possible comparator to carvedilol, but due to patent protection on the new formulation its use was not possible. Data from a number of pathophysiological studies were used to choose the trial doses of carvedilol and metoprolol [14,17]. A 2:1 ratio of 50 mg twice daily of metoprolol to 25 mg twice daily of carvedilol was chosen. Undoubtedly some patients would have tolerated higher doses of either agent.

Could the formulation of metoprolol used be responsible for the difference observed?

Clearly, there are powerful data to show that metoprolol succinate is superior to placebo in patients with heart failure [3]. It is not clear that there is a difference in the efficacy of metoprolol succinate and metoprolol tartrate [19]. The tartrate delivers about

Table 1
The effects of adopting a variety of possible changes in treatment on survival

Trial [Ref.]	Numbers	Main entry criteria	Follow-up (mo)	Placebo mortality (%)	Reduction in mortality (%)	Lives saved per thousand by adopting change[a]
ACE Inhibitors						
SOLVD-Treatment	2569	Age < 80 y				
[40]		NYHA II-IV	41.4	39.72	4.54	45
		LVEF ≤35%	12	15.65	3.28	33
HOPE [41]	9297	Age 55 y	60	12.23	1.85	19
		CVS disease				
		CVS risk factors				
		LVEF > 40%				
Beta-Blockers						
USCT [1]	1094	NYHA II-IV	6.5	7.79	4.63	46
		LVEF ≤ 35%				
COPERNICUS [4]	2289	NYHA III-IV	10.4	16.77	5.52	55
		LVEF < 25%				
CIBIS-II [2]	2647		16	17.27	5.51	55
MERIT-HF [3,37]	3991	NYHA II-IV	12	10.84	3.55	36
		LVEF ≤40%				
Aldosterone antagonists						
RALES [42]	1663	NYHA III-IV	24	45.90	11.35	114
		LVEF ≤35%				
EPHESUS [43]	6632	Post-MI	16	16.72	2.32	23
		NYHA I-IV				
		LVEF ≤ 40%				
Devices						
COMPANION [44]	1520	NYHA III-IV	12	19	7	70
					(4% CRT alone)	(40 CRT alone)
		QRS > 120 msec				
		LVEF ≤35%				
MADIT-II [45]	1232	Late post-MI	20	19.80	5.65	57
		LVEF ≤30%				
				Metoprolol mortality	Reduction with carvedilol	
COMET [14]	3029	NYHA II-IV	58	39.53	5.65	57
		LVEF ≤ 35%	12	10.21	0.81	8
		Prior CVS hosp				

Data on 1-year and long-term follow-up are shown for the SOLVD-treatment and COMET studies. Note that the short-term effect of carvedilol and metoprolol are similar and then diverge, suggesting that both treatments were similarly effective in the short-term consistent with the known data from previous trials of beta-blockers that had all stopped around 1 year. The overall long-term treatment difference between metoprolol and carvedilol was large and appears similar in magnitude to that of an ACE inhibitor compared to placebo or a defibrillator compared to control.

Abbreviations: CVS, cardiovascular; hosp, hospitalization; LVEF, left ventricular ejection fraction; MI, myocardial infarction.

[a] Note that lives saved reflects the risk of the population and the duration of follow-up (very short and very long follow-up are generally not associated with substantial differences using this outcome measure—unfortunately trials are not reported in a way that allows simple assessment of the impact of treatment on longevity).

50% more metoprolol than does the succinate preparation. Tartrate was used in many large postinfarction and hypertension studies. Meta-analysis of 13 studies of metoprolol tartrate in heart failure including 903 patients suggests no statistical heterogeneity with the mortality benefit observed in the four randomized controlled trials with succinate that included 4532 patients. This strongly suggests that it is the metoprolol in these preparations that is important for efficacy and not the formulation.

Studies of the effects of different formulations of metoprolol indicate that twice-daily, immediate-release and once-daily, extended-release metoprolol exert similar reductions in peak and trough heart rate at rest [20] and during exercise [21]. The long-term hemodynamic effects are also similar at peak and trough plasma drug concentrations [21].

In conclusion, there is compelling evidence that metoprolol tartrate (given at least twice daily) and succinate (once daily) exert similar beta-blocking effects and similar benefit on prognosis. Metoprolol tartrate is licensed for the treatment of heart failure in several countries. There is no evidence that the effect of metoprolol tartrate is inferior to metoprolol succinate for the treatment of heart failure.

Could the dose of metoprolol used be responsible for the difference observed?

There are three aspects to this question. First, would a higher dose of metoprolol be more effective? Second, if higher doses are more effective, would they be tolerated? Third, if higher doses of metoprolol are more effective, might this not also be true of carvedilol?

Dose and efficacy

More patients in the US Carvedilol Trials and in COPERNICUS were taking 25 mg twice daily of carvedilol than any other dose, indicating that this is an effective dose [1,4]. Most studies of metoprolol tartrate used a target dose of 50 mg twice daily, and the 100 mg twice daily dose appeared poorly tolerated [22]. The MDC trial [23] used a slightly higher target dose of metoprolol, but the patients in this study were young (mean age 49 years versus 62 years in COMET), all had dilated cardiomyopathy (versus 22% in COMET [24]), and their rate of comorbidity was low. The degradation of metoprolol may be delayed in older patients with comorbid conditions and therefore lower and more cautious dosing is recommended by regulatory authorities. In summary, there is strong evidence that both doses of beta-blocker used in COMET were effective.

There are no adequate dose-ranging studies of beta-blockers in heart failure. The MOCHA trial compared carvedilol titrated to 6.25 mg twice daily, 12.5 mg twice daily, and 25 mg twice daily and suggested that patients with dilated cardiomyopathy, but not those with ischemic heart disease, had a dose-related improvement in left ventricular ejection fraction [25]. All three doses of carvedilol reduced mortality and hospitalization. There was only one death in the 80 patients randomized to the highest dose of carvedilol, which was less than that observed at other doses, but this was not significantly different. On the other hand, there were only two hospitalizations for worsening heart failure with the lowest dose of carvedilol, which was less than for any of the other groups. Data from two other small studies of other beta-blockers also show inconclusive evidence of a dose-response [26,27]. It is possible that smaller doses of beta-blockers are just as effective but might have fewer side effects than larger doses and therefore, when risk and benefit are considered, could be considered optimal.

Sub-group analysis of studies using the doses of drug tolerated are confounded because patients who are less sick are more likely to tolerate higher doses and less likely to have events. However, the MERIT-HF study suggested that the benefits of metoprolol were similar in patients who could or could not tolerate doses of metoprolol succinate >100 mg/d [28] (see Fig. 2B). This further suggests that the dose of beta-blocker may not be a critically important determinant of beta-blocker effect.

Dose, weight, and tolerability

There is a consistent relationship between weight and the dose of beta-blocker tolerated. In MERIT-HF, the mean weight of patients who could tolerate >100 mg/d of metoprolol succinate (n = 1202) was 82 kg and for those only able to tolerate 100 mg/d or less (n = 604) it was 78 kg [28]. The US Carvedilol Trials also recognized the importance of weight from the outset and used a target dose of 25 mg twice daily for patients <85 kg or 50 mg twice daily if the patient weighed >85 kg in the two main component trials. Patients in the US are, on average, larger than Europeans. In the US carvedilol and the COMET trials, respectively, 60% and 29% of patients weighed > 85 kg [1,24]. Accordingly, as the COMET study was conceived as a simple pragmatic study, it was decided to have a simple 25 mg twice-daily target dose of carvedilol for all patients.

The mean dose of metoprolol tartrate in COMET was 85 mg/d and of carvedilol 41.8 mg/d, and about 75% of patients were taking the specified target doses of each therapy at end of titration and at 1 year of follow-up. The mean weight of patients in COMET was 78.6 kg, very similar to the mean weight of patients who could not tolerate doses of metoprolol succinate > 100 mg (equivalent to about 67 mg/d of metoprolol tartrate). If the dose of metoprolol had been effectively less than that of carvedilol, then metoprolol should have been better tolerated. It was not. By inference, had a higher target dose of metoprolol been chosen, then poorer tolerability, more side effects, and potentially an even worse outcome would have been observed with metoprolol.

Finally, higher doses of metoprolol start to block the beta-2-receptor. COMET was designed to test whether or not beta-1-selective blockade was as effective as comprehensive adrenergic blockade. Higher doses of metoprolol would have led to loss of beta-1-selectivity and undermined the hypothesis being tested.

Observations on the differences in heart rate and blood pressure in the COMET trial

The reductions in heart rate and blood pressure were slightly greater on carvedilol compared with metoprolol, and this has been interpreted by some as evidence of a difference in the effectiveness of beta-1-blockade and in turn an explanation for the difference in mortality. The greater reduction in heart rate with carvedilol could reflect the chronotropic effects of blocking the beta-2 receptor [29,30] rather than any subtle difference in effect on beta-1 receptors. The greater fall in arterial pressure could reflect the vasodilating effects of alpha-blockade, although this has been hard to prove. There is no evidence that any difference between carvedilol and metoprolol reflects greater beta-1-receptor blockade [31].

It seems implausible that a small, short-lived difference in heart rate would lead to a large difference in mortality. The reduction in heart rate with beta-blockers has averaged about 14 bpm in clinical trials (MDC 15 bpm, US carvedilol 13 bpm, MERIT-HF 14 bpm, CIBIS-II 10 bpm versus, in COMET, 12 bpm on metoprolol and 13 bpm on carvedilol [1–3,14]. The reduction in heart rate with metoprolol in COMET was similar to or greater than that observed in other studies of beta-1-selective agents. It has also been suggested that had heart rate been measured throughout 24 hours, greater differences would have been observed during periods of trough drug effect. However, as the pharmacokinetics of carvedilol and metoprolol tartrate are rather similar, this seems unlikely [32], and a small, independent study (n = 40) showed that the 24-hour heart rate profile with metoprolol tartrate (50 mg twice daily and carvedilol (25 mg twice daily) were superimposable [33]. Pharmacodynamic studies of metoprolol tartrate 100 mg once daily and 50 mg twice daily [21] in healthy subjects also suggest similar heart rate reductions at peak plasma concentrations and 12 hours after dosing.

Finally, it seems implausible that a small difference in arterial pressure could account for the differences in outcome, as studies of agents that have produced much greater reductions in arterial pressure (eg, prazosin, omapatrilat, and moxonidine) have been ineffective or harmful [24,34,35].

Is the difference between carvedilol and metoprolol due to greater effects on the myocardium or the periphery?

Indirect and direct comparisons suggest that carvedilol causes a greater improvement in left ventricular systolic function than metoprolol [36]. No serial measurements of cardiac function were made in COMET and so this cannot be confirmed from this trial. There was no clear evidence of a reduction in vascular events in MERIT-HF although, since mortality was reduced, an effect cannot be excluded [37]. However, there was a striking reduction in the rate of vascular events, both myocardial infarction and stroke, on carvedilol compared with metoprolol in COMET. These data suggest that differences in peripheral as well myocardial effects between carvedilol and metoprolol are important. Of course, metoprolol was designed to spare the beta-2 receptor in order not to have effects on the peripheral circulation, and that may be its weakness. Carvedilol and metoprolol both have favorable metabolic effects such as reducing plasma renin. However, blockade of beta-2 receptors may also prevent hypokalaemia [30]. This may be especially important during stress, when sympathetic activation causes a fall in serum potassium. Metoprolol blocks the beta-1 receptor but does not reduce peripheral sympathetic activity and will offer little protection from stimulation of peripheral and myocardial beta-2 or alpha-1 receptors.

Observations on the differences in morbidity in the COMET trial

It has been suggested that the lack of a difference in effect on hospitalization weakens the argument in favor of carvedilol. However, an increase in hospitalization might have been expected given the improved survival and therefore increased time at risk. Patients receiving carvedilol gained an extra 50,000 days survival but spent slightly fewer days in hospital overall [15]. In other words, all the survival gain with carvedilol was associated with a good enough health state for people not to require additional hospital care. Also, if an analysis is conducted looking at well-being and time spent with poor health, this favors carvedilol over metoprolol. Patients not only lived longer, they also lived *better* on carvedilol. Carvedilol truly prolonged life rather than prolonging death.

Observations on the differences in mortality in the COMET trial

COMET is unique for many reasons, including being one of the few large trials of beta-blockers not to be stopped early, either for efficacy or futility. All four large trials compared beta-blockers with placebo and showed benefit, including MERIT-HF. The reduction in mortality in these trials was obvious by 6 months and their mean duration was only about 1 year. In COMET, the mortality curves did not separate for 12 to 18 months. In other words, none of the previous trials can be compared with the difference between agents observed in COMET. What can be compared amongst these trials is the effect of beta-blockers compared with placebo during the first year of therapy. As there was no difference between carvedilol or metoprolol, given the robustness of the pre-existing data, both metoprolol tartrate and carvedilol must have been effective in COMET. However, although carvedilol was not superior in the short term, it did show medium and long-term superiority.

Trials of other agents

The scientific community has accepted that all beta-blockers are not equally effective. Xamoterol was associated with an excess mortality, either because it is a partial agonist of the beta-receptor or because it was introduced abruptly in large doses or because of some unknown property [7]. Bucindolol is a nonselective beta-blocker that may also have alpha-blocking activity and, controversially, partial agonist activity [6]. A large trial of this agent failed to show a significant reduction in mortality and was abandoned for futility. Some speculated that its pharmacological profile was rather similar to carvedilol and that COPERNICUS and COMET, neither of which had been presented when the results of BEST were announced, would be similarly neutral or worse after the previous success of beta-1-selective agents in CIBIS-II and MERIT-HF. These considerations emphasize that speculation is no substitute for clinical scientific evidence. Some humility in admitting that we do not fully understand the often subtle but important differences between therapeutic agents is required. No amount of basic science experimentation can be a substitute for hard clinical facts.

The effects of racial origin and genetics of participants

The BEST and MERIT studies both suggested that African Americans did not benefit from bucindolol and metoprolol, but carvedilol has been found to be similarly effective in all racial groups studied [38].

Genetic Arg/Gly389 polymorphisms of the beta-1-adrenergic receptor were reported to predict response to bucindolol in the BEST study [5]. Arg389 is associated with a greater response to norepinephrine and a greater reduction in contractility when propranolol is administered and is the more common polymorphism, especially in the Caucasian population. About 500 patients were homozygous for the Arg389 variant in the BEST study. In these patients, mortality was reduced by 38% ($P < 0.02$) and death or hospitalization by 34% ($P = 0.004$) with bucindolol. However, in a substudy of MERIT, the same polymorphism was not shown to alter prognosis or to interact with the effects of therapy [39].

Summary

COMET clearly shows that carvedilol is superior to metoprolol tartrate. There is no evidence that any other beta-1 selective agent or formulation of metoprolol would have been superior to metoprolol tartrate. It is possible that metoprolol succinate is better tolerated than metoprolol tartarte although, in contrast to large placebo controlled trials of carvedilol, the MERIT-HF trial showed an excess number of withdrawals compared with placebo in the first 3 months of therapy [37]. Unless substantial new comparative data suggests differences amongst beta-1-selective blockers, then carvedilol should be considered the beta-blocker of choice in patients with heart failure due to left ventricular systolic dysfunction.

References

[1] Packer M, Bristow MR, Cohn JN, et al for the US carvedilol study group. The effect of carvedilol on morbidity and mortality in patients with chronic heart failure. N Engl J Med 1996;334:1349–55.

[2] CIBIS-II Investigators and Committee. The Cardiac insufficiency Bisoprolol Study II (CIBIS-II): a randomised trial. Lancet 1999;353:9–13.

[3] MERIT-HF Study Group. Effect of metoprolol CR/XL in chronic heart failure: Metoprolol CR/XL Randomised Intervention Trial in Congestive Heart Failure (MERIT-HF). Lancet 1999;353:2001–7.

[4] Packer M, Coats AJS, Fowler MB, et al for the carvedilol prospective randomized cumulative survival study group. Effect of carvedilol on survival in severe chronic heart failure. N Engl J Med 2001;344:1651–8.

[5] Cleland JGF, Loh PH, Freemantle N, et al. Clinical trials update from the European Society of Cardiology. Eur J Heart Failure 2004;6:787–91.

[6] The beta-blocker evaluation of survival trial investigators. A trial of the beta-blocker bucindolol in patients with advanced chronic heart failure. N Engl J Med 2001;344:1659–67.

[7] Nicholas G, Oakley C, Pouleur H, et al. Xamoterol in severe heart failure. Lancet 1990;336:1–6.

[8] Cice G, Ferrara L, D'Andrea A, et al. Carvedilol increases two-year survival in dialysis patients with dilated cardiomyopathy. J Am Coll Cardiol 2003;41:1438–44.

[9] Dargie HJ. The CAPRICORN Steering Committee. Design and methodology of the CAPRICORN trial—a randomised double-blind, placebo-controlled study of the impact of carvedilol on morbidity and mortality in patients with left ventricular dsyfunction after myocardial infarction. Eur J Heart Fail 2000;2:325–32.

[10] The CAPRICORN Investigators. Effects of carvedilol on outcome after myocardial infarction in patients with left ventricular dysfunction: the CAPRICORN randomised trial. Lancet 2001;357:1385–90.

[11] Aronow WS, Ahn C, Kronzon I. Effect of propranolol versus no propranolol on total mortality plus non fatal myocardial infarction in older patients with prior myocardial infarction, congestive heart failure, and left ventricular ejection fraction $\geq$ 40% treated with diuretics plus angiotensin-converting enzyme inhibitors. Am J Cardiol 1997;80:207–9.

[12] Houghton T, Freemantle N, Cleland JGF. Are beta-blockers effective in patients who develop heart failure soon after myocardial infarction? A meta-regression analysis of randomised trials. Eur J Heart Fail 2000;2:333–40.

[13] Freemantle N, Cleland JGF, Young S, et al. Beta blockade after myocardial infarction:systematic review and meta regression analysis. BMJ 1999;318:1730–7.

[14] Poole-Wilson PA, Swedberg K, Cleland JGF, et al for the COMET Investigators. Comparison of carvedilol and metoprolol on clinical outcomes in patients with chronic heart failure in the Carvedilol Or Metoprolol European Trial (COMET): randomised controlled trial. Lancet 2003;362:7–13.

[15] Cleland JGF, Swedberg K, Torp Pedersen C, et al on behalf of the COMET Committees and Investigators. Comparison of the effects of metoprolol and carvedilol on symptoms, well-being and quality-adjusted life-years: a description of the "Patient-Journey" in COMET [abstract]. JACC 2004;43:206A.

[16] Bristow MR, Feldman AM, Adams KFJ, et al. Selective versus nonselective B-blockade for heart failure therapy: are there lessons to be learned from the COMET trial? J Card Failure 2003;9:444–53.

[17] Poole-Wilson PA, Cleland JGF, Hanrath P, et al on behalf of the COMET Study Investigators. Rationale and design of the Carvedilol or Metoprolol European Trial in patients with chronic heart failure; the COMET trial. Eur J Heart Fail 2002;4:321–9.

[18] Doughty RN, Rodgers A, Sharpe N, et al. Effects of beta-blocker therapy on mortality in patients with heart failure—a systematic overview of randomised controlled trials. Eur Heart J 1997;18:560–5.

[19] Herlitz J, Dellborg M, Karlson BW, et al. Similar risk reduction of death of extended-release etoprolol once daily and immediate-release metoprolol twice daily during 5 years after myocardial infarction. Cardiovasc Drugs Ther 1999;13:127–35.

[20] Kukin ML, Mannino MM, Freudenberger RS, et al. Hemodynamic comparison of twice daily metoprolol tartrate with once daily metoprolol succinate in congestive heart failure. J Am Coll Cardiol 2000;1:45–50.

[21] Sandberg A, Blomqvist I, Jonsson UE, et al. Pharmacokinetic and pharmacodynamic properties of a new controlled-release formulation of metoprolol: a comparison with conventional tablets. Eur J Clin Pharmacol 1988;33:S9–14.

[22] Currie PJ, Kelly MJ, McKenzie A, et al. Oral beta-adrenergic blockade with metoprolol in chronic severe dilated cardiomyopathy. J Am Coll Cardiol 1984;3:203–9.

[23] Waagstein F, Bristow MR, Swedberg K, et al. Beneficial effects of metoprolol in idiopathic dilated cardiomyopathy. Lancet 1993;342:1441–6.

[24] Packer M, Califf RM, Konstam MA, et al. Comparison of omapatrilat and enalapril in patients with chronic heart failure: the Omapatrilat Versus Enalapril Randomized Trial of Utility in Reducing Events (OVERTURE). Circulation 2002;106:920–6.

[25] Bristow MR, Gilbert EM, Abraham WT, et al for the MOCHA Investigators. Carvedilol produces dose-related improvements in left ventricular function and survival in subjects with chronic heart failure. Circulation 1996;94:2807–16.

[26] Bristow MR, O'Connell JB, Gilbert EM, et al. Dose-response of chronic Β-blocker treatment in heart failure from either idiopathic dilated or ischemic cardiomyopathy. Circulation 1994;89:1632–42.
[27] Uhlir O, Dvorak I, Gregor F, et al. Nebivolol in the treatment of cardiac failure: a double-blind controlled clinical trial. J Card Fail 1997;3:271–5.
[28] Wikstrand J, Hjalmarson A, Waagstein F, et al for the MERIT-HF study group. Dose of metoprolol CR/XL and clinical outcomes in patients with heart failure: analysis of the experience in metoprolol CR/XL randomised intervention trial in chronic heart failure (MERIT-HF). J Am Coll Cardiol 2002;40:491–8.
[29] Brown JE, McLeod AA, Shand DG. Evidence for cardiac beta 2-adrenoceptors in man. Clin Pharmacol Ther 1983;33:424–8.
[30] Gullestad L, Birkeland K, Nordby G, et al. Effects of selective beta-2-adrenoceptor blockade on serum potassium and exercise performance in normal men. Br J Clin Pharmacol 1991;32:201–7.
[31] Hryniewicz K, Androne AS, Hudaihed A, et al. Comparative effects of carvedilol and metoprolol on regional vascular response to adrenergic stimuli in normal subjects and patients with chronic heart failure. Circulation 2003;108:971–6.
[32] Morgan T. Clinical pharmacokinetics and pharmacodynamics of carvedilol. Clin Pharmacokinet 1994; 26:335–46.
[33] Sanderson JE, Leung LYC, Chan SKW, et al. Do metoprolol and carvedilol have equivalent heart rate effects in chronic heart failure? A comparative ambulatory 24-hour ECG study. Eur J Heart Fail, in press.
[34] Cohn JN, Archibald DG, Ziesche S, et al. Effect of vasodilator therapy on mortality in chronic congestive heart failure: results of a Veterans Administration Cooperative Study. N Engl J Med 1986;314:1547–52.
[35] Cohn JN, Pfeffer MA, Rouleau J, et al for the MOXCON Investigators. Adverse mortality effect of central sympathetic inhibition with sustained-release moxonidine in patients with heart failure (MOXCON). Eur J Heart Fail 2003;5:659–67.
[36] Packer M, Antonopoulos GV, Berlin JA, et al. Comparative effects of carvedilol and metoprolol on left ventricular ejection fraction in heart failure: results of a meta-analysis. Am Heart J 2001;141:899–907.
[37] Hjalmarson A, Goldstein S, Fagerberg B, et al. Effects of controlled-release metoprolol on total mortality, hospitalization, and well-being in patients with heart failure: the metoprolol CR-XL randomized intervention trial in congestive heart failure (MERIT-HF). JAMA 2000;283:1295–302.
[38] Yancy CW, Fowler MB, Colucci WS, et al for the US Carvedilol Heart Failure Study Group. Race and the response to adrenergic blockade with carvedilol in patients with chronic heart failure. N Engl J Med 2001; 344:1358–65.
[39] On behalf of the MERIT-HF study group, White HL, de Boer RA, Maqbool A, et al. An evaluation of the beta-1-adrenergic receptor Arg389Gly polymorphism in individuals with heart failure: a MERIT-HF sub-study. Eur J Heart Fail 2003;5:463–8.
[40] Yusuf S. Effect of enalapril on survival in patients with reduced left ventricular ejection fractions and congestive heart failure. N Engl J Med 1991;325: 293–302.
[41] Yusuf S, Sleight P, Pogue J, et al. Effects of the angiotensin converting enzyme inhibitor, ramipril, on cardiovascular events in high risk patients. The Heart Outcomes Prevention Evaluation study investigators. N Engl J Med 2000;342:145–53.
[42] Pitt B, Zannad F, Remme WJ, et al. The effect of spironolactone on morbidity and mortality in patients with severe heart failure. N Engl J Med 1999;341: 709–17.
[43] Pitt B, Remme W, Zannad F, et al for the Eplerenone Post-Acute Myocardial Infarction Heart Failure Efficacy and Survival Study Investigators. Eplerenone, a selective aldosterone blocker, in patients with left ventricular dysfunction after myocardial infarction. N Engl J Med 2003;348:1309–21.
[44] Bristow MR, Feldman AM, Saxon LA, for the Companion Steering Committee and Companion Clinical Investigators. Heart Failure Management Using Implantable Devices for Ventricular Resynchronization: Comparison of Medical Therapy, Pacing and Defibrillation in Chronic Heart Failure (COMPANION) Trial. J Card Fail 2000;6:276–85.
[45] Moss AJ, Zareba W, Hall WJ, et al for the Multicenter Automatic Defibrillator Implantation Trial II Investigators. Prophylactic implantation of a defibrillator in patients with myocardial infarction and reduced ejection fraction. N Engl J Med 2002;346:877–83.

ELSEVIER
SAUNDERS

Heart Failure Clin 1 (2005) 67 – 75

HEART
FAILURE
CLINICS

Could β-Blockers Precede or Replace Angiotensin-Converting Enzyme Inhibitors in Heart Failure?

Willem J. Remme, MD, PhD*

Sticares Cardiovascular Research Foundation, Rhoon, The Netherlands

Neurohormonal activation contributes greatly to the development and progression of heart failure. Neuroendocrine systems, the most relevant in this respect, include the renin–angiotensin system (RAS), the sympathetic nervous system (SNS), aldosterone, and endothelins. They play a pivotal role in cardiac remodeling, an essential mechanism underlying the development of ventricular dysfunction and heart failure, and contribute to structural and functional changes in the cardiovascular system, such as cellular hypertrophy, apoptosis, and fibrosis.

Although some systems become activated later in the development of heart failure, the SNS is an early contributor, reportedly preceding activation of the RAS. In the Studies of Left Ventricular Dysfunction (SOLVD), plasma measurements of neurohormones indicated an earlier activation of the SNS than the RAS [1].

In heart failure, sympathetic overactivation occurs particularly in the heart and the kidney. As a consequence, increased cardiac norepinephrine production stimulates the β_1-, β_2-, and α_1-adrenergic receptors, each of which are linked to pathways leading to cardiac cellular remodeling signals (Fig. 1). Although some pathways also can be modulated by the RAS, other β-adrenergic intracellular signaling pathways are independent. Consequently, full β-adrenergic receptor blockade would modulate the remodeling process more completely than inhibition of the RAS.

The change in the β-adrenergic receptor population in the cardiovascular system during heart failure—from a predominant β_1 profile to more β_2 and α_1 adrenoceptors—underscores the importance of blocking all adrenergic receptors rather than the β_1 receptor only. Because adrenergic activation happens early, this blockade should be initiated as soon as possible. Moreover, because adrenergic activation may precede that of the RAS, a case could be made for initiating β-blockade before inhibiting the latter system through angiotensin-converting enzyme (ACE) inhibition.

Angiotensin-converting enzyme inhibition in heart failure: should it always be first-line therapy?

Current heart failure guidelines indicate the use of ACE inhibition with or without diuretics as first-line therapy, before treatment with β-blockade [2]. This recommendation is based on evidence from several large, controlled, clinical trials conducted in the mid- to late-1980s and early 1990s indicating that ACE inhibition significantly reduces mortality and cardiovascular hospitalization in symptomatic heart failure, and hospitalizations for cardiovascular reasons and worsening heart failure in patients who have asymptomatic left ventricular (LV) dysfunction, compared with placebo or the vasodilator combination hydralazine-isosorbide dinitrate [3–9].

ACE inhibitors thus became the first-line choice in treating heart failure. This choice, however, was based on historical grounds, because ACE inhibitors were the first class of neurohormonal modulators to be investigated in well-designed, sufficiently large

* Sticares Cardiovascular Research Foundation, "Albrandssate", Oever 1-5, 3161 KC, Rhoon, The Netherlands.
E-mail address: w.j.remme@sticares.org

1551-7136/05/$ – see front matter
doi:10.1016/j.hfc.2004.12.001

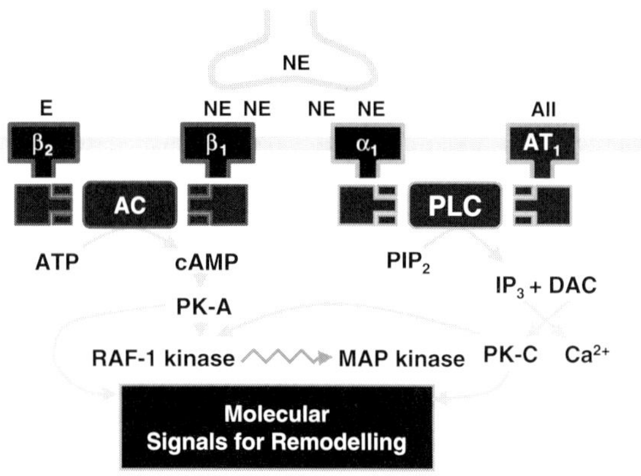

Fig. 1. Simplified representation of subcellular pathways leading to remodeling processes following α_1-, β_1-, and β_2-adrenoceptor and angiotensin-II (AII) type-I receptor (AT_1) stimulation. AC, adenylate cyclase; DAC, diacylglycerol; E, epinephrine; IP3, inositol triphosphate; MAP kinase, mitogen-activated protein kinase; NE, norepinephrine; PIP2, phosphatidyl inositol biphosphate; PK-A, protein kinase A; PK-C, protein kinase C; PLC, phospholipase C.

and controlled studies. Most important, these studies were performed before a general understanding of the importance of another class of neurohormonal agents, β-blocking drugs, in cardiac dysfunction and heart failure. Indeed, β-blocking drugs may have become the cornerstone of heart failure therapy had their efficacy in decreasing deaths and hospitalizations, improving clinical well-being and cardiac function, and reversing cardiac remodeling in heart failure patients been understood. Unfortunately, it took the medical community a long time to understand that β-blocking agents should be viewed not as contraindicated, but as mandatory therapy in heart failure.

Several large, controlled trials, including the United States carvedilol program, the Cardiac Insufficiency Bisoprolol Study II, Metoprolol CR/XL Randomised Intervention Trial in Congestive Heart Failure, and Carvedilol Prospective Randomized Cumulative Survival Study [10–13], have shown the benefit of β-blockade to ACE inhibition in mild, moderate, and severe but stable heart failure. Because this benefit occurred on top of ACE inhibition, β-blocking drugs are presented as mandatory but second-line drugs in heart failure guidelines, a position which is difficult to change.

Although proving better efficacy as a first-line drug compared with ACE inhibitors would require large, controlled, head-to-head comparisons of β-blockade and ACE inhibition on clinical endpoints, such as mortality and hospitalizations for cardiovascular reasons, such trials would be resisted because half the study population would not receive either an ACE inhibitor or a β-blocker for some time: an obvious ethical problem. This concern would be lessened if smaller, shorter studies were conducted. This would require a different endpoint, however; one considered sufficient as a surrogate endpoint or at least to support the hypothesis that β-blockade is as good or better than ACE inhibition as heart failure therapy. Cardiac remodeling may be such an endpoint.

Cardiac remodeling and β-blockade

The most important contributing factors to cardiac remodeling include mechanical stretch, ischemia, apoptosis, neurohormonal and cytokine activation, oxidative stress, and inducible nitric oxide (NO) production (Box 1). Neurohormonal systems, which promote remodeling, include the SNS, the RAS, aldosterone, and endothelins. Their effect may be modulated by bradykinin, prostaglandins, and natriuretic peptides.

These mechanisms leading to cardiac remodeling interrelate. Thus, mechanical stretch activates several neurohormonal pathways, such as the α_1-adrenergic system, angiotensin-II production, and endothelin [14]. Cytokines, such as TNF-α, increase inducible NO [15]. Excess NO may lead to oxyradicals, which,

Box 1. Factors influencing cardiac remodeling

Activating factors

- (Local) neurohormonal activation: angiotensin II, endothelins, aldosterone, sympathetic activation (norepinephrine)
- Mechanical stretch
- Activation mechanosensitive ion channels: Na/H exchanger – calcium uptake
- Cytokine activation (tumor necrosis factor-α [TNF-α], interleukins)
- Inducible nitric oxide synthase activation/NO production
- Oxidative stress
- Apoptosis, necrosis
- Ischemia

Modulating factors

- Bradykinin
- Prostaglandins
- Natriuretic peptides

in addition to cytokines and stretch, may trigger apoptosis.

Cytokine activation is influenced by the SNS and angiotensin II. Thus, β-blockade and ACE inhibition could modulate cardiac remodeling by their effect on different mechanisms leading to remodeling. The possibility that early activation of the sympathetic system compared with the RAS would favor β-blockade as first-line therapy to stop or revert the remodeling process is attractive, although speculative.

Other reasons to consider β-blockade specifically in remodeling and heart failure progression relate to the fact that high cardiac sympathetic drive may lead to myocardial necrosis. Norepinephrine at concentrations present in the failing heart is toxic for cardiomyocytes [16]. β-Adrenergic desensitization can ameliorate catecholamine-induced necrosis [17], suggesting a specific role for β-blockade in modulating the remodeling process. In addition, excess catecholamines may trigger apoptosis [18], which is reduced by β-blockade [19]. β-Blockade may upregulate the expression of Bcl-2, a protein that inhibits apoptosis, and downregulate myocardial expression of Bak, a proapoptotic protein, and the apoptotic-inducing factor [20], supporting its role in suppressing the occurrence of apoptosis.

Another specific factor of β-blockade is reduced heart rate, which is beneficial in reducing myocardial oxygen consumption. In addition, it lengthens the diastolic period and extends the time of calcium uptake in the sarcoplasmatic reticulum. In heart failure, the expression of the sarcoplasmatic reticulum Ca^{2+}-ATPase (SERCA-2a) pump is reduced and calcium uptake is decreased. β-blockade, besides lengthening the diastolic filling time, also increases phosphorylation of phospholamban, a protein involved in the expression of Ca^{2+}-ATPase [21]. A further consequence of the hyperadrenergic state of the heart in heart failure is a hypermetabolic state with increased levels and use of free fatty acids because of enhanced lipolysis. This leads to ATP waste, limiting the availability of ATP for cardiac contraction. β-Blockade increases the dependency on carbohydrate use instead of free fatty acid use with better preservation of available ATP.

β-Blockade and remodeling: why carvedilol?

Carvedilol may be preferable than more selective β-blocking agents in modulating cardiac remodeling for several reasons. Because β_2- and α_1-adrenoceptors activate subcellular pathways leading to remodeling, it does not make sense to leave these receptors unprotected, which occurs with selective β_1-blockade, particularly because in heart failure these receptors increase relative to the β_1-receptor.

Myocardial stretch, a typical factor of remodeling, increases α-adrenergic activation, and α_1-blockade would seem a logical countermeasure. Further negative effects of α-adrenergic activation include cardiac hypertrophy, myocardial toxicity, and peripheral and renal vasoconstriction. β_2-receptor activation facilitates presynaptic norepinephrine release. Furthermore, β_2 stimulation results in cyclic AMP-mediated positive inotropic and chronotropy effects, myocardial fibrosis [22], arrhythmias [23], and hypokalemia. It therefore seems reasonable to expect better modulation of cardiac remodeling with more complete blockade of all adrenergic receptors in heart failure, as occurs with carvedilol, which blocks the β_1-, β_2-, and α_1-receptor.

Also, carvedilol, through combined β_1- and β_2-blockade, more markedly reduces cardiac sympathetic activity than the β_1-selective blocker metoprolol [24]. Furthermore, carvedilol reportedly has additional characteristics, including antioxidant and antiendothelin properties, which may contribute to its effect on remodeling.

Several studies in heart failure patients support carvedilol's better effect on remodeling and function than metoprolol. Metra and colleagues [25] observed in a relatively large study that after a prolonged period of treatment carvedilol increased LV ejection fraction more than metoprolol, and decreased LV volumes to a greater extent. Sanderson and colleagues [26] found that carvedilol decreased LV volumes more than metoprolol in heart failure patients. Packer and colleagues [27] reported from a meta-analysis of studies comparing both β-blockers directly that carvedilol significantly improved LV ejection fraction better than metoprolol. Finally, the Carvedilol or Metoprolol European Trial (COMET), which compared carvedilol and metoprolol tartrate head-to-head in a 5-year study in patients who had New York Heart Association (NYHA) class-II to -IV heart failure, indicated that in clinical endpoints including death and heart-failure hospitalizations, carvedilol was significantly better than metoprolol [28]. Thus, of the available β-blocking drugs evaluated clinically in heart failure, carvedilol seems the most likely agent to confer antiremodeling effects. Is it reasonable, however, to expect a better effect on remodeling compared with ACE inhibition?

Cardiac remodeling: carvedilol versus angiotensin-converting enzyme inhibition

Comparing the pharmacologic profiles of ACE inhibition and carvedilol in terms of their potential effects on mechanisms leading to remodeling, carvedilol seems to affect remodeling more comprehensively than ACE inhibition (Table 1). Although ACE inhibition may diminish sympathetic tone, carvedilol more profoundly blocks the effect of increased sympathetic tone in heart, kidney, and other organs affected by heart failure. ACE inhibition, however, affects angiotensin-II production and possibly aldosterone to a larger extent than carvedilol, which may modulate the RAS by decreasing renin formation. ACE inhibitors increase bradykinin levels, a strong vasodilator and antiremodeling agent. Carvedilol, however, reduces heart rate with an important reduction in myocardial oxygen demand, has stronger anti-ischemic effects than ACE inhibition, and has antioxidant and antiendothelin properties. Whether these multiple actions of carvedilol would produce stronger antiapoptotic effects is unclear, but likely. These reasons favor a stronger antiremodeling effect of carvedilol than ACE inhibition. Has this been confirmed in the clinical setting?

Table 1
Comparative effects of angiotensin-converting enzyme inhibition and carvedilol on mechanisms in the remodeling process

Mechanism	Carvedilol	ACE inhibition
Neurohormonal modulation	SNS activates RAS	RAS activates SNS
Cardiac antiadrenergic effects	+ +	+/–
β_2-Blockade	+	–
α_1-Blockade	+	–
Bradykinin/NO	–	+ +
Antioxidant	+ +	+
Apoptosis	+	+?
Anti-ischemic	+ +	+?
Heart rate reduction	+	–

Abbreviations: +, effect; + +, marked effect; +?, questionable effect; –, no effect.

Remodeling studies in heart failure using angiotensin-converting enzyme inhibitors and carvedilol

A SOLVD echocardiographic substudy compared the effects of enalapril and placebo in patients who had asymptomatic LV dysfunction or heart failure [29]. Treatment over 1 year indicated that although LV volumes increased in placebo-treated patients, enalapril prevented further dilatation. In this study, however, there was no reduction in size (ie, no reverse remodeling). In contrast, in the Australia and New Zealand (ANZ) study, which compared carvedilol with placebo in patients who had mild heart failure and LV systolic dysfunction, the β-blocker significantly reduced LV volumes compared with placebo treatment [30]. This does not suggest, however, that β-blockade with carvedilol provides better antiremodeling than ACE inhibition.

Apart from comparative efficacy requiring a direct comparison between the two treatments, as in all studies after the establishment of ACE inhibition as mandatory therapy for heart failure, in the ANZ study the β-blocker was administered on top of ACE inhibition in most patients. The additive antiremodeling effects of both treatments may account for the reversed remodeling observed with carvedilol in that study. A direct comparison between carvedilol and ACE inhibition was required to answer whether β-blockade with carvedilol provides better protection against remodeling than ACE inhibition.

Carvedilol Remodeling in Mild Heart Failure Evaluation

The Carvedilol Remodeling in Mild Heart Failure Evaluation (CARMEN) [31] was designed to evaluate whether β-blockade with carvedilol as monotherapy would provide better antiremodeling effects than ACE inhibition as monotherapy in patients who had early or mild-to-moderate heart failure. Furthermore, the study aimed to confirm earlier observations that adding carvedilol to ACE inhibition would provide reverse remodeling compared with ACE inhibition alone. Consequently, the study had three arms: one with the combination carvedilol and enalapril, one with carvedilol and placebo, and one with enalapril and placebo (Fig. 2). In the arms containing carvedilol, carvedilol was uptitrated before enalapril or placebo. In the enalapril arm, enalapril was uptitrated before placebo. Target dosages for carvedilol were 25 mg twice daily for patients weighing less than 85 kg and 50 mg twice daily for patients weighing 85 kg or more. The target dose of enalapril was 10 mg twice daily. Following the two uptitration phases was a maintenance phase of 18 months' duration. Echocardiograms were performed at baseline, and at 6, 12, and 18 months of blinded maintenance treatment.

The primary endpoint was the absolute change in left ventricular end-systolic volume (LVESV) between baseline and month 18, comparing carvedilol alone versus enalapril alone, and comparing the combination arm with the enalapril-alone arm. Secondary endpoints included the comparison of changes in LVESV between baseline and month 18 between the combination and carvedilol-alone arm, and within-group changes in LVESV from baseline to months 6, 12, and 18.

Of the 572 patients randomized in the study, 93 did not have an evaluable postbaseline echocardiogram. The remaining 479 patients in the intention-to-treat evaluation were well divided among the three arms. Nearly all were white, mostly male, and relatively young (average age 62 years); 62% to 68% were in NYHA class II, 25% to 31% were in NYHA class III, and 47% to 57% had a history of a previous myocardial infarction. Approximately two thirds were on ACE-inhibitor therapy before inclusion. ACE inhibitors were stopped between 2 and 14 days before entering the study. β-Blocking agents, which were taken by 4% to 8% of patients, had to be stopped 4 weeks before inclusion.

The results [32] showed that the combination arm was superior to enalapril alone and carvedilol alone (Fig. 3). No changes occurred in the enalapril-alone arm, whereas LVESV decreased in the carvedilol-alone arm. The difference between both groups between baseline and month 18 were not significant, although they were at months 6 and 12. When within-group changes from baseline were compared, however, carvedilol alone and the combination arm significantly reduced LVESV, but the enalapril-alone arm did not (Fig. 4). Similar directional findings as LVESV were observed with LV end-diastolic volumes and LV ejection fraction.

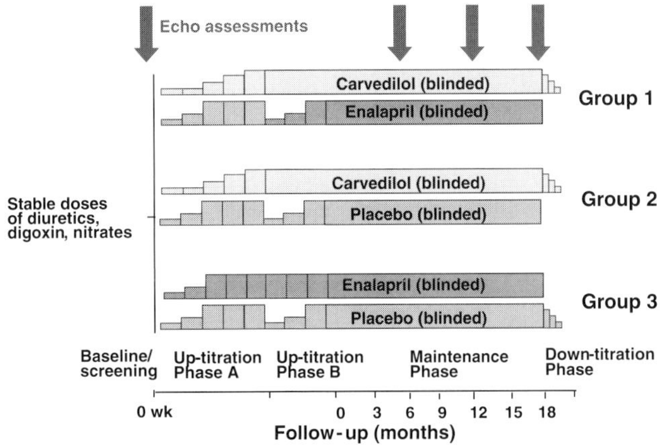

Fig. 2. Overview of the CARMEN study design. In the combined treatment arm, carvedilol is uptitrated before enalapril.

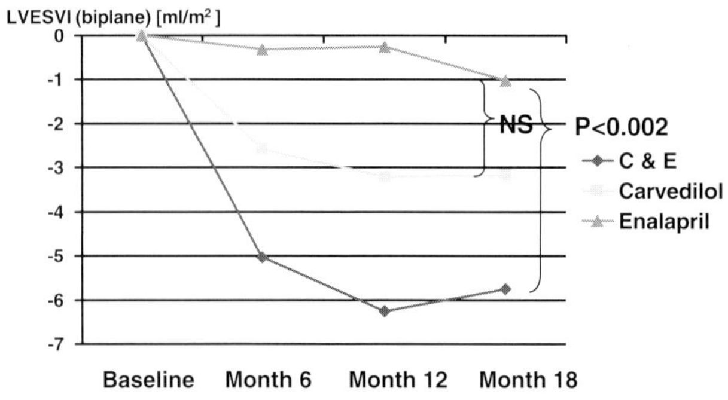

Fig. 3. Primary endpoint: comparison of LVESVI between treatments; mean change from baseline (intention-to-treat population). Differences between groups, *P* values valid for comparisons at all time points. C, carvedilol; E, enalapril; NS, not significant.

The safety profile was similar in all treatment groups. Withdrawal rates were comparable, as were serious adverse events and mortality (Table 2) [33]. All-cause and cardiovascular hospitalizations were not significantly different, although there was a tendency to higher incidence in the enalapril-alone arm. Importantly, uptitration with carvedilol in the absence of ACE inhibition was well tolerated and did not lead to a greater withdrawal rate or adverse event rate than observed during enalapril uptitration.

Lessons from the Carvedilol Remodeling in Mild Heart Failure Evaluation

The CARMEN study was the first to demonstrate that early combination of ACE inhibition and carvedilol significantly reverses cardiac remodeling. Because the effect in the combination arm was greater than in either monotherapy arm, early combination of the two treatment regimens is necessary when heart failure is detected in a patient. Moreover, because carvedilol alone reduced cardiac volumes, in contrast to enalapril alone, and was well tolerated as first drug during uptitration, the order in which the drugs are administered may be carvedilol followed by the ACE inhibitor. The patients for whom this may be considered will depend on baseline characteristics, such as heart rate.

The findings of CARMEN support a strategic strategy in which the prescription of β-blockade in heart failure should not be delayed. Current guidelines recommend adding a β-blocker to ACE inhibition only if patients remain symptomatic, which may

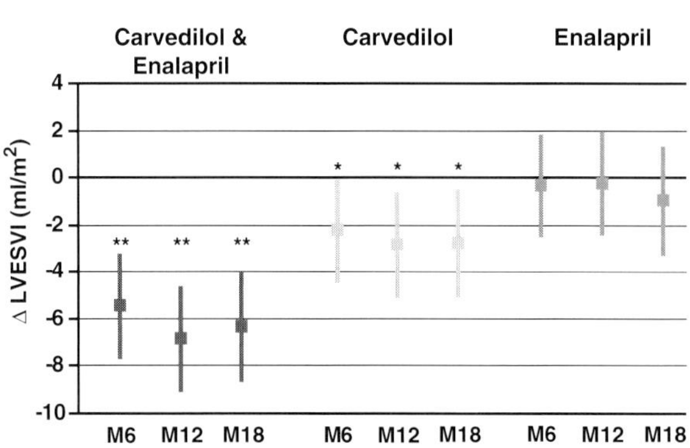

Fig. 4. Mean change from baseline within treatment-arm comparison in LVESVI (intention-to-treat population). Bars represent 95% confidence intervals. *P* values for within-group changes are depicted (*$P < .05$, **$P < .01$). M, month.

Table 2
Adverse events and withdrawal rates in Carvedilol Remodeling in Mild Heart Failure Evaluation

		Monotherapy	
Guideline	Carvedilol + enalapril (N = 191)	Carvedilol (N = 191)	Enalapril (N = 190)
Patients who have any AEs (%)	79	77	75
Total no. AEs	497	426	461
Patients who have serious AEs (%)	28	29	34
Total no. serious AEs	81	101	94
Patients who have AEs leading to withdrawal (%)	18	18	21
Total no. AEs leading to withdrawal	45	43	48

Abbreviation: AEs, adverse events.
Data from Remme WJ, on behalf of the CARMEN Steering Committee and Investigators. The Carvedilol and ACE-Inhibitor Remodeling Mild Heart Failure Evaluation trial (CARMEN)—rationale and design. Cardiovasc Drugs Ther 2001;15:69–77.

affect a timely prescription of a β-blocker in clinical practice.

β-Blockers are underused grossly. CARMEN indicates that early administration of β-blockade with carvedilol in addition to ACE inhibition is mandatory to modulate cardiac remodeling, and possibly progression of heart failure. Moreover, the study's findings that β-blockade can be administered safely as first-line therapy may remove concerns for physicians, remnants of the historical view that these agents are contraindicated and dangerous for heart failure patients.

CARMEN was set up to test the superiority of carvedilol over ACE inhibition. Although there was a tendency toward a better effect of carvedilol, it did not reach significance at the end of the study, although it did at earlier time points. Also, in the within-group comparisons, carvedilol but not enalapril decreased cardiac volumes.

One reason for the diminished effect of enalapril could be that approximately two thirds of patients had been on an ACE inhibitor, and that the (initial) remodeling effect of the ACE inhibitor was no longer present. In the patients who had never received an ACE inhibitor, however, there was no superior effect of de novo enalapril over carvedilol. In contrast, in the patients who had received an ACE inhibitor before the study but received only carvedilol, a highly significant reversal of cardiac remodeling was observed during 18 months of carvedilol monotherapy [34].

Recently, Sliwa and colleagues [35] published data from a smaller, randomized, single-center open-label study comparing carvedilol as first-dose treatment versus perindopril as first-dose administration in newly diagnosed heart failure. In that study, patients stayed on single therapy for 6 months before the comparator drug was added. After 12 months LV volumes were reduced more significantly from baseline in the carvedilol-first patients compared with the perindopril-first patients, which support the observations in CARMEN that the lesser effect of the ACE inhibitor may not result from patients having received ACE inhibition already and thereby becoming immune to its effect, but could relate to differential pharmacologic properties favoring carvedilol to ACE inhibition.

The lessons from CARMEN are clear in that combined treatment of β-blockade with carvedilol and ACE inhibition should be considered when heart failure is detected in a patient. The order of administration is at the discretion of the clinician, and may relate to baseline characteristics such as heart rate and blood pressure. The observations of CARMEN, supported by the findings of Sliwa and colleagues [35], are important because they indicate that mandatory first-line therapy with ACE inhibition—the result of these agents being studied before β-blockade—needs to be reconsidered. Therapy for heart failure need not be dogmatic, and the order can be adjusted in the individual patient.

References

[1] Francis GS, Benedict C, Johnston DE, et al. Comparison of neuroendocrine activation in patients with left ventricular dysfunction with and without congestive heart failure: a substudy of the Studies Of Left Ventricular Dysfunction (SOLVD). Circulation 1990;82:1724–9.

[2] Remme WJ, Swedberg K. Task Force for the Diagnosis and Treatment of Chronic Heart Failure, European Society of Cardiology Guidelines for the diagnosis and treatment of chronic heart failure. Eur Heart J 2001;22:1527–60.

[3] CONSENSUS Trial Study Group. Effect of enalapril on mortality in severe congestive heart failure. Results

of the North Scandinavian enalapril survival study. N Engl J Med 1987;316:1429–35.

[4] The SOLVD Investigators. Effects of enalapril on survival in patients with reduced left ventricular ejection fractions and congestive heart failure. N Engl J Med 1991;325:293–302.

[5] The SOLVD Investigators. Effects of enalapril on mortality and the development of heart failure in asymptomatic patients with reduced left ventricular ejection fractions. N Engl J Med 1992;327:685–91.

[6] Cohn JN, Johnson G, Ziesche S, et al. A comparison of enalapril with hydralazine-isosorbide dinitrate in the treatment of chronic congestive heart failure. N Engl J Med 1991;325:303–10.

[7] Acute Infarction Ramipril Efficacy (AIRE) Investigators. Effects of ramipril on mortality and morbidity of survivors of acute myocardial infarction with clinical evidence of heart failure. Lancet 1993;342:821–8.

[8] Pfeffer MA, Braunwald E, Moyé LA, on behalf of the SAVE investigators. Effect of captopril on mortality and morbidity in patients with left ventricular dysfunction after myocardial infarction. N Engl J Med 1992; 327:669–77.

[9] Køber L, Torp-Pederson C, Carlsen JE, et al, for the TRACE Study Group. A clinical trial of the angiotensin-converting-enzyme inhibitor trandolapril in patients with left ventricular dysfunction after myocardial infarction. N Engl J Med 1995;333: 1670–6.

[10] Packer M, Bristow MR, Cohn JN, et al. The effect of carvedilol on morbidity and mortality in patients with chronic heart failure. US Carvedilol Heart Failure Study Group. N Engl J Med 1996;334:1349–55.

[11] CIBIS II Investigators and Committees. The Cardiac Insufficiency Bisoprolol Study II (CIBIS II): a randomised trial. Lancet 1999;353:9–13.

[12] Hjalmarson A, Goldstein S, Fagerberg B, et al. Effect of metoprolol CR/XL in chronic heart failure: metoprolol CR/XL randomized intervention trial in congestive heart failure (MERIT-HF). Lancet 1999;353: 2001–7.

[13] Packer M, Coats AJS, Fowler MB, et al, for the Carvedilol Prospective Randomized Cumulative Survival Study Group (COPERNICUS). Effect of carvedilol on survival in severe chronic heart failure. N Engl J Med 2001;344:1651–8.

[14] Yamazaki T, Komuro I, Kudoh S, et al. Role of ion channels and exchangers in mechanical stretch-induced cardiomyocyte hypertrophy. Circ Res 1998;82:430–7.

[15] Ungureanu-Longrois D, Balligand JL, Simmons SW, et al. Induction of nitric oxide synthase activity by cytokines in ventricular myocytes is necessary but not sufficient to decrease contractile responsiveness to β-adrenergic agonists. Circ Res 1995;77:494–502.

[16] Mann DL, Kent RL, Parsons B, et al. Adrenergic effects on the biology of the adult mammalian cardiocyte. Circulation 1992;24:549–64.

[17] Tan LB, Benjamin IJ, Clark WA. Beta-adrenergic receptor desensitization may serve a cardioprotective role. Cardiovasc Res 1992;26:608–14.

[18] Communal C, Singh K, Pimentel DR. Norepinephrine stimulates apoptosis in adult rat ventricular myocytes by activation of beta-adrenergic pathway. Circulation 1998;98:1329–34.

[19] Sabbah HN, Sharov VG, Todor A, et al. Chronic therapy with metoprolol attenuates cardiomyocyte apoptosis in dogs with heart failure. J Am Coll Cardiol 2000;36:1698–705.

[20] Todor AV, Sharov VG, Suzuki G, et al. Chronic therapy with metoprolol CR/XL prevents apoptosis inducing factor and downregulates the pro-apoptotic protein Bak in cardiomyocytes of dogs with heart failure (abstr). J Am Coll Cardiol 2002;39:165A.

[21] Gupta RC, Mishra S, Imai M, et al. Chronic monotherapy with extended release metoprolol succinate improves sarcoplasmic reticulum phospholamban phosphorylation in dogs with chronic heart failure [abstract]. Circulation 2003;108(Suppl IV):IV–370.

[22] Du XJ, Autelitano D, Dilley RJ, et al. β_2-adrenergic overexpression exacerbates development of heart failure after aortic stenosis. Circulation 2000;101:71–7.

[23] Billman GE, Castillo LC, Hensley J, et al. β_2-adrenergic receptor antagonists protect against ventricular fibrillation. In vivo and in vitro evidence for enhanced sensitivity to β_2-adrenergic stimulation in animals susceptible to sudden death. Circulation 1997;96: 1914–22.

[24] Azevedo ER, Kubo T, Mak S, et al. Nonselective versus selective beta-adrenergic receptor blockade in congestive heart failure: differential effects on sympathetic activity. Circulation 2001;104(18):2194–9.

[25] Metra M, Gibbini R, Nodari S, et al. Differential effects of beta-blockers in patients with heart failure. A prospective, randomized, double-blind comparison of the long-term effects of metoprolol versus carvedilol. Circulation 2000;102:546–51.

[26] Sanderson JE, Chan SKW, Yip G, et al. Beta-blockade in heart failure. A comparison of carvedilol with metoprolol. J Am Coll Cardiol 1999;34:1522–8.

[27] Packer M, Antonopoulos GV, Berlin JA, et al. Comparative effects of carvedilol and metoprolol on left ventricular ejection fraction in heart failure: results of a meta-analysis. Am Heart J 2001;141:899–907.

[28] Poole-Wilson PA, Swedberg K, Cleland JGF, et al. Comparison of carvedilol and metoprolol on clinical outcomes in patients with chronic heart failure. Results of the Carvedilol Or Metoprolol European Trial (COMET). Lancet 2003;362:7–13.

[29] Greenberg B, Quinones MA, Koilpillai C, et al. Effects of long term enalapril therapy on cardiac structure and function in patients with left ventricular dysfunction. Results of the SOLVD echocardiographic study. Circulation 1995;91:2573–81.

[30] Doughty RN, Whalley GA, Gamble G, et al. Left ventricular remodeling with carvedilol in patients with congestive heart failure due to ischemic heart dis-

ease. Australia-New Zealand Heart Failure Research Collaborative Group. J Am Coll Cardiol 1997;29: 1060–6.

[31] Remme WJ, on behalf of the CARMEN Steering Committee and Investigators. The Carvedilol and ACE-Inhibitor Remodeling Mild Heart Failure EvaluatioN trial (CARMEN)—rationale and design. Cardiovasc Drugs Ther 2001;15:69–77.

[32] Remme WJ, Riegger G, Hildebrandt P, et al, on behalf of the CARMEN investigators. The benefits of early combination treatment of carvedilol and an ACE-inhibitor in mild heart failure and left ventricular systolic dysfunction. The Carvedilol and Ace-inhibitor Remodeling Mild heart failure EvaluatioN trial (CARMEN). Cardiovasc Drugs Ther 2004;18:57–66.

[33] Komajda M, Lutiger B, Madeira H, on behalf of the CARMEN investigators and coordinators. Tolerability of carvedilol and ACE-inhibition in mild heart failure. Results of CARMEN. Eur J Heart Fail 2004;6: 467–75.

[34] Remme WJ, Soler-Soler J, Ryden L, on behalf of the CARMEN investigators. Replacement of angiotensin converting enzyme inhibition by carvedilol results in long-term reversed left ventricular remodeling in mild heart failure and is well tolerated: results of the CARMEN study. J Am Coll Cardiol 2003; 41(Suppl A):205A.

[35] Sliwa K, Norton GR, Kone N, et al. Impact of initiating carvedilol before angiotensin converting enzyme inhibitor therapy on cardiac function in newly diagnosed heart failure. J Am Coll Cardiol 2004;44: 1825–30.

ELSEVIER
SAUNDERS

Heart Failure Clin 1 (2005) 77 – 93

HEART
FAILURE
CLINICS

Role of Neurohormonal Modulators in Heart Failure with Relatively Preserved Systolic Function

Jonathan A. Rapp, MD[a], Mihai Gheorghiade, MD[b,*]

[a]*Northwestern University, Chicago, IL, USA*
[b]*Northwestern University Feinberg School of Medicine, Chicago, IL, USA*

Cardiovascular disease remains the leading cause of mortality in the developed world and is responsible for nearly 1 million deaths per year in the United States [1]. Although the age-adjusted rates of death secondary to coronary artery disease (CAD) and stroke have decreased by approximately 50% in the last 10 years, there has been a large increase in the prevalence of heart failure (HF) [2,3].

It is estimated that 5 million Americans suffer from HF, and roughly 550,000 new cases are diagnosed annually [1]. HF was responsible for nearly 1 million hospital admissions in 2001 and is the most common discharge diagnosis in patients over 65 years of age. Furthermore, it is the primary cause of readmission within 60 days of discharge [1,4]. Approximately 330,000 patients die each year from HF, and the 1-year mortality rate of newly diagnosed patients approximates 20%. The total direct and indirect cost of managing this disease is expected to exceed $25 billion for 2004 [1].

Several echocardiographic cross-sectional studies have found that 40% to 71% of patients who have HF have relatively preserved systolic functions, a condition referred to as *diastolic heart failure* (DHF) [5–15]. In the last 15 years, several hospital-based studies have found that approximately 40% of patients admitted with worsening HF had DHF [16,17]. The most recently published database of patients who have HF found that approximately 40% of patients had an ejection fraction (EF) greater than 0.40 [18]. Although there are abundant data to guide the treatment of HF and systolic dysfunction (systolic heart failure, or SHF), evidence-based data are lacking in the management of DHF. This article examines the role of neurohormonal modulators in the management of DHF.

Definition and diagnosis

Definition

HF is a clinical syndrome that results from any functional or structural cardiac disorder that impairs the ability of the ventricles to fill with or eject blood. Symptoms include fatigue, poor exercise tolerance, dyspnea (exertional or resting), and signs and radiographic evidence of pulmonary and systemic congestion [19]. Standardized criteria for the diagnosis of HF have been described, such as those from the Framingham study [20]. Other tools, such as echocardiography and measurement of B-natriuretic peptide (BNP), also are used for diagnosis. BNP is a neurohormone secreted by the ventricles in response to muscle stretch caused by volume or pressure overload. Although it is a valuable marker of HF, it cannot be used to distinguish SHF from DHF [21,22] because patients often have components of both [23]. DHF is caused by diastolic dysfunction or, more specifically, abnormalities in active relaxation or passive stiffness of the left ventricle that result in

* Corresponding author. Feinberg Cardiovascular Research Institute, Northwestern University Feinberg School of Medicine, Galter 10-240, 201 East Huron Street, Chicago, IL 60611.

E-mail address: m-gheorghiade@northwestern.edu (M. Gheorghiade).

1551-7136/05/$ – see front matter
doi:10.1016/j.hfc.2004.10.003

abnormal left ventricular (LV) filling and elevated filling pressures [24,25].

Diagnosis

The Working Group of the European Society of Cardiology first published diagnostic criteria for DHF in 1998. It suggested that DHF could be diagnosed if (1) the patient had HF symptoms, (2) there was evidence of a normal left ventricular ejection fraction (LVEF), and (3) there was evidence of abnormal LV diastolic stiffness, relaxation, or filling [26]. Vasan and Levy [27] modified these criteria and proposed categorizing DHF diagnosis as definite, probable, and possible. All patients were required to have signs and symptoms of HF as well as an LVEF greater than 0.50. Diagnosis of definite and probable DHF required LVEF to be measured within 72 hours of the HF event. Furthermore, diagnosis of definite DHF required evidence of diastolic dysfunction measured by catheterization.

Gandhi and colleagues [28] found that, among patients hospitalized for acute pulmonary edema, there was no significant difference in LVEF between the time of presentation and 72 hours later after compensation was achieved. This proved to be true in the presence of SHF and DHF and indicated that a measurement of systolic function during an acute setting may not be necessary to establish the diagnosis of DHF. Moreover, a study by Smith and colleagues [17] demonstrated that outcomes were similar in patients who had DHF whose LVEFs were examined on index admission or 6 to 12 months previously. Therefore, as long as no intervening event had occurred, DHF can be diagnosed using an LVEF greater than 0.50 within 6 to 12 months before the initial presentation of HF [17,25]. Piccini and colleagues [21] also stated that DHF can be diagnosed without a measurement of diastolic function if the patient has (1) HF symptoms, (2) LVEF greater than 0.50, and (3) no significant valvular or pericardial disease. Clinically, SHF and DHF often coexist, and their managements are similar.

A comparison of the clinical characteristics of patients who have diastolic heart failure and systolic heart failure

Patients who have DHF and SHF have differing clinical characteristics. In a recent hospital-based study examining the differences between patients who have HF, 55% of women with HF had relatively preserved systolic functions compared with 29% of men. Patients who had DHF also tended to be older than their counterparts with SHF (71 years versus 67 years of age) [29]. The Acute Decompensated Heart Failure National Registry (ADHERE), the largest HF registry, also found that patients who had DHF were older (74.2 versus 69.9 years of age) and more likely to be women (62% versus 39%) than patients who had SHF [18]. These data are consistent with prior studies that showed that women comprise 70% to 75% of patients who have DHF, and such patients have a mean age of 70 to 75 years [30–32].

Patients who have SHF and DHF also differ in their associated comorbidities. The ADHERE registry documented that a higher percentage of patients who have DHF are diabetic (46% versus 42%) and have atrial fibrillation (AF) (21% versus 17%) when compared with patients who have SHF, but CAD was more frequent in patients who have SHF (61% versus 47%) [18].

Lenzen and colleagues [29] found generally similar results (Table 1). Patients who had DHF had a higher prevalence of AF (25% versus 23%), hypertension (59% versus 50%), renal insufficiency (69% versus 59%), and history of stroke (28% versus 26%) than patients who had SHF. Although diabetes mellitus and ischemic heart disease were prevalent in both populations, they were more so in patients who had SHF.

Treatment differences, which have been studied, are quite striking. Patients who have DHF are less likely to receive angiotensin-converting enzyme (ACE) inhibitors, angiotensin II receptor–blockers (ARBs), β-blockers, digoxin, or diuretics than are patients who have SHF. They are, however, more likely to receive calcium-channel blockers [29–32].

Prognosis

Unfortunately, prognosis is poor for patients who have either SHF or DHF. Among hospitalized patients, mortality is similar between the two groups. It is almost certain that any difference favoring DHF becomes insignificant 3 to 6 months after hospital discharge [17,33–35]. Community-based studies showed similar mortality rates between the two groups in patients more than 65 years of age. In patients less than 65 years of age, however, DHF carries a lower 1-year mortality rate than SHF (7%–9% versus 12%–19%, respectively) [36–40].

Mortality seems to be related to age and the degree of accompanying CAD. The DIG trial found that the 3-year mortality for DHF was as low as 9% in patients less than 50 years of age but as high as 39% in patients more than 80 years of age [41]. The

Table 1
Comorbidities of patients with heart failure and with or without systolic dysfunction

	Patients with known left ventricular function			Patients not in this analysis
Characteristic	PLVF n = 31,348	LVSD n = 3658	*P* value[a]	n = 3895
Age (mean, SD)	71 ± 12 y	67 ± 13 y	< .001	76 ± 11.6 y
Women	1739 (55%)	1065 (29%)	< .001	2216 (57%)
Men > 70 y	666 (21%)	961 (26%)	< .001	1039 (27%)
Women > 70 y	1099 (35%)	607 (17%)	< .001	1748 (45%)
Comorbidity				
Hypertension	1845 (59%)	1829 (50%)	< .001	2005 (52%)
Diabetes mellitus	816 (26%)	1016 (28%)	.09	1075 (28%)
Ischemic heart disease	1851 (59%)	2508 (69%)	< .001	2060 (53%)
Previous revascularization	377 (12%)	674 (18%)	< .001	291 (8%)
Renal insufficiency	155 (5%)	220 (6%)	.05	296 (8%)
Prior stroke	492 (16%)	501 (14%)	.02	814 (21%)
Chronic atrial fibrillation	795 (25%)	827 (23%)	.01	860 (22%)
LVEF (mean, SD)	56 ± 9.8%	33 ± 10.9%	< .001	NA
Specialty at admission				
General internal medicine	1299 (42%)	1164 (32%)	< .001	2659 (68%)
Cardiology/cardiovascular surgery	1615 (51%)	2288 (63%)	< .001	769 (20%)
Duration of index hospitalization (median, IQR)	10 d (6–16)	10 d (6–15)	.26	9 d (5–14)
Contribution of heart failure to index admission	1189 (38%)	1904 (52%)	< .001	1141 (29%)

Abbreviations: IQR, interquartile range; LVEF, left ventricular ejection fraction; LVSD, left ventricular systolic dysfunction; NA, not available; PLVF, preserved left ventricular function; SD, standard deviation.

[a] Statistical difference between PLVF and LVSD.

From Lenzen MJ, Scholte op Reimer WJM, Boersma E, et al. Differences between patients with a preserved and a depressed left ventricular function: a report from the EuroHeart Failure Survey. Eur Heart J 2004;25:1214–20; with permission.

Coronary Artery Surgery Study (CASS) found that the number of diseased vessels in patients who have DHF correlated with 3-year mortality (8% with no disease, 17% in one- or two-vessel disease, and 32% with triple-vessel disease) [42]. Results of morbidity studies mirror those of mortality studies. In community-based studies, the hospitalization rate for HF or a cardiovascular cause is lower in patients who have DHF than in those who have SHF [38,40]. Among hospitalized patients, the all-cause or HF readmission rates are similar in patients less than 80 years of age, regardless of type of HF (the all-cause readmission rate is approximately 45% at 6 months) [17,34,35]. In patients over 80 years of age, readmission rates for those who have SHF are higher than for those who have DHF [17].

Pathophysiology

The pathophysiology of DHF is understood best by dividing the disease into (1) intrinsic processes that describe the pathologic changes in the myocardium itself and include mechanical, molecular, and neurohormonal factors, and (2) extrinsic processes that consist of the morbidities that cause the intrinsic changes. These morbidities include age, hypertension, CAD, AF, and diabetes mellitus (Fig. 1). Understanding the intrinsic processes is important because research into them may provide novel approaches to future therapy. The importance of the extrinsic factors cannot be overstated, however, because they create and worsen DHF and serve as the primary targets of current medical therapy. DHF also can be caused by infiltrative or restrictive cardiomyopathies (eg, amyloidosis, sarcoidosis, and hemochromatosis), but this article does not discuss these conditions [43].

Intrinsic processes

Ventricular relaxation

During systole, the left ventricle contracts and twists on its own axis. While blood is ejected, potential energy is stored in the ventricular myofibrils that creates the torsion forces necessary for the ensuing ventricular suction and diastolic filling [44,45]. Echocardiographic studies have demonstrated that the extent of ventricular systolic twist highly correlates with mitral inflow acceleration and early diastolic filling [46]. Oblique fiber shortening is the most significant factor contributing to systolic twist and consequent filling [47]. During isovolumic relaxa-

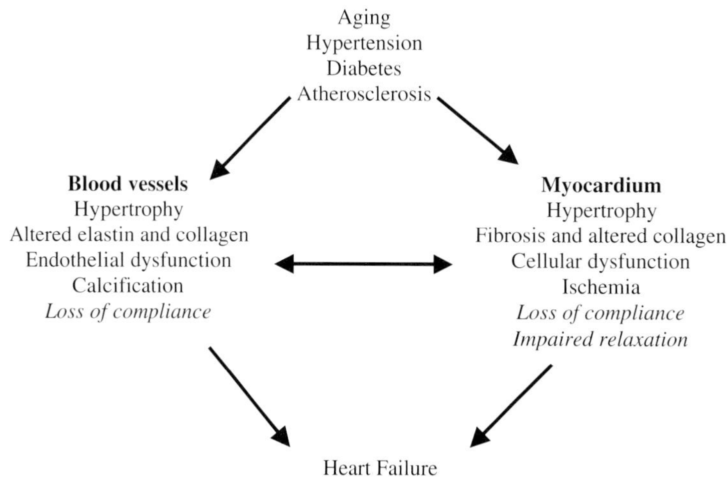

Fig. 1. Extrinsic diseases that bring about diastolic heart failure. Hypertension, coronary artery disease, atrial fibrillation, and diabetes mellitus serve as the primary targets of therapy for diastolic heart failure. (*From* Massie BM. Natriuretic peptide measurements for the diagnosis of "nonsystolic" heart failure: good news and bad. J Am Coll Cardiol 2003;41: 2018–21; with permission.)

tion, the left ventricle untwists about its axis without any blood movement between the cardiac chambers. This creates an intraventricular pressure gradient whose suction effect assists blood entry from the atrium into the ventricle once the mitral valve opens [48]. This process is normally responsible for roughly 70% of transmitral flow. β-Adrenergic stimulation may enhance the suction effect by increasing the rate and degree of ventricular pressure decline [49]. This effect is most critical during exercise, when it allows for increased diastolic filling volume without increased filling pressures. This effect is obtained while shortening the diastolic filling time [43].

Intracellular calcium handling seems to play a major role in ventricular relaxation. For contracted myocytes to relax and return to their resting length, actin-myosin bonds must be lysed through ATP-mediated processes in which calcium first dissociates from troponin-c and is then sequestered into the sarcoplasmic reticulum. This latter process is performed by the sarcoplasmic reticulum-calcium ATPase (SERCA) pump. The rate and degree of these cellular processes dictate the rate and degree of ventricular active relaxation [50]. Decreases in either the levels or activity of SERCA or increased levels of the SERCA inhibitor protein phospholamban can increase the amount of cytosolic calcium, thereby inhibiting the molecular processes required for myocyte relaxation and lengthening. Such events can occur in myocardial ischemia [51–53] or hypertrophy [54,55], two common circumstances in which diastolic dysfunction and failure occur.

Heart rate influences intracellular calcium concentration and transport [21]. In a patient who has defective calcium metabolism, increased heart rate can result in the accumulation of intracellular calcium ions and eventual calcium overload. This may yield prolonged interaction between actin and myosin, thus resulting in a state of prolonged myocardial contraction and possible impairment of diastolic function [56]. Additionally, tachycardia per se may hinder diastolic filling as a simple function of time: a faster heart rate results in less time for blood to enter the ventricles.

Ventricular compliance

Ventricular compliance is a function of mass and myocardial composition. Intracellular and extracellular structures influence compliance [50]. Titin is an intracellular protein component of the myocyte cytoskeleton. It is compressed during systole, and potential energy is stored. It returns to its resting length during diastole, like a spring, and contributes to the heart's diastolic relaxation. The degree of relaxation of titin is limited, thus protecting the sarcomere from excessive stretching. A change in titin isoform decreases compliance [57,58].

Alterations in collagen, an extracellular protein, also can impair diastolic function through its effects on ventricular compliance. Changes in the amount, distribution, type, degree of cross-linking, or geometry can be implicated [59–61]. Collagen synthesis can be altered by many physiologic circumstances, including neurohormonal activation, changes in preload or afterload, and changes in growth factor concentrations [21].

Neurohormonal factors in diastolic heart failure

In addition to the systemic renin–angiotensin–aldosterone system (RAAS), growing evidence supports the existence of a RAAS within the heart that may contribute to diastolic dysfunction [62–64]. Several observations have been made in hypertrophied hearts regarding the RAAS. For example, an infusion of angiotensin I in rats immediately impaired diastolic relaxation in hypertrophied, but not nonhypertrophied, hearts [64]. The hypertrophied hearts also had a greater ability to convert angiotensin I to angiotensin II [64]. Furthermore, after exposure to angiotensin II, hypertrophied hearts showed an exaggerated diastolic dysfunction during low-flow ischemia and a greater degree of ischemic diastolic dysfunction compared with nonhypertrophied hearts [65]. ACE inhibitors reduce the ischemia-mediated exaggeration of diastolic dysfunction in hypertrophied, but not in nonhypertrophied, hearts [65]. Angiotensin II, however, increases ischemic diastolic dysfunction even in nonhypertrophied hearts [66].

Aldosterone has deleterious effects on cardiac remodeling, specifically those that cause myocardial fibrosis. Cardiomyocytes, endothelial cells, and fibroblasts of the human heart all contain mineralocorticoid receptors that can be activated by aldosterone [67]. Such activation results in several events that increase myocardial fibrosis. There is up-regulation of the Na+/K+ ATPase in the heart that promotes events to induce fibroblast growth and collagen synthesis [68,69]. Aldosterone stimulates translation of the genes for types I and III collagen and fibrillar collagen [70]. It also alters coronary vascular permeability that may result in the exposure of fibroblasts to growth factors such as platelet-derived growth factor, which would increase collagen synthesis further [71,72]. Fibrosis begins as an accumulation of fibrillar collagen within the adventitia of the intramuscular coronary arteries, but eventually extends into the intracellular spaces [59,71]. Ultimately, aldosterone causes interstitial and perivascular myocardial fibrosis.

Extrinsic processes

Age

As noted, age is a major risk factor for DHF. Aging is associated with an increase in myocardial collagen, decreased β-receptor responsiveness [73], and impaired calcium ion handling because of decreased levels of SERCA [74], all of which lead to abnormal relaxation or altered myocardial elasticity. Aortic stiffness also increases with age, increasing afterload and causing LV hypertrophy, which may add to ventricular stiffness [75].

Hypertension

Hypertension is the most common risk factor for the development of DHF [21]. Hypertension has been associated with irregular myocardial high-energy phosphate metabolism [76] that may lower cytosolic concentrations of ATP [77]. This may cause malfunction of the SERCA, calcium overload, and impaired diastolic relaxation [43,78]. Hypertension also creates a high LV afterload that can retard relaxation and cause elevated filling pressures and a decreased end-diastolic volume [79]. This leads to increased ventricular wall tension that induces myocardial stretching and activation of neurohormonal systems, such as those that increase production of angiotensin II [80]. These events trigger altered gene expression with subsequent cell growth and extracellular matrix changes that further contribute to increased LV mass and stiffness [81].

Coronary artery disease

CAD can induce diastolic dysfunction in two major ways. First, infarcted muscle can result in scarring, fibrosis, and compensatory hypertrophy of healthy myocardium, all of which yield noncompliant tissue. Second, ischemia can cause calcium ion sequestration into the sarcoplasmic reticulum during ATP-dependent relaxation [43,51]. Notably, when diastolic dysfunction is present in the early phases of an acute myocardial infarction (MI), there is an increased association between the development of in-hospital HF and cardiac death within 1 year [82].

Atrial fibrillation

AF is of special concern in patients who have DHF. Atrial contraction is usually responsible for less than 30% of the forward flow from the atrium to the ventricle but can become critically important when LV filling pressures are high secondary to diastolic dysfunction. Loss of coordinated atrial contraction can lead to decreased ventricular filling, particularly when associated with a rapid ventricular response, and may lead rapidly to pulmonary congestion [83].

Diabetes mellitus

Diabetes mellitus is associated with diastolic dysfunction and HF. Several studies have identified diabetes mellitus as a major risk factor for the development of HF, including the Studies of Left Ventricular Dysfunction (SOLVD), the Heart Outcomes

Prevention Evaluation (HOPE) trial, and the Cardiovascular Health Study [84–86]. Recent work examining the relationship between diabetes mellitus and DHF has found that diastolic dysfunction may be the first stage of diabetic cardiomyopathy [87,88]. Zalbalgoitia and colleagues [89] found that over 40% of patients who had diabetes mellitus had some form of diastolic dysfunction, and abnormal LV relaxation seems to correlate with hemoglobin A_{1C} levels [90,91]. Similar findings were confirmed in the Strong Heart Study, which found that Native Americans who had diabetes mellitus tended to have higher rates of echocardiographic evidence of diastolic dysfunction independent of age, systolic function, blood pressure, or LV mass [90].

The pathologic changes seen in the diabetic heart consist of increased matrix collagen, myocyte hypertrophy, intramyocardial microangiopathy, and interstitial fibrosis [92]. These morphologic abnormalities likely result from altered myocardial glucose and fatty acid metabolism associated with diabetes mellitus [21]. Diabetes mellitus causes advanced glycosylated end products (AGEs) that affect several aspects of cardiac microanatomy and physiology. Once AGEs develop in the arterial walls and myocardial tissue, they form cross-links to local collagen fibers, thereby decreasing distensbility of the blood vessels and myocardium [93]. Furthermore, AGEs and reactive oxygen species can affect calcium handling, ion channels, mitochondrial function, and apoptosis; these processes lead to diastolic and systolic dysfunction [93]. Additional changes noted in patients who have diabetes mellitus include impaired β-receptor signal transduction and induction of the fetal gene pattern [94,95]. This gene pattern favors expression of an isoform of the α-myosin heavy chain (β-myosin heavy chain) that has slower ATPase activity than its adult isoform [96]. There is also down-regulation of the SERCA gene resulting in abnormal calcium homeostasis [97,98]. This further contributes to diastolic dysfunction [99].

Treatment

With the exception of the Candesartan in Heart Failure: Assessment of Reduction in Mortality and Morbidity (CHARM)-Preserved [100] and Digitalis Investigation Group (DIG) studies [41], no large, randomized, double-blind, placebo-controlled trial results are available to direct the management of patients who have DHF. Therefore, treatment is based largely on results from smaller clinical studies, personal experience, and, most important, the control of the extrinsic processes known to create and exacerbate DHF (ie, hypertension, CAD, AF/tachycardia, and diabetes mellitus) [50]. Fortunately, there is a wealth of clinical data to guide the latter therapy, much of which focuses on neurohormonal modulation. After briefly discussing symptom control, this article reviews the evidence-based literature in the treatment of DHF and then focuses on the role of neurohormonal modulators in the management of the conditions that contribute to DHF.

Symptom control

The initial goal in the treatment of DHF is symptomatic relief, which is achieved by decreasing pulmonary congestion. Therapeutic goals may include diastolic volume reduction (with the objective of lowering LV diastolic pressure), maintenance of sinus rhythm, or increasing the duration of diastole by slowing the ventricular rate [50].

Diastolic volume and, thereby, LV diastolic filling pressure can be lowered in several ways. First, total body volume can be reduced with the use of diuretics and fluid or sodium restriction. Second, preload can be reduced with the use of nitrates. Third, blockade of the RAAS by ACE inhibitors, ARBs, or aldosterone antagonists may be employed [50].

Because of the dependence on atrial contraction for ventricular filling in patients who have DHF, AF must be treated aggressively. Optimally, sinus rhythm can be maintained, but if this is not possible, rate control is a necessity [19]. Preventing tachycardia is important for symptom control because it may lead to incomplete ventricular relaxation, pulmonary congestion, and, therefore, symptoms [50]. Blood pressure should be kept below 130/80 in accordance with current American College of Cardiology/American Heart Association guidelines [19]. All patients suspected of having an ischemic etiology of HF should be treated appropriately medically and investigated for revascularization [19]. Anti-ischemic medications such as nitrates, β-blockers, and calcium channel blockers should be used as necessary.

Evidence-based review of treatment for diastolic heart failure

DIG, the first large randomized study, evaluated the effects of digoxin on mortality (the primary endpoint) and cardiovascular death, death from worsening HF, HF hospitalization, and hospitalization for other causes (the secondary endpoints) in patients who had HF [41]. The study was conducted over 3 to 5 years in patients who had HF and normal sinus rhythm. There were two trials: the main trial included patients with LVEF of 0.45 or less, and the ancillary trial studied patients with LVEF greater than 0.45. This discussion focuses on the ancillary trial.

Patients were assigned to receive digoxin (n = 492) or placebo (n = 496). Dosing was calculated by an algorithm according to the patient's age, sex, weight, and renal function. The two groups shared similar baseline characteristics. Examples of recorded statistics were age, sex, LVEF, New York Heart Association (NYHA) class, number of signs or symptoms of HF, dose of study medication, and concomitant medications (diuretics, ACE inhibitors, nitrates, or other vasodilators). There were 115 deaths (23.4%) in the digoxin group and 116 deaths (23.4%) in the placebo group, yielding a risk ratio of 0.99. With respect to the combined outcome of death and hospitalization from worsening HF, the risk ratio was 0.82 in favor of the digoxin group; most of the benefit was seen in rates of hospitalization. The results of this study indicate that digoxin provides a benefit in HF morbidity but not in mortality.

The CHARM-Preserved trial [100] studied the effects of an angiotensin-receptor blocker, candesartan, on the composite outcome of cardiovascular mortality or hospital admission caused by worsening HF. Several secondary outcomes were assessed, including nonfatal MI, nonfatal stroke, and coronary revascularization. Three thousand twenty-three patients were randomized to either candesartan therapy or placebo. Mean follow-up was 36.6 months. LVEF was required to be greater than 0.40. The mean age was 67 years, and approximately 26% of patients were 75 or more years of age. The mean LVEF was 54%. Approximately 60% of patients were NYHA class II. Roughly 56% of patients had an ischemic cause of their HF, and over 28% had coexisting diabetes mellitus. Most patients were treated with β-blockers, diuretics, and antiplatelet agents, whereas less than half received ACE inhibitors, spironolactone, calcium channel blockers, digoxin, or lipid-lowering agents. The target dose of study drug was 32 mg/d.

The primary outcome occurred in 22% of patients in the candesartan group compared with 24% of patients in the placebo group (Fig. 2). Most of the benefit was from a 29% reduction in the number of congestive heart failure (CHF) hospitalizations in the candesartan group. The cardiovascular mortality was 11% in both groups. The low mortality likely was related to patient selection, with most patients having NYHA class II HF. Ultimately, the investigators described a trend in favor of using candesartan for the prevention of cardiovascular outcomes in their study population, but the difference in the primary outcome was modest and of borderline significance. Secondary outcomes did not reach statistical significance.

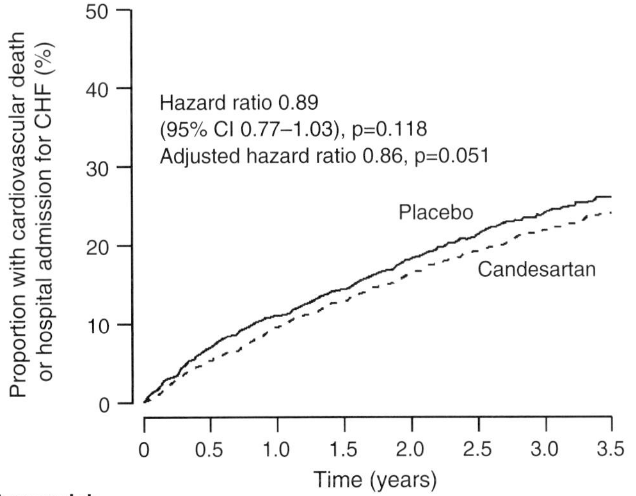

Number ar risk

	0	1.0	2.0	3.0	3.5
Candesartan	1514	1458	1377	833	182
Placebo	1509	1441	1359	824	195

Fig. 2. Results of the CHARM-Preserved trial. There was no statistically significant benefit in primary outcome in the study: cardiovascular death or hospital admission for congestive heart failure. (*From* Yusuf S, Pfeffer MA, Swedberg K, et al. Effects of candesartan in patients with chronic HF and preserved left-ventricular ejection fraction: the CHARM-Preserved Trial. Lancet 2003;362:777–81; with permission.)

There was a 40% reduction in the diagnosis of new-onset diabetes mellitus in the candesartan group. This finding has implications for the future treatment of DHF and longer-term follow-up is perhaps necessary. Notably, DIG [41] and CHARM-Preserved [100] demonstrated that much of the morbidity and mortality associated with DHF patients was unrelated to DHF per se, a fact thay may have contributed to the negative results in these trials.

Neurohormonal modulation in the treatment of conditions that contribute to diastolic heart failure

ACE-inhibitors, ARBs, β-blockers, and aldosterone antagonists are neurohormonal modulators that influence hypertension, CAD, atrial fibrillation, diabetes mellitus, or have direct effects on myocardium. These medications form the backbone of treatment for DHF because they are effective in the treatment of the underlying cardiovascular diseases that can lead or contribute to DHF.

Angiotensin-converting enzyme inhibitors

Hypertension. ACE inhibitors are considered the cornerstone of therapy in many patients who have cardiovascular disease. The antihypertensive effect of ACE inhibitors is accepted widely, which is of primary importance in their role in the treatment of DHF. Although studies such as the Antihypertensive and Lipid-Lowering Treatment to Prevent Heart Attack Trial [101] and those discussed below document blood pressure reduction with use of these agents, this article focuses on trials that have demonstrated other beneficial effects of ACE inhibitors on the conditions that contribute to DHF.

Coronary artery disease. HOPE is one of many studies showing the benefits of ACE inhibitors [102]. In this study, over 9200 patients at high risk for cardiovascular events were assigned to receive either ramipril, 10 mg/d orally, or placebo to assess the effects of ramipril on cardiovascular outcomes. Patients were followed for up to 5 years and were 55 or more years of age with a history of CAD, stroke, peripheral vascular disease, or diabetes mellitus plus at least one other cardiovascular risk factor (hypertension, elevated cholesterol levels, low high-density lipoprotein levels, cigarette smoking, or documented microalbuminuria).

The investigators found a statistically significant reduction in the ramipril group compared with the placebo group for the primary endpoint of MI, stroke, or death caused by cardiovascular causes (14% versus 17.8%) as well as death from cardiovascular causes (6.1% versus 8.1%), MI (9.9% versus 12.3%), stroke (3.4% versus 4.9%), and all-cause mortality (10.4% versus 12.2%). The need for revascularization also was decreased in the ramipril group (16% versus 18.3%). HF occurred in 9% of the ramipril group and 11.5% of the placebo group. The investigators noted that the results were independent of blood pressure–lowering effects alone because most patients did not have hypertension at baseline and the mean blood pressure reduction was only 3/2 mm Hg. They speculated that the benefits of ACE inhibition may result from blocking angiotensin II–mediated vasoconstriction [103], inhibiting vascular smooth muscle cell proliferation [103], preventing plaque rupture [104], or reducing LV hypertrophy [102,103].

More recently, the European Trial on Reduction of Cardiac Events with Perindopril in Stable Coronary Artery Disease (EUROPA) investigated a similar question with a different ACE inhibitor [105]. This trial included patients 18 or more years of age without evidence of HF and with a history of stable CAD—defined as a history of MI (64%), percutaneous or surgical coronary revascularization (55%), or angiographic evidence of at least 70% stenosis of at least one major coronary artery (61%). Men were included if they had a positive stress test (5%). The investigators compared the ability of perindopril, 8 mg/d orally, with placebo in preventing death, MI, or cardiac arrest in patients without HF or excessive hypertension. The mean follow-up was 4.2 years. Cardiovascular mortality, MI, or cardiac arrest was reduced in the perindopril group (8.0% versus 9.9%). The reduction in frequency of clinical MI and cardiovascular death was similar to that found in HOPE (20% versus 21%, respectively). Both trials allowed concomitant treatment with medications such as β-blockers, diuretics, aspirin, and others.

Atrial fibrillation. A substudy of the Trandolapril Cardiac Evaluation (TRACE) was the first to suggest that ACE inhibitors prevent AF in some patients [106]. Patients were assigned to receive either trandolapril or placebo on day 3 to 7 after an acute MI. Trandolapril was titrated up to 4 mg/d as tolerated, and patients were followed for 2 to 4 years. The patients had normal sinus rhythm at baseline, were over 18 years of age, were admitted to the hospital for an acute MI, and displayed impaired LV dysfunction by echocardiography (LVEF < 0.36). The investigators found that placebo-treated patients were more than twice as likely to develop AF than trandolapril-treated patients (5.3% versus 2.3%).

Vermes and colleagues [107] reported a similar finding in their retrospective analysis of patients from the Montreal Heart Institute included in the SOLVD trial. Patients who had AF on a baseline electrocardiogram were excluded. The average length of follow-up was 3 years. Of the 55 patients who developed AF, there was a statistically significant difference: 10 (5.4%) were in the enalapril group and 45 (24%) were in the placebo group.

Diabetes mellitus. ACE inhibitors also have an effect on the development of diabetes mellitus. The HOPE trial demonstrated a statistically significant reduction in new-onset diabetes mellitus in those taking ramipril (3.6% versus 5.4%) [102]. Although there was no comment on the reduction of diabetes mellitus in the EUROPA trial, the CAPPP study demonstrated that captopril, like ramipril, was associated with a statistically significant reduction in the diagnosis of new-onset diabetes mellitus [108].

Direct effects on myocardium. Several studies have documented a reduction in myocardial mass with ACE inhibitor therapy, such as the 4E study discussed below [109]. More recently, however, Brilla and colleagues [110] described the lisinopril-mediated regression of myocardial fibrosis in patients who have hypertensive heart disease. This study examined 35 patients who had primary hypertension, left ventricular hypertrophy (LVH), and LV diastolic dysfunction. Patients were randomized to receive either lisinopril or hydrochlorothiazide (HCTZ). Left heart catheterization with endomyocardial biopsy, Doppler echocardiography, and 24-hour blood pressure monitoring were performed at baseline and at 6 months. The primary endpoint was myocardial fibrosis (directly measured by the collagen volume fraction and myocardial hydroxyproline concentration), and the secondary endpoints were blood pressure, LVH as determined by LV mass index and myocyte diameter, and LV diastolic function assessed using parameters to measure relaxation and myocardial stiffness.

In the lisinopril group, the collagen volume fraction was reduced from a mean of 6.9% to a mean of 6.3% and the myocardial hydroxyproline concentration decreased from an average of 9.9 μg/mg to 8.3 μg/mg of LV weight ($P < .05$ and $P < .00001$ compared with the HCTZ group, respectively). This was associated with an increase in the ratio of early to late diastolic filling (E:A ratio) from a mean of 0.72 to a mean of 0.91 ($P < .05$ versus HCTZ) and a decrease in isovolumic relaxation time from a mean of 123 milliseconds to a mean of 81 milliseconds ($P < .00002$ versus HCTZ). The A-wave duration of transmitral flow during atrial contraction was improved significantly in the lisinopril group compared with the HCTZ group ($P < .0002$), indicating that there was a reduction in ventricular stiffness in the lisinopril group, but there was no statistically significant change in either group when the stiffness constant k was assessed. Normalized blood pressure did not alter the results significantly. No regression in LVH occurred in the lisinopril-treated patients, whereas the HCTZ group experienced a decrease in myocyte diameter from a mean of 22.1 μm to a mean of 20.7 μm ($P < .01$ compared with lisinopril). The important finding is that lisinopril altered myocardial fibrosis and concomitantly improved diastolic function [110].

Clearly, ACE inhibitors play a significant role in the treatment and prevention of entities that contribute to DHF, specifically hypertension, CAD, AF, diabetes mellitus, and unhealthy ventricular remodeling and myocardial fibrosis.

Angiotensin II–receptor blockers

Hypertension. Like ACE inhibitors, ARBs modify several of the disease processes that contribute to DHF. Their power to reduce hypertension has been documented in several trials [111–113], and the current discussion will focus on trials that demonstrate other beneficial effects.

Coronary artery disease. The Valsartan Antihypertensive Long-Term Use Evaluation (VALUE) tested the hypothesis that, despite similar blood pressure reduction, valsartan would reduce cardiac morbidity and mortality more effectively than amlodipine [111]. Patients were 50 or more years of age, had treated or untreated baseline hypertension, and had a combination of predefined risk factors, including diabetes mellitus, smoking, proteinuria by urine dipstick, and elevated total cholesterol. Patients were followed for 4 to 6 years. The primary outcome of time to first major cardiac event and the development of HF were not significantly different between the two groups. The valsartan group did, however, demonstrate a statistically significant difference in the rate of MI compared with the amlodipine group, 4.1% versus 4.8%, respectively. Blood pressure was reduced by both medications, although more so for amlodipine.

The Losartan Intervention for Endpoint Reduction in Hypertension (LIFE) study investigated if blocking the angiotensin-II receptor with losartan would improve LVH beyond blood pressure reduction and, subsequently, lower cardiovascular morbidity and mortality [112]. The investigators included patients 55 to 80 years of age who had previously treated or untreated hypertension and LVH, as determined by electrocardiogram. Patients who had an MI or stroke within the last 6 months, angina requiring treatment with β-blockers or calcium channel blockers, CHF, or LVEF less than 0.40 were excluded. Mean follow-up was 4.8 years.

The study found that a composite endpoint of stroke, MI, or cardiovascular death was decreased in the losartan patients compared with those who were assigned atenolol for a similar blood pressure reduction (23.8% versus 27.9%, respectively). Additionally, a new diagnosis of diabetes mellitus was made more frequently in the atenolol group compared with the losartan group (17.4% versus 13%, respectively). There was no statistically significant difference in admission for HF. Importantly, blood pressure was reduced similarly in the losartan and atenolol groups (reductions of 30.2/16.6 and 29.1/16.8, respectively); therefore it is likely that the beneficial effects of the ARB extended beyond blood pressure control.

Atrial fibrillation. Like ACE inhibitors, ARBs may help prevent AF. Madrid and colleagues [114] investigated irbesartan in maintaining sinus rhythm following conversion from AF. Patients were 18 or more years of age, had AF for more than 7 days, and were randomized to either amiodarone, 400 mg/d orally, or amiodarone plus irbesartan, 150 to 300 mg/d orally. There were several exclusion criteria, including cardiac surgery within 3 months, MI during the previous 6 months, unstable angina, and NYHA class IV HF. Medical therapy was started after anticoagulation to an international normalized ratio above 2.0 and electrical cardioversion was scheduled for 3 weeks later. At 2-month follow-up, 84.79% of the amiodarone group had AF compared with only 63.16% of the dual therapy group. Results were statistically significant.

Diabetes mellitus. Similar to ACE inhibitors, ARBs may be beneficial in the prevention of diabetes mellitus. The VALUE trial found that new-onset diabetes mellitus was far less frequent in the valsartan group than the amlodipine group (32.1% versus 41.1%) [111].

Direct effects on myocardium. The LIFE study demonstrated a final benefit of ARBs. Losartan-based therapy reduced LVH (and to a greater degree than the atenolol-based therapy) based on electrocardiogram criteria and echocardiographic studies [112,115]. The mean Cornell voltage-duration product was reduced by 290 and 124 mm/ms in the losartan and atenolol groups, respectively. The Sokolow-Lyon voltage was reduced by 4.6 and 2.7 mm, respectively [112]. Reduced hypertrophy may be yet another way in which ARBs can improve diastolic dysfunction. Thus, compared with ACE inhibitors, ARBs are acceptable alternatives for the treatment for DHF because of their effects on LVH and on the underlying conditions of DHF.

β-Blockers

Hypertension. A wealth of literature supports the use of selective and nonselective β-receptor antagonists in many conditions, making them one of the most important classes of medications in cardiology. The blood-pressure lowering effects of β-blockers have been well documented and are generally accepted [116–119]. These agents have been used to treat hypertension for over 30 years [119].

Coronary artery disease. β-Blockers also play a role in the treatment of CAD. In the Norwegian Multicenter Study Group trial, 1884 post-MI patients were assigned randomly to timolol, 5 mg/d orally starting dose, with a goal of 20 mg/d orally, or placebo [120]. Therapy was started 7 to 28 days after infarction, and patients were followed for 12 to 33 months. All-cause mortality was reduced by 39%, sudden death by 45%, and nonfatal reinfarction by 28% in the timolol group.

In the Beta-blocker Heart Attack Trial (BHAT), over 3800 patients were monitored following an acute MI [121,122]. Five to twenty-one days post-MI, patients were assigned randomly to receive either propranolol, 180 to 240 mg/d orally, or placebo. Patients were followed for an average of 24 months (the study was ended 9 months prematurely). The propranolol group showed a 26% reduction in all-cause mortality, a 28% reduction in sudden death, and a 23% reduction in all-cause mortality and reinfarction (all reductions were statistically significant). Although not statistically significant, the propranolol group had lower rates of reinfarction than the placebo group when this endpoint was measured independently (10% versus 13%).

Although the Norwegian and BHAT studies were done before the modern era of treatments for CAD such as ACE inhibitors, statins, or interventional techniques, their benefits in post-MI patients have been confirmed in other trials, such as the Survival and Ventricular Enlargement (SAVE) and Acute Infarction Ramipril Efficacy (AIRE) trials [123,124].

Atrial fibrillation. β-Blockers are useful in patients who have AF or other tachycardic states. Maintaining a resting heart rate between 60 and 70 beats per minute and blunting exercise-induced tachycardia may prevent LV pressure elevation and pulmonary congestion by mechanisms previously discussed, thereby providing symptomatic relief [21,50]. Recent studies have validated that rate control is an acceptable, if not preferable, goal of therapy in AF and that β-blockers are effective rate-controlling agents in AF [125,126]. Furthermore, after cardioversion, β-blockers are effective agents for maintaining sinus rhythm [127].

Direct effects on myocardium. As with the other medications in this article, β-blockers reduce LVH, although by a lesser degree than other antihypertensive medications [128]. In their meta-analysis of 50 studies, Schmieder and colleagues [128] found that β-blockers were associated with a 4.5% reduction in LV mass index. ACE inhibitors and diuretics, however, were associated with 11.8% and 8.6% reductions in LV mass index, respectively.

Three recent studies have demonstrated that carvedilol has a beneficial effect on diastolic function. In 27 patients who had LV systolic dysfunction, carvedilol therapy favorably modified diastolic filling, independent of systolic function. A restrictive filling pattern, related to an unfavorable prognosis, changed to pseudonormal or altered relaxation during treatment with carvedilol. The results of Doppler ultrasound after 4 months showed a significant increase of A wave, deceleration time, and isovolumic relaxation time. These improvements were increased to a greater extent at 1 year and were not seen in the placebo group [129].

A study that treated 45 patients who had HF (LVEF = 0.24) with carvedilol showed that long-term therapy with this β-blocker prevented or partially reversed progressive LV dilatation. The effects on LV remodeling were associated with a concomitant significant recovery of diastolic reserve and a significant decrease of mitral regurgitation [130].

Finally, a study including 113 patients who had preserved systolic dysfunction and DHF showed that carvedilol significantly improved the E/A ratio versus placebo. Carvedilol improved diastolic filling compared with placebo, and patients with higher heart rates showed particular benefit [131]. Further investigation into the beneficial effects of β-blockers in DHF should be pursued.

Aldosterone-receptor antagonists

Hypertension. Aldosterone receptor-blockers, such as spironolactone and eplerenone, are potassium-sparing diuretics that have blood pressure–lowering effects in addition to other effects [132]. Eplerenone, which differs from spironolactone in that it has reduced progesterone and androgen-receptor effects, reduces blood pressure an average of 6/4 to 24/14 mm Hg, depending on the dose [132]. Comparative trials have shown that eplerenone has similar antihypertensive effects to those of enalapril, amlodipine, losartan, and spironolactone [132–135].

Direct effects on myocardium. Spironolactone reduces the density of angiotensin-I receptors brought about by aldosterone, suppresses vascular angiotensin-II conversion, improves endothelial function hindered by aldosterone, and inhibits aldosterone-induced interstitial and perivascular fibrosis [136–140]. Spironolactone also can prevent cardiac and arterial fibrosis, improving the overall hemodynamic circumstances that create diastolic dysfunction [141]. Chronic treatment with spironolactone reduces LV mass and plasma markers of myocardial fibrosis [142,143].

Eplerenone has similar effects to those of spironolactone. It significantly reduces cardiac hypertrophy in experimental models [144] as well as improves ventricular remodeling in HF [145]. Studies such as the 4E-Left Ventricular Hypertrophy Study have confirmed eplerenone's beneficial effects in reducing LV mass in patients who have hypertension, similar to the effects seen with spironolactone [109]. In that study, patients who received eplerenone, 200 mg/d orally, were compared with those who received enalapril, 40 mg/d orally, and patients who received a combination of eplerone 200 mg/d orally and enalapril 10 mg/d orally. The primary endpoint was change from baseline LV mass at either 9 months or at the time of study discontinuation. LV mass was assessed using MRI. The investigators found that eplerenone resulted in an adjusted mean decrease of 14.5 g in LV mass compared with 19.7 g for enalapril and 27.2 g for the combination group. The changes in LV mass and hypertrophy have important implications for the treatment of diastolic dysfunction. Moreover, although ACE inhibitors and ARBs reduce blood aldosterone levels initially, there is a rebound effect in which aldosterone levels increase over time after the initiation of blockade of the angiotensin system [146]. Therefore, aldosterone-blocking agents may prove to be key players in the treatment of DHF.

Although the role of neurohormonal modulators in the treatment of DHF needs to be studied in dedicated randomized, placebo-controlled trials, these medications have been well studied in the treatment of conditions that contribute to DHF. These medications are therefore state-of-the-art therapy for the treatment of DHF and should be used whenever necessary. Several trials evaluating treatment options in patients who have DHF are underway. The Perindopril for Elderly People With Chronic Heart Failure study is studying the effect of the ACE inhibitor perindopril in patients who have DHF. Two trials are examining the effects of ARBs (irbesartan and losartan), and another study is comparing perindopril with irbesartan and placebo in patients who have DHF. Finally, one trial is investigating the role of an agent that may improve calcium uptake in the sarcoplasmic reticulum (MCC-135) in the treatment of DHF [21]. The management of this increasingly prevalent disease will be defined better when the results of these trials are published and new trials are developed.

Additional treatment options

Several primary [147,148] and secondary [149–151] prevention trials have shown that statins reduce CAD morbidity and mortality rates and increase overall survival in patients who have cardiovascular disease. Through their influence in decreasing the rate of MI and their beneficial effects on CAD, they contribute to the treatment of DHF.

Given the significance of diabetes mellitus in DHF, glycemic control should be managed tightly in diabetic patients. Iribarren and colleagues [152] found that glycemic control reduces the risk of HF in patients who have diabetes mellitus. Unfortunately, there are no data available describing which glucose-altering medications provide the best reduction in HF [21].

Summary

Approximately 40% to 50% of patients who have clinical HF have DHF. DHF carries a significant burden of morbidity and mortality as well as cost to society. The major conditions associated with it are advanced age, hypertension, CAD, AF, and diabetes mellitus. Currently, there is a paucity of evidence-based data guiding the treatment of HF with a relatively preserved systolic function although several studies are in progress. The data from the two large, randomized trials that are available indicate that a significant percentage of these patients' morbidity and mortality stems from causes other than heart failure. The challenge for future researchers is to develop trials that overcome the age-associated morbidities and mortality of these patient's thereby producing studies that may yield positive results, thus improving the way DHF is managed.

Neurohormonal modulators such as ACE inhibitors, ARBs, β-blockers, and aldosterone-receptor antagonists are important tools in the treatment of DHF because of their indispensable roles in treating the underlying conditions known to cause diastolic dysfunction. As clinical and basic science research mounts, clinicians will have better defined options to attack this prevalent problem and, it is hoped, will change the poor prognosis that faces these patients.

References

[1] American Heart Association. Heart disease and stroke statistics—2004 update. Dallas (TX): American Heart Association; 2003.

[2] American Heart Association. 2002 heart and stroke statistical update. Dallas (TX): American Heart Association; 2003.

[3] Miller LW, Missov ED. Epidemiology of heart failure. Cardiol Clin 2001;19:547–55.

[4] Haldeman GA, Croft JB, Giles WH, et al. Hospitalization of patients with heart failure: National Hospital Discharge Survey, 1985 to 1995. Am Heart J 1999;137:352–60.

[5] Hogg K, Swedlberg K, McMurray J. Heart failure with preserved left ventricular systolic function: epidemiology, clinical characteristics, and prognosis. J Am Coll Cardiol 2004;43:317–27.

[6] Cortina A, Reguero J, Segovia E, et al. Prevalence of heart failure in Asturias (a region in the north of Spain). Am J Cardiol 2001;87:1417–9.

[7] Mosterd A, Hoes AW, de Bruyne MC, et al. Prevalence of heart failure and left ventricular dysfunction in the general population: the Rotterdam Study. Eur Heart J 1999;20:447–55.

[8] Nielsen OW, Hilden J, Larsen CT, et al. Cross-sectional study estimating prevalence of heart failure and left ventricular systolic dysfunction in community patients at risk. Heart 2001;86:172–8.

[9] Hedberg P, Lonnberg I, Jonason T, et al. Left ventricular systolic dysfunction in 75-year-old men and women; a population-based study. Eur Heart J 2001;22:676–83.

[10] Morgan S, Smith H, Simpson I, et al. Prevalence and clinical characteristics of left ventricular dysfunction among elderly patients in general practice setting: cross-sectional survey. BMJ 1999;318:368–72.

[11] Kupari M, Lindroos M, Iivanainen AM, et al. Congestive heart failure in old age: prevalence, mechanisms and 4-year prognosis in the Helsinki Ageing Study. J Intern Med 1997;241:387–94.

[12] Ceia F, Fonseca C, Mota T, et al, and the EPICA Investigators. Prevalence of chronic heart failure in Southwestern Europe: the EPICA study. Eur J Heart Fail 2002;4:531–9.

[13] Kitzman DW, Gardin JM, Gottdiener JS, et al. Importance of heart failure with preserved systolic

function in patients > or = 65 years of age. CHS Research Group. Cardiovascular Health Study. Am J Cardiol 2001;87:413–9.

[14] Devereux RB, Roman MJ, Liu JE, et al. Congestive heart failure despite normal left ventricular systolic function in a population-based sample: the Strong Heart Study. Am J Cardiol 2000;86:1090–6.

[15] Redfield MM, Jacobsen SJ, Burnett Jr JC, et al. Burden of systolic and diastolic ventricular dysfunction in the community: appreciating the scope of the heart failure epidemic. JAMA 2003;289:194–202.

[16] Vasan RS, Benjamin EJ, Levy D. Prevalence, clinical features and prognosis of diastolic heart failure: an epidemiologic perspective. J Am Coll Cardiol 1995;26:1565–74.

[17] Smith GL, Masoudi FA, Vaccarino V, et al. Outcomes in heart failure patients with preserved ejection fraction: mortality, readmission, and functional decline. J Am Coll Cardiol 2003;41:1510–8.

[18] Fonarow GC for the ADHERE Scientific Advisory Committee. The Acute Decompensated Heart Failure National Registry (ADHERE): opportunities to improve care of patients hospitalized with acute decompensated heart failure. Rev Cardiovasc Med 2003; 4(Suppl 7):S21–30.

[19] Hunt SA, Baker DW, Chin MH, et al. ACC/AHA guidelines for the evaluation and management of chronic heart failure in the adult: executive summary. A report of the American College of Cardiology/ American Heart Association Task Force on Practice Guidelines (Committee to revise the 1995 Guidelines for the Evaluation and Management of Heart Failure). J Am Coll Cardiol 2001;38:2101–13.

[20] McKee PA, Castelli WP, McNamara PM, et al. The natural history of congestive heart failure: the Framingham study. N Engl J Med 1971;285:1441–6.

[21] Piccini JP, Klein L, Gheorghiade M, et al. New insights into diastolic heart failure: role of diabetes mellitus. Am J Med 2004;116(5A):64S–75S.

[22] Maisel AS, McCord J, Nowak RM, et al. Bedside B-type natriuretic peptide in the emergency diagnosis of heart failure with reduced or preserved ejection fraction. Results from the Breathing not Properly Multinational Study. J Am Coll Cardiol 2003;41: 2018–21.

[23] Zile MR, Brutsaert DL. New concepts in diastolic dysfunction and diastolic heart failure: part I: diagnosis, prognosis, and measurements of diastolic function. Circulation 2002;105:1387–93.

[24] Zile MR, Catalin FB, Gaasch WH. Diastolic heart failure—abnormalities in active relaxation and passive stiffness of the left ventricle. N Engl J Med 2004;350:1953–9.

[25] Zile MR. Heart failure with preserved ejection fraction: is this diastolic heart failure? J Am Coll Cardiol 2003;41:1519–22.

[26] European Study Group on Diastolic Heart Failure. How to diagnose diastolic heart failure. Eur Heart J 1998;19:990–1003.

[27] Vasan RS, Levy D. Defining diastolic heart failure: a call for standardized diagnostic criteria. Circulation 2000;101:2118–21.

[28] Gandhi SK, Powers JC, Nomeir AM, et al. The pathogenesis of acute pulmonary edema associated with hypertension. N Engl J Med 2001;344:17–22.

[29] Lenzen MJ, Scholte op Reimer WJM, Boersma E, et al. Differences between patients with a preserved and a depressed left ventricular function: a report from the EuroHeart Failure Survey. Eur Heart J 2004; 25:1214–20.

[30] Kitzman DW, Little WC, Brubaker PH, et al. Pathophysiological characterization of isolated diastolic heart failure in comparison to systolic heart failure. JAMA 2002;288:2144–50.

[31] Chen HH, Lainchbury JG, Senni M, et al. Diastolic heart failure in the community: clinical profile, natural history, therapy, and impact of proposed diagnostic criteria. J Card Fail 2002;8:279–87.

[32] McDermott MM, Feinglass J, Sy J, et al. Hospitalized congestive heart failure patients with preserved versus abnormal left ventricular systolic function: clinical characteristics and drug therapy. Am J Med 1995;99:629–35.

[33] Philbin EF, Rocco TA, Lindenmuth NW, et al. Systolic versus diastolic heart failure in the community practice: clinical features, outcomes, and the use of angiotensin-converting enzyme inhibitors. Am J Med 2000;109:605–13.

[34] Pernenkil R, Vinson JM, Shah AS, et al. Course and prognosis in patients > or = 70 years of age with congestive heart failure and normal versus abnormal left ventricular ejection fraction. Am J Cardiol 1997;79:216–9.

[35] McDermott MM, Feinglass J, Lee PI, et al. Systolic function, readmission rates, and survival among consecutively hospitalized patients with congestive heart failure. Am Heart J 1997;134:728–36.

[36] Vasan RS, Larson MG, Benjamin EJ, et al. Congestive heart failure in subjects with normal versus reduced left ventricular ejection fraction: prevalence and mortality in a population-based cohort. J Am Coll Cardiol 1999;33:1948–55.

[37] McAlister FA, Teo KK, Taher M, et al. Insights into the contemporary epidemiology and outpatient management of congestive heart failure. Am Heart J 1999;138:87–94.

[38] Senni M, Tribouilloy CM, Rodeheffer RJ, et al. Congestive heart failure in the community: a study of all incident cases in Olmsted County, Minnesota, in 1991. Circulation 1998;98:2282–9.

[39] Rich MW, McSherry F, Williford WO, et al. Effect of age on mortality, hospitalizations and response to digoxin in patients with heart failure: the DIG Study. J Am Coll Cardiol 2001;38:806–13.

[40] Tarantini L, Faggiano P, Senni M, et al. Clinical features and prognosis associated with a preserved left ventricular systolic function in a large cohort of congestive heart failure outpatients managed by

cardiologists: data from the Italian Network on Congestive Heart Failure. Ital Heart J 2002;3: 656–64.
[41] The Digitalis Investigation Group. The effect of digoxin on mortality and morbidity in patients with heart failure. N Engl J Med 1997;336:525–33.
[42] Judge KW, Pawitan Y, Caldwell J, et al. Congestive heart failure symptoms in patients with preserved left ventricular systolic function: analysis of the CASS registry. J Am Coll Cardiol 1991;18:377–82.
[43] Bonow RO, Udelson JE. Left ventricular diastolic dysfunction as a cause of congestive heart failure: mechanisms and management. Ann Intern Med 1992; 117:502–10.
[44] McDonald IG. The shape and movements of the human left ventricle during systole: a study by cineangiography and by cineradiography of epicardial markers. Am J Cardiol 1970;26:221–30.
[45] Ingels NB, Daughters GT, Stinson EB, et al. Measurement of midwall myocardial dynamics in intact man by radiography of surgically implanted markers. Circulation 1975;52:859–67.
[46] Rothfeld JM, LeWinter MM, Tischler MD. Left ventricular systolic torsion and early diastolic filling by echocardiography in normal humans. Am J Cardiol 1998;81:1465–9.
[47] Michelfelder EC, Khoury P, Witt SA, et al. Noncircumferential myofiber function: impact on early diastolic filling in children. J Am Soc Echocardiogr 2001;14:1065–9.
[48] Rademakers FE, Buchalter MB, Rogers WJ, et al. Dissociation between left ventricular untwisting and filling: accentuation by catecholamines. Circulation 1992;85:1572–81.
[49] Udelson JE, Bacharach SL, Cannon III RO, et al. Minimum left ventricular pressure during beta-adrenergic stimulation in human subjects: evidence for elastic recoil and diastolic "suction" in the normal heart. Circulation 1990;82:1174–82.
[50] Zile MR, Brutsaert DL. New concepts in diastolic dysfunction and diastolic heart failure II. Causal mechanisms and treatment. Circulation 2002;105:1503–8.
[51] Nayler WG, Poole-Wilson PA, Williams A. Hypoxia and calcium. J Mol Cell Cardiol 1979;11:683–706.
[52] Henry PD, Schuchleib R, Davis J, et al. Myocardial contracture and accumulation of mitochondrial calcium in ischemic rabbit heart. Am J Physiol 1977; 233:H677–84.
[53] Weisfeldt ML, Armstrong P, Scully HE, et al. Incomplete relaxation between beats after myocardial hypoxia and ischemia. J Clin Invest 1974;53: 1626–36.
[54] Sordahl LA, McCollum WB, Wood WG, et al. Mitochondria and sarcoplasmic reticulum function in cardiac hypertrophy and failure. Am J Physiol 1973;224:497–502.
[55] Ito Y, Suko J, Chidsey CA. Intracellular calcium and myocardial contractility. V. Calcium uptake of sarcoplasmic reticulum fractions in hypertrophied and failing rabbit hearts. J Mol Cell Cardiol 1974; 6:237–47.
[56] Gwathmey JK, Copelas L, MacKinnon R, et al. Abnormal intracellular calcium handling in myocardium from patients with end-stage heart failure. Circ Res 1987;61:70–6.
[57] Bell SP, Nyland L, Tischler MD, et al. Alterations in the determinants of diastolic suction during pacing tachycardia. Circ Res 2000;87:235–40.
[58] Cazorla O, Freiburg A, Helmes M, et al. Differential expression of cardiac titin isoforms and modulation of cellular stiffness. Circ Res 2000;86:59–67.
[59] Jalil JE, Doering CW, Janicki JS, et al. Fibrillar collagen and myocardial stiffness in the intact hypertrophied rat left ventricle. Circ Res 1989;64: 1041–50.
[60] Weber KT, Janicki JS, Pick R, et al. Myocardial fibrosis and pathologic hypertrophy in the rat with renovascular hypertension. Am J Cardiol 1990;65: G1–7.
[61] Kato S, Spinale FG, Tanaka R, et al. Inhibition of collagen cross-linking: effects on fibrillar collagen and ventricular diastolic function. Am J Physiol 1995;269:H863–8.
[62] Raman VK, Lee YA, Lindpaintner K. The cardiac renin-angiotensin-aldosterone system and hypertensive cardiac hypertrophy. Am J Cardiol 1995;76: 18D–23D.
[63] Dzau VJ. Tissue renin-angiotensin system in myocardial hypertrophy and failure. Arch Intern Med 1993;153:937–42.
[64] Schunkert H, Dzau VJ, Tang SS, et al. Increased rat cardiac angiotensin converting enzyme activity and mRNA expression in pressure overload left ventricular hypertrophy: effects on coronary resistance, contractility and relaxation. J Clin Invest 1990;86: 1913–20.
[65] Eberli FR, Apstein CS, Ngoy S, et al. Exacerbation of left ventricular ischemic diastolic dysfunction by pressure-overload hypertrophy: modification by specific inhibition of cardiac angiotensin converting enzyme. Circ Res 1992;70:931–43.
[66] Mochizuki T, Eberli FR, Apstein CS, et al. Exacerbation of ischemic dysfunction by angiotensin II in red cell-perfused rabbit hearts: Effects of coronary flow, contractility, and high-energy phosphate metabolism. J Clin Invest 1992;89:490–8.
[67] Zennaro MC, Farman N, Bonbalet JP, et al. Tissue-specific expression of alpha and beta messenger ribonucleic acid isoforms of the human mineralocorticoid receptor in normal and pathological states. J Clin Endocrinol Metab 1997;82:1345–52.
[68] Weber KT. Aldosterone in congestive heart failure. N Engl J Med 2001;345:1689–97.
[69] Horisberger JD, Rossier BC. Aldosterone regulation of gene transcription leading to control of ion transport. Hypertension 1992;19:221–7.
[70] Robert V, Van Thiem N, Cheav SL, et al. Increased cardiac types I and III collagen mRNAs in

aldosterone-salt hypertension. Hypertension 1994;24: 30–6.
[71] Khan NU, Movahed A. The role of aldosterone and aldosterone-receptor antagonists in heart failure. Rev Cardiovasc Med 2004;5:71–81.
[72] Laine GA. Microvascular changes in the heart during chronic arterial hypertension. Circ Res 1988;62: 953–60.
[73] White M, Leenen FH. Aging and cardiovascular responsiveness to beta-agonist in humans: role of changes in beta-receptor responses versus baroreflex activity. Clin Pharmacol Ther 1994;56:543–53.
[74] Lakatta EG, Yin FC. Myocardial aging: functional alterations and related cellular mechanisms. Am J Physiol 1982;242:H927–41.
[75] O'Rourke MF. Diastolic heart failure, diastolic left ventricular dysfunction and exercise intolerance. J Am Coll Cardiol 2001;38:803–5.
[76] Lamb HJ, Beyerbacht HP, van der Laarse A, et al. Diastolic dysfunction in hypertensive heart disease is associated with altered myocardial metabolism. Circulation 1999;99:2261–7.
[77] Zhang J, McDonald KM. Bioenergetic consequences of left ventricular remodeling. Circulation 1995;92: 1011–9.
[78] Yelamarty RV, Moore RL, Yu FT, et al. Relaxation abnormalities in single cardiac myocytes from renovascular hypertensive rats. Am J Physiol 1992;262: C980–90.
[79] Leite-Moreira AF, Correia-Pinto J, Gillebert TC. Afterload induced changes in myocardial relaxation: a mechanism for diastolic dysfunction. Cardiovasc Res 1999;43:344–53.
[80] Sadoshima J, Xu Y, Slayter HS, et al. Autocrine release of angiotensin II mediates stretch-induced hypertrophy of cardiac myocytes in vitro. Cell 1993; 75:977–84.
[81] Van Heugten HA, De Jonge HW, Bezstarosti K, et al. Intracellular signaling and genetic reprogramming during agonist-induced hypertrophy of cardiomyocytes. Ann N Y Acad Sci 1995;752:343–52.
[82] Poulsen SH, Jensen SE, Egstrup K. Longitudinal changes and prognostic implications of left ventricular diastolic function in first acute myocardial infarction. Am Heart J 1999;137:910–8.
[83] Pardaens K, Van Cleemput J, Vanhaecke J, et al. Atrial fibrillation is associated with a lower exercise capacity in male chronic heart failure patients. Heart 1997;78:564–8.
[84] Gottdiener JS, Arnold AM, Aurigemma GP, et al. Predictors of congestive heart failure in the elderly: the Cardiovascular Health Study. J Am Coll Cardiol 2000;35:1628–37.
[85] Parker AB, Yusuf S, Naylor CD. The relevance of subgroup-specific treatment effects: the Studies of Left Ventricular Dysfunction (SOLVD) revisited. Am Heart J 2002;144:941–7.
[86] Arnold JM, Yusuf S, Young J, et al. Prevention of heart failure in patients in the Heart Outcomes Prevention Evaluation (HOPE) study. Circulation 2003;107:1284–90.
[87] Seneviratne BI. Diabetic cardiomyopathy: the preclinical phase. BMJ 1977;1:1444–6.
[88] Raev DC. Which left ventricular function is impaired earlier in the evolution of diabetic cardiomyopathy?: an echocardiographic study of young type I diabetic patients. Diabetes Care 1994;17:633–9.
[89] Zabalgoitia M, Ismaeil MF, Anderson L, et al. Prevalence of diastolic dysfunction in normotensive, asymptomatic patients with well-controlled type 2 diabetes mellitus. Am J Cardiol 2001;87:320–3.
[90] Liu JE, Palmieri V, Roman MJ, et al. The impact of diabetes on left ventricular filling pattern in normotensive and hypertensive adults: the Strong Heart Study. J Am Coll Cardiol 2001;37:1943–9.
[91] Uusitupa M, Siitonen O, Aro A, et al. Effect of correction of hyperglycemia on left ventricular function in non-insulin-dependent (type 2) diabetics. Acta Med Scand 1983;213:363–8.
[92] Hardin N. The myocardial and vascular pathology of diabetic cardiomyopathy. Coron Artery Dis 1996; 7:99–108.
[93] Young ME, McNulty P, Taegtmeyer H. Adaptation and maladaptation of the heart in diabetes. II. Potential mechanisms. Circulation 2002;105:1861–70.
[94] Rupp H, Elimban V, Dhalla NS. Modification of myosin isozymes and SR Ca(2 +)-pump ATPase of the diabetic rat heart by lipid-lowering interventions. Mol Cell Biochem 1994;132:69–80.
[95] Bristow MR. Why does the myocardium fail?: insights from basic science. Lancet 1998;352:S8–14.
[96] Depre C, Young ME, Ying J, et al. Streptozotocin-induced changes in cardiac gene expression in the absence of severe contractile dysfunction. J Mol Cell Cardiol 2000;32:985–96.
[97] Golfman L, Dixon IM, Takeda N, et al. Differential changes in cardiac myofibrillar and sarcoplasmic reticular gene expression in alloxan-induced diabetes. Mol Cell Biochem 1999;200:15–25.
[98] Flarsheim CE, Grupp IL, Matlib MA. Mitochondrial dysfunction accompanies diastolic dysfunction in diabetic rat heart. Am J Physiol 1996;271:H192–202.
[99] Bristow M. Etomoxir: a new approach to treatment of chronic heart failure. Lancet 2000;356:1621–2.
[100] Yusuf S, Pfeffer MA, Swedberg K, et al. Effects of candesartan in patients with chronic HF and preserved left-ventricular ejection fraction: the CHARM-Preserved Trial. Lancet 2003;362:777–81.
[101] Officers ALLHAT and Coordinators for the ALLHAT Collaborative Research Group. Major outcomes in high-risk hypertensive patients randomized to angiotensin-converting enzyme inhibitor or calcium channel blocker vs diuretic: the Antihypertensive and Lipid-Lowering Treatment to Prevent Heart Attack Trial (ALLHAT). JAMA 2002;288:2981–97.
[102] The Heart Outcomes Prevention Evaluation Investigators. Effects of an angiotensin-converting-enzyme inhibitor, ramipril, on cardiovascular events

in high-risk patients. N Engl J Med 2000;342: 145–53.
[103] Lonn EM, Yusuf S, Jha P, et al. Emerging role of angiotensin-converting enzyme inhibitors in cardiac and vascular protection. Circulation 1994;90: 2056–69.
[104] Schieffer B, Schieffer E, Hilfiker-Kleiner D, et al. Expression of angiotensin II and interleukin 6 in human coronary atherosclerotic plaques: potential implications for inflammation and plaque instability. Circulation 2000;101:1372–8.
[105] The European trial on reduction of cardiac events with perindopril in stable coronary artery disease Investigators. Efficacy of perindopril in reduction of cardiovascular events among patients with stable coronary artery disease: randomised, double-blind, placebo-controlled, multicentre trial (the EUROPA study). Lancet 2003;362:782–8.
[106] Pedersen OD, Bagger H, Kober L, et al. Trandolapril reduces the incidence of atrial fibrillation after acute myocardial infarction in patients with left ventricular dysfunction. Circulation 1999;100:376–80.
[107] Vermes E, Tardif JC, Bourassa MG, et al. Enalapril decreases the incidence of atrial fibrillation in patients with left ventricular dysfunction: insight from the Studies Of Left Ventricular Dysfunction (SOLVD) trials. Circulation 2003;10:2926–31.
[108] Hansson L, Lindholm LH, Niskanen L, et al. Effect of angiotensin-converting- enzyme inhibition compared with conventional therapy on cardiovascular morbidity and mortality in hypertension: the Captopril Prevention Project (CAPPP) randomised trial. Lancet 1999;353:611–6.
[109] Pitt B, Reichek N, Willenbrock R, et al. Effects of eplerenone, enalapril, and eplerenone/enalapril in patients with essential hypertension and left ventricular hypertrophy. The 4E-left ventricular hypertrophy study. Circulation 2003;108:1831–8.
[110] Brilla CG, Funck RC, Rupp H. Lisionpril-mediated regression of myocardial fibrosis in patients with hypertensive heart disease. Circulation 2000;102: 1388–93.
[111] Julius S, Kjeldsen SE, Weber M, et al, for the VALUE trial group. Outcomes in hypertensive patients at high cardiovascular risk treated with regimens based on valsartan or amlodipine: the VALUE randomised trial. Lancet 2004;363:2022–31.
[112] Dahlof B, Devereux RB, Kjeldsen SE, et al, for the LIFE Study Group. Cardiovascular morbidity and mortality in the Losartan Intervention For Endpoint reduction in hypertension study (LIFE): a randomised trial against atenolol. Lancet 2002;359:995–1003.
[113] Lithell H, Hansson L, Skoog I, et al. The Study on Cognition and Prognosis in the Elderly (SCOPE): principal results of a randomized double-blind intervention trial. J Hypertens 2003;21:875–86.
[114] Madrid AH, Bueno MG, Rebollo JM, et al. Use of irbesartan to maintain sinus rhythm in patients with long-lasting persistent atrial fibrillation: a prospective and randomized study. Circulation 2002;106: 331–6.
[115] Devereux RB, Gerdts E, Wachtell K, et al. Regression of hypertensive left ventricular hypertrophy by angiotensin receptor blockade versus beta-blockade: the LIFE trial (abstract). Am J Hypertens 2002;15:15A.
[116] Coope J, Warrender TS. Randomised trial of treatment of hypertension in elderly patients in primary care. BMJ 1986;293:1145–51.
[117] Ekbom T, Dahlof B, Hansson L, et al. Antihypertensive efficacy and side effects of three beta-blockers and a diuretic in elderly hypertensives: a report from the STOP-Hypertension study. J Hypertens 1992;10: 1525–30.
[118] MRC Working Party. Medical Research Council trial of treatment of hypertension in older adults: principal results. BMJ 1992;304:405–12.
[119] Messerli F, Grossman E. Beta-blockers in hypertension: is carvedilol different? Am J Cardiol 2004; 93(Suppl):7B–12B.
[120] Norwegian Multicenter Study Group. Timolol-induced reduction in mortality and reinfarction in patients surviving acute myocardial infarction. N Engl J Med 1981;304:801–7.
[121] Beta-Blocker Heart Attack Trial Research Group. A randomized trial of propranolol in patients with acute myocardial infarction: I. Mortality results. JAMA 1982;247:1707–14.
[122] Beta-Blocker Heart Attack Trial Research Group. A randomized trial of propranolol in patients with acute myocardial infarction: II. Morbidity results. JAMA 1983;250:2814–9.
[123] Vantrimpont P, Rouleau JL, Wun CC, et al. Additive beneficial effects of beta-blockers to angiotensin-converting enzyme inhibitors in the Survival and Ventricular Enlargement (SAVE) Study. SAVE Investigators. J Am Coll Cardiol 1997;29:229–36.
[124] Spargias KS, Hall AS, Greenwood DC, et al. Beta-blocker treatment and other prognostic variables in patients with clinical evidence of heart failure after acute myocardial infarction: evidence from the AIRE study. Heart 1999;81:25–32.
[125] Wyse DG, Waldo AL, DiMarco JP, et al. A comparison of rate control and rhythm control in patients with atrial fibrillation. N Engl J Med 2002; 347:1825–33.
[126] Olshansky B, Rosenfeld LE, Warner AL, et al. The Atrial Fibrillation Follow-Up Investigation of Rhythm Management (AFFIRM) study approaches to control rate in atrial fibrillation. J Am Coll Cardiol 2004;43:1201–8.
[127] Kuhlkamp V, Schirdewan A, Stangl K, et al. Use of metoprolol CR/XL to maintain sinus rhythm after conversion from persistent atrial fibrillation: a randomized, double-blind, placebo-controlled study. J Am Coll Cardiol 2000;36:139–46.
[128] Schmieder RE, Schlaich MP, Klingbeil AU, et al. Update on reversal of left ventricular hypertrophy in essential hypertension (a meta-analysis of all ran-

domized double-blind studies until December 1996). Nephrol Dial Transplant 1998;13:564–9.
[129] Palazzuoli A, Carrera A, Calabria P, et al. Effects of carvedilol therapy on restrictive diastolic filling pattern in chronic heart failure. Am Heart J 2004; 147:1–7.
[130] Capomolla S, Febo O, Gnemmi M, et al. Beta-blockade therapy in chronic heart failure: diastolic function and mitral regurgitation improvement by carvedilol. Am Heart J 2000;139:596–608.
[131] Bergstrom A, Andersson B, Edner M, et al. Effect of carvedilol on diastolic function in patients with diastolic heart failure and preserved systolic function. Results of the Swedish Doppler-echocardiographic study (SWEDIC). Eur J Heart Fail 2004;6:453–61.
[132] Taylor CT. Eplerenone (Inspra) for hypertension. Am Fam Physician 2004;69:915–6.
[133] Williams GH, Burgess E, Kolloch RE, et al. Efficacy of eplerenone versus enalapril as monotherapy in systemic hypertension. Am J Cardiol 2004;93:990–6.
[134] White WB, Duprez D, St. Hillaire R, et al. Effects of the selective aldosterone blocker eplerenone versus the calcium antagonist amlodipine in systolic hypertension. Hypertension 2003;41:1021–6.
[135] Flack JM, Oparil S, Pratt JH, et al. Efficacy and tolerability of eplerenone and losartan in hypertensive black and white patients. J Am Coll Cardiol 2003;41: 1148–55.
[136] Robert V, Heymes C, Silvestre JS, et al. Angiotensin AT1 receptor subtype as a cardiac target of aldosterone: role in aldosterone-salt induced fibrosis. Hypertension 1999;33:981–6.
[137] Duprez DA, DeBuyzere ML, Rietzschel ER, et al. Inverse relationship between aldosterone and large artery compliance in chronically treated heart failure patients. Eur Heart J 1998;19:1371–6.
[138] Bauersachs J, Heck M, Fraccarollo D, et al. Addition of spironolactone to angiotensin-converting enzyme inhibition in heart failure improves endothelial vasomotor dysfunction: role of vascular superoxide anion formation and endothelial nitric oxide synthase expression. J Am Coll Cardiol 2002;39:351–8.
[139] Brilla CG, Matsubara LS, Weber KT. Antifibrotic effects of spironolactone in preventing myocardial fibrosis in systemic arterial hypertension. Am J Cardiol 1993;71:12A–6A.
[140] Brilla CG, Matsubara LS, Weber KT. Anti-aldosterone treatment and prevention of myocardial fibrosis in primary and secondary hyperaldosteronism. J Mol Cell Cardiol 1993;25:563–75.
[141] Lacolley P, Safar ME, Lucet B, et al. Prevention of aortic and cardiac fibrosis by spironolactone in old normotensive rats. J Am Coll Cardiol 2001;37: 662–7.
[142] Zannad F, Alla F, Dousset B, et al. Limitation of excessive extracellular matrix turnover may contribute to survival benefit of spironolactone therapy in patients with congestive heart failure. Circulation 2000;102:2700–6.
[143] Querejeta R, Varo N, Lopez B, et al. Serum carboxy-terminal propeptide of procollagen type I is a marker of myocardial fibrosis in hypertensive heart disease. Circulation 2000;101:1729–35.
[144] Frierdich G, Schuh J, Brown M, et al. Effects of the selective mineralocorticoid receptor antagonist, eplerenone, in a model of aldosterone-induced hypertension and cardiac fibrosis [abstract]. Am J Hypertens 1998;11:94.
[145] Suzuki G, Morita H, Mishima T, et al. Effects of long-term monotherapy with eplerenone, a novel aldosterone blocker, on progression of left ventricular dysfunction and remodeling in dogs with heart failure. Circulation 2002;106:2967–72.
[146] Struthers AD, MacDonald TM. Review of aldosterone- and angiotensin II-induced target organ damage and prevention. Cardiovasc Res 2004;61:663–70.
[147] Shepherd J, Cobbe SM, Ford I, et al. Prevention of coronary heart disease with pravastatin in men with hypercholesterolemia. West of Scotland Coronary Prevention Study Group. N Engl J Med 1995; 333:1301–7.
[148] Heart Protection Study Collaborative Group. MRC/BHF Heart Protection Study of cholesterol lowering with simvastatin in 20,536 high-risk individuals: a randomised placebo-controlled trial. Lancet 2002; 360:7–22.
[149] Randomised trial of cholesterol lowering in 4444 patients with coronary heart disease: the Scandinavian Simvastatin Survival Study (4S). Lancet 1994;344: 1383–9.
[150] Sacks FM, Pfeffer MA, Moye LA, et al. The effect of pravastatin on coronary events after myocardial infarction in patients with average cholesterol levels. Cholesterol and Recurrent Events Trial investigators. N Engl J Med 1996;335:1001–9.
[151] Prevention of cardiovascular events and death with pravastatin in patients with coronary heart disease and a broad range of initial cholesterol levels. The Long-Term Intervention with Pravastatin in Ischaemic Disease (LIPID) Study Group. N Engl J Med 1998; 339:1349–57.
[152] Iribarren C, Karter AJ, Go AS, et al. Glycemic control and heart failure among adult patients with diabetes. Circulation 2001;103:2668–73.

ELSEVIER
SAUNDERS

Heart Failure Clin 1 (2005) 95 – 102

HEART
FAILURE
CLINICS

Neutral Endopeptidase Inhibitors and Endothelin Antagonists: Why Did the Clinical Trials Not Demonstrate Beneficial Effects?

Srinivas Iyengar, MD*, William T. Abraham, MD

Ohio State University, Columbus, OH, USA

Over the last 15 years, the deleterious effects of the neurohormonal cascade on the failing heart have been documented increasingly. Treatment algorithms for patients who have systolic heart failure revolve around offsetting the effects of this hormonal barrage. The use of angiotensin-converting enzyme (ACE) inhibitors [1], beta-blockers [2], aldosterone antagonists [3], and angiotensin II–receptor blockers [4] have formed the cornerstone of heart failure therapy. Using this theory of hormonal antagonism, additional therapeutic agents have been developed. Two newer classes, neutral endopeptidase (NEP) inhibitors and endothelin (ET) antagonists, are medications that showed promise in initial studies, but, as a possible indication that the pathoetiology of heart failure is more complex than is understood, larger clinical trials with these agents fell short of expected results.

Neutral endopeptidase inhibitors

Background

NEP is a membrane-bound metallopeptidase that functions to cleave endogenous peptides at the amino side of hydrophilic residues [5]. NEP is found in various cell lines, including endothelial cells and vascular smooth muscle cells [6,7], as well as in various organs. Natriuretic hormones, such as atrial natriuretic peptide, brain natriuretic peptide, and C-type natriuretic peptide, are peptides whose degradation is facilitated by the actions of NEP [8,9]. In addition, NEP catalyzes the degradation of endothelin-1 (ET-1) and angiotensin II [10]. NEP inhibitors, as their name suggests, counteract the functions of NEP. This dual antagonism of the degradation process for vasoconstrictive and vasodilatory peptides has led to questions about how NEP inhibition affects the vascular system given its effects on these two seemingly opposite entities.

Experimental data

This idea of nonselective (between constrictive versus dilatory peptides) degradation inhibition has resulted in studies with mixed conclusions about which action is predominant in NEP inhibition. Studies examining patients who have essential hypertension have shown improvement and worsening during treatment with NEP inhibitors [11,12]; it is theorized that the response to NEP inhibition is linked to the amounts of predominant substrate present, whether vasoconstrictive or vasodilatory. This could explain why NEP inhibitors have shown beneficial hemodynamic effects in hypertensive patients but not in normotensive patients [13].

In the area of heart failure, NEP inhibitors have had varying results. Although Kahn and colleagues [14] demonstrated the natriuretic effects of NEP inhibition with the lowering of pulmonary capillary wedge pressure (PCWP) and Good and colleagues

* Corresponding author. Division of Cardiovascular Medicine, Ohio State University, 473 West 12th Avenue, Room 110P DHLRI, Columbus, OH 43210-1252.
E-mail address: iyengar-1@medctr.osu.edu (S. Iyengar).

1551-7136/05/$ – see front matter
doi:10.1016/j.hfc.2004.11.001

Table 1
Overture trial results

Endpoint	Enalapril n = 2884	Omapatrilat n = 2886	*P* value
Primary			
Death and/or HF hospitalization	973	914	.187
Secondary			
All-cause mortality	509	477	.339
CV death and/or CV hospitalization	1275	1178	.024

Abbreviations: CV, cardiovascular; HF, heart failure.

[15] showed a dose-dependent diuresis with candoxatrilat in moderate to severe heart failure patients, chronic treatment with these medications has not produced similar results.

Recently, several trials have investigated a modified form of NEP inhibitor: the vasopeptidase inhibitors. These compounds are composed of dual metalloprotease inhibitors that simultaneously block ACE and NEP. The drive for this new therapeutic agent stemmed from the idea that these agents together could have a beneficial synergistic effect on vascular hemodynamics and renal function not seen with individual use [16,17].

Several vasopeptide inhibitors have been studied, in small animal and human models, and the initial results were particularly favorable regarding the treatment of hypertension [18,19]. The most thoroughly studied vasopeptide inhibitor, omapatrilat, had a beneficial effect on blood pressure in hypertensive rats [20] as well as in heart-failure hamster models, even compared with an ACE inhibitor [21]. Although many of the clinical trials in which omapatrilat was used were in the antihypertensive arena, it also was examined for potential use in heart failure.

McClean and colleagues [22] published data on a study of 48 patients who had New York Heart Association (NYHA) class-II to -III heart failure treated with omapatrilat who reported improvement in functional class, as well as increases in left ventricular function. These data were bolstered by the IMPRESS trial [23], which sought to determine the long-term effects of omapatrilat on exercise tolerance and morbidity compared with lisinopril. Five hundred seventy-three patients who had NYHA class-II to -IV chronic heart failure were assigned randomly to receive either omapatrilat at a target dose of 40 mg/d or lisinopril at a target dose of 20 mg/d for 24 weeks, with the primary endpoints focusing on improvement in exercise tolerance at week 12. Secondary endpoints such as death and comorbid events indicative of worsening heart failure also were examined. At week 12, no significant difference in exercise tolerance was seen between the two groups. At the end of the study, there were no statistical differences between omapatrilat and lisinopril in the frequencies of death or hospitalization, but omapatrilat significantly decreased the composite endpoint of death, hospitalization, or discontinuation of study treatment for worsening heart failure compared with lisinopril (6% versus 10%, $P = .035$). Improvement in NYHA functional class also was related more closely to omapatrilat than to lisinopril therapy.

The largest trial investigating omapatrilat's role in heart failure was the Omapatrilat Versus Enalapril Randomized Trial of Utility in Reducing Events (OVERTURE) trial, which randomized 5770 patients who had NYHA class-II to -IV heart failure to either omapatrilat, 40 mg, or an uptitrated dose of enalapril, 10 mg twice daily [24]. Primary endpoints (death or hospitalization for chronic heart failure requiring intravenous medication) were not significantly different between the drugs (Table 1). In addition, there was an increased incidence of hypotension, dizziness, cough, and angioedema with omapatrilat therapy compared with patients treated with enalapril, although impaired renal function and fatigue were seen more frequently in the enalapril arm (Table 2). A post hoc analysis, however, which defined hospitalization for heart failure as any hospitalization for heart failure requiring a change in regimen, whether oral or intravenous, showed omapatrilat to be superior to enalapril. In subgroup analyses, an advantage of omapatrilat over enalapril was found among women, those who had hypertension (systolic pressure > 140 mm Hg) at the start of the study, and those without diabetes mellitus. Among patients who had pre-existing hypertension, the incidence of renal impairment was lower for the omapatrilat group (3.9% versus 7.1%).

McClean and colleagues [25] followed up their initial work with a study investigating different dosing regimens of omapatrilat. In a randomized,

Table 2
Overture trial adverse events

Event	Enalapril n = 2884 (%)	Omapatrilat n = 2886 (%)
Dizziness	401 (13.9)	561 (19.4)
Hypotension	332 (11.5)	564 (19.5)
Renal impairment	291 (10.1)	196 (6.8)
Fatigue	276 (9.6)	233 (8.1)
Cough	259 (9.0)	279 (9.7)
Angioedema	14 (0.5)	24 (0.8)

double-blind, multicenter trial, 369 patients who had NYHA class II- to IV heart failure and ejection fractions of less than 40% were assigned randomly to receive 12 weeks of omapatrilat, 2.5 to 40 mg/d, as a replacement to ACE inhibitor therapy. ACE inhibitors were discontinued at least 4 days before randomization. Hemodynamic and neurohormonal parameters were evaluated at baseline and at the end of the study. Treatment with omapatrilat resulted in a dose-related reduction of PCWP, systolic and diastolic blood pressure, and systemic vascular resistance. In addition, a dose-dependent increase in left ventricular ejection fraction was reported, but no significant changes in cardiac index were noted. On a neurohormonal level, treatment with omapatrilat resulted in decreased NEP activity, whereas no significant changes in trough plasma epinephrine, norepinephrine, or ET-1 levels were seen during treatment. In addition, improvement in NYHA functional class correlated more strongly with patients being treated with higher dosages of omapatrilat. Despite the encouraging data, the initial results of the OVERTURE trial loom large, and the debate over the applicability of using vasopeptide inhibitors to treat heart failure continues.

Discussion

There are three main theories for NEP inhibition alone and its lack of clinical efficacy for heart failure: (1) the dual inhibition of peptide degradation by NEP inhibitors can increase disproportionately the activity of the renin-angiotensin-aldosterone system (RAAS) and ET over time, (2) tolerance to natriuretic peptides might develop with chronic treatment, and (3) downregulation of natriuretic peptide receptors in response to the decreased degradation of natriuretic peptides may be a factor. Alone or in combination, these theories could explain the lack of clinical benefit seen with these agents.

NEP and ACE-inhibition combinations have not been demonstrated more effective than other standard agents for treating heart failure. Omapatrilat, the vasopeptidase inhibitor most extensively studied, did not demonstrate any incremental benefit over ACE inhibition alone, and had more side effects in relation to angioedema [24]. There are two possible explanations: (1) these results could be limited to the actions of omapatrilat, not all vasopeptidase inhibitors and (2) the effects of bradykinin. Although bradykinin can be related to the positive effects of ACE inhibitors by accentuating some of their blood pressure–reducing actions, too much bradykinin (through NEP and ACE inhibition) may tip the scales in the opposite direction. The end result might be the best explanation for the increase in angioedema seen with vasopeptide inhibitor use [26].

Although there may be several factors responsible for omapatrilat's failure to distinguish itself as a superior or equal therapy to ACE inhibitors, it has widened the knowledge base of researchers focused on the development of hormone-specific therapies for heart failure.

Endothelin antagonists

Background

ET is a 21–amino acid peptide that is produced by endopeptidase cleavage of preproendothelin [27]. Yanagisawa [28] first described it in 1988 as an exceptionally potent vasoconstrictor. Various types of cells in the heart, lung, and other organs produce ET [29]. ET-1 to -4 are produced from big ET by an ET-converting enzyme. The formation of ET is stimulated by cytokines, catecholamines, and hormones, as well as by vasoactive agents [30,31]. The effects of ET include vasoconstriction of vascular smooth muscle, increased production of cardiac fibroblasts, and hypertrophy of cardiac myocytes [32]. Furthermore, in patients with intact cardiac function, ET seems to have a positive inotropic effect, although its inotropic effect in heart failure is questionable [33]. ET has been associated with two main receptor types: type A (ET-A) and type B (ET-B) [34]. ET-A receptor has been associated with potent vasoconstriction and cell hypertrophy, whereas ET-B receptor has been associated with more vasodilatory effects, although its exact role is not known. Elevated serum levels of ET have been found in patients who have decompensated heart failure, and these levels have been associated with negative clinical parameters and poorer overall prognosis [35–37]. With the consequences of the pathologic effects of ET increasingly being realized, creating agents that could inhibit the production of ET or antagonize its ability to interact with its receptors was appealing. After the introduction of ET-receptor antagonists for the treatment of pulmonary hypertension [38], it was believed to be only a matter of time before the indications of these agents would be extended to heart failure.

Experimental data

ET-receptor antagonists first were investigated in various animal models of heart failure. Sakai and colleagues [39] demonstrated that long-term treatment with a selective ET-A receptor antagonist in the treatment of post–myocardial infarction heart failure rat models could decrease mortality and increase ventricular function. Studies using nonselective ET-receptor antagonists with the same type of rat model have demonstrated similar results [40]. Although early administration (within 3–6 hours) of an ET-receptor antagonist, selective or nonselective, post–myocardial infarction has been associated with increased left ventricular dysfunction and mortality in animal models [41,42], the weight of positive evidence from additional animal studies pointed to an overall favorable effect of these agents for the treatment of heart failure [43–45]. The beneficial effects of ET-receptor antagonists in animal models initially were demonstrated using intravenous formulations, but these effects also were seen with oral preparations [46].

Although bolstered by the strength of several experimental animal trials, researchers still questioned: how would ET antagonists fare in the human heart failure population? Small, short-term trials examining the use of ET antagonists in patients who had heart failure were initially promising [47,48]. These first results encouraged larger studies. The effect of long-term bosentan use on the primary endpoint of all-cause mortality or hospitalization for heart failure was examined in the Research on Endothelin Antagonist in Chronic Heart Failure (REACH-1) study, which revealed improvements in reducing the combined endpoints of death and worsening heart failure after 6 months, but was associated with an increase in liver enzymes [49]. In addition, bosentan was associated with more heart failure events during the first 6 months. This study was conducted with a bosentan dose of 500 mg twice daily, and it was believed that the elevated enzymes were a dose-dependent phenomenon.

This trial was followed by the Endothelin Antagonist Bosentan for Lowering Cardiac Events in Heart Failure (ENABLE) study, which used a lower dose of bosentan, 125 mg twice daily, in patients who had NYHA class-IIIB to -IV heart failure [50]. Despite fewer adverse enzyme interactions than in the REACH-1 study, no overall mortality benefit was revealed with this therapy. The Heart Failure ET-A Receptor Blockade Trial examined the effects of darusentan, a selective ET-A receptor antagonist, in 157 NYHA class-II heart failure patients. Patients were treated for 3 weeks, and certain hemodynamic parameters (cardiac output, systemic vascular resistance) improved, but others (PCWP) did not change significantly [51].

The Randomized Intravenous Tezosentan (RITZ) study groups examined the hemodynamic and clinical effects of tezosentan, a nonselective ET-receptor antagonist, for the treatment of heart failure. Although RITZ-2 demonstrated an improvement in cardiac index and lowering of PCWP compared with placebo [52], RITZ-1 failed to demonstrate any difference in the primary endpoint of change in dyspnea compared with placebo [53]. In addition, RITZ-4 revealed that treatment with tezosentan did not improve significantly any of the major clinical endpoints, including death or worsening heart failure [54]. RITZ-5 evaluated oxygen saturations in patients who had heart failure and pulmonary edema and found no significant difference between the placebo and medication arms [55].

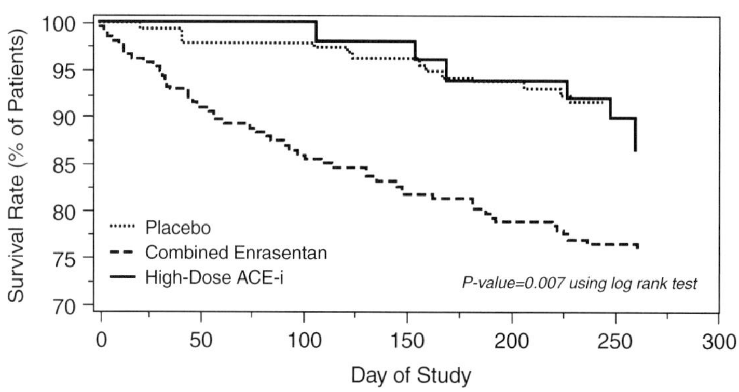

Fig. 1. Results of the ENCORE Trial showing time to death, heart failure hospitalization, or withdrawal caused by worsening heart failure. ACE-I, ACE inhibitor. (*Data from* Abraham WT. Results of the ENCORE Trial. Presented at: Scientific Sessions of the American College of Cardiology, 2001.)

The Enrasentan Clinical Outcomes Randomized (ENCORE) study compared the nonselective ET-receptor antagonist enrasentan (at varying doses) with placebo or high-dose ACE inhibition for 9 months in 419 patients who had NYHA class-II or -III heart failure [52]. Negative trends seen with the enrasentan arm included worsening heart failure and excess mortality (Fig. 1).

The Endothelin-A Receptor Antagonist Trial in Heart Failure (EARTH) trial examined the effects of darusentan (at varying doses) compared with placebo in NYHA class-II to -IV heart failure patients who also had depressed ejection fractions and were on stable oral heart failure therapy [56]. The primary endpoint of the study was the effect these therapies had on left ventricular remodeling, as determined by cardiac MRI; in addition, 6-minute walk tests and quality-of-life assessments were performed. Although there was a weak positive trend for darusentan at higher doses for reduction of left ventricular end-systolic volumes, it was not statistically significant. It also was reported that darusentan did not reduce the incidence of death, all-cause hospitalizations, or hospitalizations caused by heart failure. No significant differences between placebo and darusentan in relation to the 6-minute walk tests or quality-of-life assessments could be discerned between the two therapies.

Discussion

Before scrutinizing the human clinical trials involving ET-antagonists, one should re-examine how ET functions in the body. Clinical agents developed for the ET arena in the past few years have focused mainly on ET-A receptor antagonism, but some agents have been nonselective. Whether it is best to antagonize the ET-A receptor, the ET-B receptor, or both is unknown. Although the ET-B receptor is associated with vasodilation, it also has been linked to aldosterone secretion in heart failure [57]. The lack of fundamental knowledge of these receptor subtypes can undermine assumptions of how specific ET receptor antagonists work. Therefore, judging a therapy as a failure mandates a closer inspection of how these receptor types might interact with one another in pathologic situations.

In relation to the post–myocardial infarction animal model experiments, the question of "therapeutic timing" is vital. The timing of administration of an ET antagonist likely is pivotal in determining positive clinical outcomes. Although many post–myocardial infarction animal models did well in relation to hemodynamic and clinical parameters, some had negative outcomes from therapy instituted early in the disease process. ET, despite having potential long-term deleterious effects on the failing heart, may help the acutely injured heart repair itself through fibroblast proliferation and tissue stability [32]. Thus timing as well as dosage may be critical when using these agents to treat post–myocardial infarction–induced heart failure.

Examining the human heart failure clinical trials, the quandary of how receptor-subtype antagonism is mediated is repeated; selective agents have not conferred significant benefits over placebo in several different clinical endpoints. The weak positive dose-related trend seen with the higher doses in the EARTH trial presents a muddled picture: with higher doses, are ET-A receptor antagonists engaged in some overlap with the ET-B receptor? Or at higher doses, is the ET-A receptor site blockaded more thoroughly? Post hoc analysis of the RITZ-5 trial revealed that patients receiving the higher dose of tezosentan had worse outcomes than patients who received placebo; patients who received the lower dose had improved outcomes compared with placebo [55]. As a nonselective agent, tezosentan is intrinsically different in function and composition than darusentan; thus, assuming that nonselective ET-receptor blockade at a low dose would be more beneficial than selective antagonism at higher doses would be inappropriate, especially given the failure of bosentan to establish this premise in the ENABLE study. Finally, blockade of ET-B receptors may have a deleterious effect on renal salt and water handling. This may explain the increased incidence of worsening heart failure seen in some trials (eg, REACH, ENABLE, ENCORE).

Summary

The number of therapeutic agents available to physicians treating patients who have heart failure seems to be expanding daily. The emphasis on receptor sites and hormonal interactions involved in the pathogenesis of heart failure results in continuous development in this area, as evidenced by the development of NEP inhibitors and ET antagonists. Unfortunately, these therapies have fallen short of their intended goal of effectively disrupting the neurohormonal cascade of heart failure. Before banishing these agents to the nether regions of the pharmaceutical spectrum, however, one should take into account the baseline knowledge, or lack thereof, of how these medications function. Is the breadth of their cellular interactions and underlying mechanisms known? Are these agents truly limited in their scope to treat heart failure because of a lack of positive results in the clinical trials? It would behoove clinicians and researchers to investigate thoroughly the basic workings of these medications because they may offer clues or further insight that could aid the development of alternative remedies. Otherwise, the future will bring repetition of the same labored steps with fruitless trials and another new class of supposed "wonder drugs."

References

[1] The CONSENSUS Trial Study Group. Effects of enalapril on mortality in severe congestive heart failure. Results of the Cooperative North Scandinavian Enalapril Survival Study (CONSENSUS). N Engl J Med 1987;316(23):1429–35.

[2] Packer M, Bristow MR, Cohn JN, et al. The effect of carvedilol on morbidity and mortality in patients with chronic heart failure. US Carvedilol Heart Failure Study Group. N Engl J Med 1996;334(21):1349–55.

[3] Pitt B, Zannad F, Remme WJ, et al. The effect of spironolactone on morbidity and mortality in patients with severe heart failure. N Engl J Med 1999;341: 709–17.

[4] Cohn JN, Tognoni G. A randomized trial of the angiotensin-receptor blocker valsartan in chronic heart failure. N Engl J Med 2001;345:1667–75.

[5] Margulies KB, Barclay PL, Burnett Jr JC. The role of neutral endopeptidase in dogs with evolving congestive heart failure. Circulation 1995;91:2036–42.

[6] Graf K, Koehne P, Grafe M, et al. Regulation and differential expression of neutral endopeptidase 24.11 in human endothelial cells. Hypertension 1995;26: 230–5.

[7] Dussaule JC, Stefanski A, Bea ML, et al. Characterization of neutral endopeptidase in vascular smooth muscle cells of rabbit renal cortex. Am J Physiol 1993; 264:F45–52.

[8] Stephenson SL, Kenny AJ. The hydrolysis of alpha-human atrial natriuretic peptide by pig kidney microvillar membranes is initiated by endopeptidase 24.11. Biochem J 1987;243:183–7.

[9] Kenny AJ, Bourne A, Ingram J. Hydrolysis of human and pig brain natriuretic peptides, urodilantin, C-type natriuretic peptide and some C-type receptor ligands by endopeptidase 24.11. Biochem J 1993;291:83–8.

[10] Skidgel RA, Engelbrecht S, Johnson AR, et al. Hydrolysis of substance P and neurotensin by converting enzyme and neutral endopeptidase. Peptides 1984;5:769–76.

[11] Ogihara T, Rakugi H, Masuo K, et al. Antihypertensive effects of the neutral endopeptidase inhibitor SCH 42495 in essential hypertension. Am J Hypertens 1994;7:943–7.

[12] Singer DR, Markandu ND, Buckley MG, et al. Dietary sodium and inhibition of neutral endopeptidase 24.11 in essential hypertension. Hypertension 1991;18:798–804.

[13] Ando S, Rahman MA, Butler GC, et al. Comparison of candoxatril and atrial natriuretic factor in healthy men. Effects on hemodynamics, sympathetic activity, heart rate variability, and endothelin. Hypertension 1995;26: 1160–6.

[14] Kahn JC, Patey M, Dubois-Rande JL, et al. Effect of sinorphan on plasma atrial natriuretic factor in congestive heart failure. Lancet 1990;335:118–9.

[15] Good JM, Peters M, Wilkins M, et al. Renal response to candoxatrilat in patients with heart failure. J Am Coll Cardiol 1995;25:1273–81.

[16] Trippodo NC, Robl JA, Asaas MM, et al. Cardiovascular effects of the novel dual inhibitor of neutral endopeptidase and angiotensin-converting enzyme BMS-182657 in experimental hypertension and heart failure. J Pharmacol Exp Ther 1995;275:745–52.

[17] Fournie-Zaluski MC, Coric P, Thery V, et al. Design of orally active dual inhibitors of neutral endopeptidase and angiotensin-converting enzyme with long duration of action. J Med Chem 1996;39:2594–608.

[18] Laurent S, Boutouyrie P, Azizi M, et al. Antihypertensive effects of fasidotril, a dual inhibitor of neprilysin and angiotensin-converting enzyme, in rats and humans. Hypertension 2000;35:1148–53.

[19] Wallis EJ, Ramsay LE, Hettiarachchi J. Combined inhibition of neutral endopeptidase and angiotensin-converting enzyme by sampatrilat in essential hypertension. Clin Pharmacol Ther 1998;64:439–49.

[20] Trippodo NC, Robl JA, Asaad MM, et al. Effects of omapatrilat in low, normal, and high renin experimental hypertension. Am J Hypertens 1998;11:363–72.

[21] Trippodo NC, Fox M, Monticello TM, et al. Vasopeptidase inhibition with omapatrilat improves cardiac geometry and survival in cardiomyopathic hamsters more than does ACE inhibition with captopril. J Cardiovasc Pharmacol 1999;34:782–90.

[22] McClean DR, Ikram H, Garlick AH, et al. The clinical, cardiac, renal, arterial and neurohormonal effects of omapatrilat, a vasopeptidase inhibitor, in patients with chronic heart failure. J Am Coll Cardiol 2000;36(2): 479–86.

[23] Rouleau JL, Pfeffer MA, Stewart DJ, et al. Comparison of vasopeptidase inhibitor, omapatrilat, and lisinopril on exercise tolerance and morbidity in patients with heart failure: IMPRESS randomized trial. Lancet 2000;356:615–20.

[24] Packer M, Cakiff RM, Konstam MA, et al. Comparison of omapatrilat and enalapril in patients with chronic heart failure. The Omapatrilat Versus Enalapril Randomized Trial of Utility in Reducing Events (OVERTURE). Circulation 2002;106:920–6.

[25] McClean DR, Ikram H, Mehta S, et al. Vasopeptidase inhibition with omapatrilat in chronic heart failure: acute and long-term hemodynamic and neurohumoral effects. J Am Coll Cardiol 2002;39(12):2034–41.

[26] Messerli FH, Nussberger J. Vasopeptidase inhibition and angioedema. Lancet 2000;356:608–9.

[27] Deedwania PC. Endothelin, the bad actor in the play: a marker or mediator of cardiovascular disease. J Am Coll Cardiol 1999;33:2007–18.
[28] Yanagisawa M, Kurihara H, Kimura S, et al. A novel potent vasoconstrictor peptide produced by vascular endothelial cells. Nature 1988;332:411–5.
[29] Giaid A, Yanagisawa M, Langleben D, et al. Expression of endothelin-1 in the lungs of patients with pulmonary hypertension. N Engl J Med 1993;328: 1732–9.
[30] Ohta K, Hirata Y, Imai T, et al. Cytokine-induced release of endothelin-1 from porcine renal epithelial cell line. Biochem Biophys Res Commun 1990;169: 578–84.
[31] Kohno M, Murakawa K, Yokokawa K, et al. Production of endothelin by cultured and porcine endothelial cells; modulation by adrenaline. J Hypertens 1989; 7(Suppl):S130–1.
[32] Piacentini L, Gray M, Honbo NY, et al. Endothelin-1 stimulates cardiac fibroblast proliferation through activation of protein kinase C. J Mol Cell Cardiol 2000;32:565–76.
[33] MacCarthy PA, Grocott-Mason R, Prendergast PD, et al. Contrasting inotropic effects of endogenous endothelin in the normal and failing human heart: studies with an intracoronary ETA receptor antagonist. Circulation 2000;101:142–7.
[34] Masaki T, Kimura S, Yanagisawa M, et al. Molecular and cellular mechanism of endothelin regulation: implications for vascular function. Circulation 1991; 84:1457–68.
[35] Pousset F, Isnard R, Lechat P, et al. Prognostic value of plasma endothelin-1 in patients with chronic heart failure. Eur Heart J 1997;18:254–8.
[36] Wei CM, Lerman A, Rodehoeffer RJ, et al. Endothelin in human congestive heart failure. Circulation 1994; 89:1580–6.
[37] McMurray JJ, Ray SG, Abdullah I, et al. Plasma endothelin in chronic heart failure. Circulation 1992; 85:1374–9.
[38] Rubin LJ, Badesch DB, Barst RJ, et al. Bosentan therapy for pulmonary arterial hypertension. N Engl J Med 2002;346:896–903.
[39] Sakai S, Miyauchi T, Kobayashi M, et al. Inhibition of myocardial endothelin pathway improves long-term survival in heart failure. Nature 1996;384:353–5.
[40] Fraccarollo D, Hu K, Galuppo P, et al. Chronic endothelin receptor blockade attenuates progressive ventricular dilatation and improves cardiac function in rats with myocardial infarction: possible involvement of myocardial endothelin system in ventricular remodeling. Circulation 1997;96:3963–73.
[41] Hu K, Gaudron P, Schmidt TJ, et al. Aggravation of left ventricular remodeling by a novel specific endothelin ET-A antagonist EMD94246 in rats with myocardial infarction. J Cardiovasc Pharmacol 1998; 32:505–8.
[42] Nguyen QT, Cernacek P, Sirois MG, et al. Long-term effects of non-selective endothelin A and B receptor antagonism in post-infarction rat: importance of timing. Circulation 2001;104:2075–81.
[43] Clozel M, Qiu C, Qiu CS, et al. Short-term endothelin receptor blockade with tezosentan has both immediate and long-term beneficial effects in rats with myocardial infarction. J Am Coll Cardiol 2002;39: 142–7.
[44] Bauersachs J, Fraccarollo D, Galuppo P, et al. Endothelin receptor blockade improves endothelial vasomotor dysfunction in heart failure. Cardiovasc Res 2000;47:142–9.
[45] Saad D, Mukherjee R, Thomas P, et al. The effects of endothelin-A receptor blockade during the progression of pacing-induced congestive heart failure. J Am Coll Cardiol 1998;32:1779–86.
[46] Teerlink J, Löffler BM, Hess P, et al. Role of endothelin in the maintenance of blood pressure in conscious rats with chronic heart failure. Circulation 1994;90:2510–8.
[47] Torre-Amione G, Young JB, Durnad JB, et al. Hemodynamic effects of tezosentan, an intravenous dual endothelin receptor antagonist, in patients with class III to IV congestive heart failure. Circulation 2001;103:973–80.
[48] Berger R, Stanek B, Hulsmann M, et al. Effects of ET-A receptor blockade on endothelial function in patients with chronic heart failure. Circulation 2001; 103:981–6.
[49] Mylona P, Cleland JG. Update of REACH-1 and MERIT-HF clinical trials in heart failure: Cardio.net Editorial Team. Eur J Heart Fail 1999;1:197–200.
[50] Kalra PR, Moon JC, Coats AJ. Do results of the ENABLE study spell the end for non-selective endothelin antagonism in heart failure? Int J Cardiol 2002;85:195–7.
[51] Luscher TF, Enseleit F, Pacher R, et al. Hemodynamic and neurohormonal effects of selective endothelin A (ET-A) receptor blockade in chronic heart failure: the Heart Failure ET-A Receptor Blockade Trial (HEAT). Circulation 2002;106:2666–72.
[52] Louis A, Cleland JG, Crabbe S, et al. Clinical trials update: CAPRICORN, COPERNICUS, MIRACLE, STAF, RITZ-2, RECOVER, and RENAISSANCE and cachexia and cholesterol in heart failure: highlights of the Scientific Sessions of the American College of Cardiology, 2001. Eur J Heart Fail 2001;3:381–7.
[53] Coletta AP, Cleland JG. Clinical trials update. Highlights of the scientific sessions of the XXIII Congress of the European Society of Cardiology: WARIS II, ESCAMI, PAFAC, RITZ-1, and TIME. Eur J Heart Fail 2001;3:747–50.
[54] O'Connor CM, Gattis WA, Adams KF, et al. Tezosentan in patients with acute heart failure and acute coronary syndromes: results of the Randomized Intravenous Tezosentan Study (RITZ-4). J Am Coll Cardiol 2003;41:1452–7.
[55] Kaluski E, Kobrin I, Zimlichman R, et al. RITZ-5: Randomized Intravenous Tezosentan for the treatment of pulmonary edema: a prospective, multicenter,

double-blind, placebo-controlled study. J Am Coll Cardiol 2003;41:204–10.

[56] Anand I, McMurray J, Cohn JN, et al. Long term effects of darusentan on left-ventricular remodeling and clinical outcomes in the ET-A Receptor Antagonist Trial in Heart Failure (EARTH): randomized, double-blind, placebo-controlled trial. Lancet 2004; 364:347–54.

[57] Wada A, Tsutamoto T, Fukai D, et al. Comparison of the effects of selective endothelin ET-A and ET-B receptor antagonists in congestive heart failure. J Am Coll Cardiol 1997;30:1385–92.

ELSEVIER
SAUNDERS

Heart Failure Clin 1 (2005) 103 – 127

HEART
FAILURE
CLINICS

Novel Neurohormonal Antagonist Strategies: Vasopressin Antagonism, Anticytokine Therapy, and Endothelin Antagonism in Patients Who Have Heart Failure

Olaf Hedrich, MD, John Finley, MD, Marvin A. Konstam, MD, James E. Udelson, MD*

Tufts–New England Medical Center and Tufts University School of Medicine, Boston, MA, USA

The evolution of the notion that neurohormonal activation is central to the progression of heart failure (HF) is based mainly on studies of the effects of inhibiting the renin–angiotensin–aldosterone system (RAAS) and sympathetic nervous system in this syndrome. The observed results have yielded pharmacologic modalities capable of reducing morbidity and mortality in this debilitating and costly condition. More recent characterization of additional, maladaptive responses in HF has identified further potential opportunities for therapeutic intervention. Among others, arginine vasopressin (AVP), inflammatory cytokines, and endothelin have been implicated in the progression of HF, and antagonists of each have undergone extensive evaluation for potential therapeutic benefit.

The role of vasopressin and vasopressin antagonists in heart failure

AVP recently has attracted attention as a potentially important neurohormonal mediator of the HF syndrome in humans [1]. A neurohypophysial hormone, vasopressin (also called *antidiuretic hormone* or ADH) helps regulate free water reabsorption, body fluid osmolality, blood volume, blood vessel vasoconstriction, and myocardial contractile function [2,3]. These biologic functions are subtended by two distinct receptors (V_{1a} and V_2), which in turn activate intracellular second messenger pathways with diverse effects [4]. Accordingly, this system represents a novel target for the treatment of HF, and several vasopressin antagonists are under development [5].

Pathophysiology

Vasopressin receptors

There are three distinct vasopressin receptors (V-R) through which vasopressin exerts its biologic effects (Table 1) [4]. V_{1a} (*vascular*) receptors are located on several diverse cell types, including vascular smooth muscle and cardiomyocytes. It is through this receptor that vasopressin assists in maintaining and regulating vascular tone and myocardial function [3]. V_2 (*renal*) receptors are expressed on the basolateral membrane of the renal collecting ducts, and mediate the antidiuretic effects of vasopressin. Intracellular events triggered by binding of vasopressin to the V_2 receptor include *shuttling* of aquaporin 2 water channels (AQP-2) from cytoplasmic vesicles to the luminal surface of the renal collecting duct cells where they are inserted into the cell membrane and facilitate water transport across the collecting duct cells (Fig. 1) [6,7]. V_2 receptor agonism also seems to promote increased de novo synthesis of AQP-2 channels. V_{1b} (*pituitary*) recep-

* Corresponding author. Division of Cardiology, Department of Medicine, Tufts–New England Medical Center and Tufts University School of Medicine, Box 70 NEMC, 750 Washington Street, Boston, MA 02111.
E-mail address: Judelson@tufts-nemc.org (J.E. Udelson).

1551-7136/05/$ – see front matter
doi:10.1016/j.hfc.2004.12.002

Table 1
Vasopressin receptor subtypes

Receptor subtypes	Alternative nomenclature	Site of action	AVP activation effects
V_{1a}	V_1-vascular receptor	Vascular smooth muscle cells	Vasoconstriction
		Platelets	Platelet aggregation
		Lymphocytes and monocytes	Coagulation factor release
		Adrenal cortex	Glycogenolysis
V_2	V_2-renal receptor	Basolateral membrane of distal nephron and renal collecting duct	Free water reabsorption
V_{1b}	V_3-pituitary receptor	Anterior pituitary	ACTH and β-endorphin release

Data from Lee CR, Watkins MI, Patterson JH, et al. Vasopressin: a new target for the treatment of heart failure. Am Heart J 2003;146:9–18.

tors are expressed on the surfaces of corticotrophic cells in the anterior pituitary, where they potentiate the release of adrenocorticotropic hormone (ACTH).

Vasopressin in heart failure

General concepts

Several studies have shown a significant elevation in plasma vasopressin concentration in the setting of heart failure [5,8–10]. In the neuroendocrine substudy of the Studies of Left Ventricular Dysfunction (SOLVD), patients who had left ventricular (LV) dysfunction had higher levels of vasopressin than control patients [10]. Patients with asymptomatic LV dysfunction (LV ejection fraction $\leq$ 35%) had higher mean vasopressin levels (AVP = 2.2 pg/mL) than their controls (AVP = 1.8 pg/mL). Individuals with mild to moderate symptoms of HF had even higher mean levels (AVP = 3.0 pg/mL) than their asymptomatic counterparts. A summary of vasopressin levels in several major HF populations is presented in Table 2. Not all studies or all patients in these studies demonstrate consistently elevated vasopressin levels compared with controls. These levels may be *inappropriately* elevated in HF relative to the state

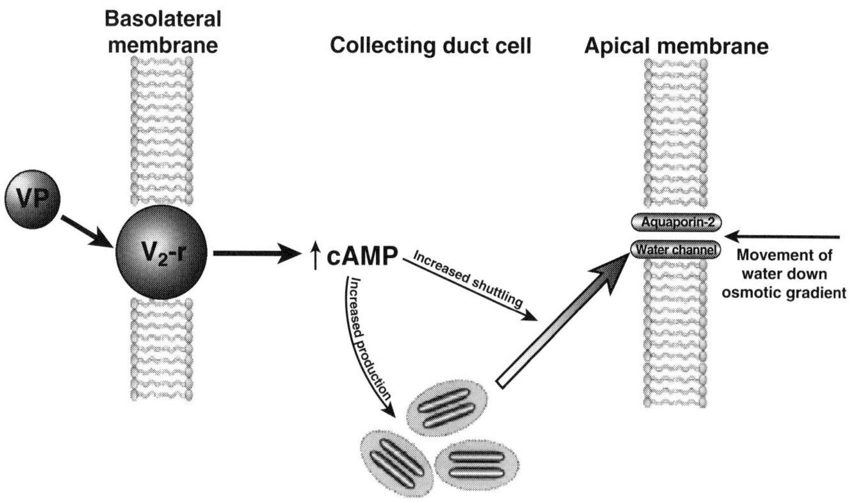

Fig. 1. Intracellular events in renal collecting duct cells in response to V_2 receptor stimulation. Upon binding with vasopressin, the V_2 receptor (on the basolateral membrane of the renal collecting duct cells) causes activation of adenylyl cyclase and subsequent synthesis of intracellular cyclic adenosine monophosphate (cAMP). AQP-2 water channels are "shuttled" from their cytoplasmic vesicles to the apical membrane, where they facilitate movement of free water across the apical membrane down an osmotic gradient. AQP-2 synthesis also is increased. (*From* Kalra PR, Anker SD, Coats AJS. Water and sodium regulation in chronic heart failure: the role of natriuretic peptides and vasopressin. Cardiovasc Res 2001;51:495–509; with permission.)

Table 2
Vasopressin levels measured by radioimunosorbent assay heart failure and other populations

Author, year [Ref.]	Patients	Mean AVP levels (pg/mL)	Comments
Creager et al, 1986 [24]	CHF, n = 10	2.4 ± 0.6	Vasodilators held at ×48 h
Nicod et al, 1985 [164]	CHF, n = 10	2.3 ± 0.8	—
Pruszczynski et al, 1984 [165]	CHF, n = 14	4.6 ± 0.3	On diuretics
	HTN, n = 8	2.9 ± 0.1	On diuretics
	CAD, n = 11	3.4 ± 0.2	Not on diuretics
Goldsmith et al, 1983 [8]	CHF, n = 31	9.5 ± 0.9	Vasodilators/diuretics held ×48 h; low-sodium diet
	NP, n = 51	4.7 ± .07	—
Goldsmith et al, 1983 [166]	CHF, n = 15	11.6 ± 5.5	Elevated baseline levels in HF patients did not increase in response to orthostatic stress
	NP, n = 9	5.3 ± 2.3	—
Szatalowicz et al, 1981 [9]	CHF, n = 9	4.6 ± 2.1	At serum (sodium) 137 mEq/L
Kramer et al, 1999 [11]	CHF, n = 20	14.5 ± 8.8[a]	—
		3.9 ± 1.0[b]	
Rouleau et al, 1993 [17]	Asx LVD, n = 534	1.8 ± 6.7	27% activated[c]
Gavras et al, 1984 [167]	NP, n = 12	1.1 ± 0.2	—
Francis et al, 1990 [10]	CHF, n = 80	3.5	Range 2.3–4.4[d]
	Asx LVD, n = 147	2.6	Range 1.7–3.0[d]
	NP, n = 54	2.9	Range 1.4–2.3[d]
Uretsky et al, 1985 [14]	CHF, n = 42	3.0 ± 2.5	—
	NP, n = 10	1.0 ± 0.4	—
Udelson et al, 2001 [42]	CHF, n = 142	2.1 ± 2.9 (median levels)	—

Abbreviations: Asx LVD, asymptomatic LV dysfunction; NP, normal patients.
[a] High AVP for plasma osmolality.
[b] Low AVP for plasma osmolality.
[c] SAVE trial population: 1.96 SD above age-matched controls.
[d] SOLVD population.

of plasma volume or osmolality, however, although studies often are not analyzed as such [11].

Although in the normal physiologic state there is a close relationship between plasma vasopressin levels and osmolality, this relationship seems to be disrupted in HF [12,13]. In a population of HF patients who received an osmotic load by means of mannitol infusion, vasopressin levels increased to a greater degree than in non-HF subjects, and baseline levels of vasopressin relative to plasma osmolality were higher in the HF patients than in their normal counterparts [14]. Although dysregulated, the overall sensitivity of the system seems to remain intact, but with an *upward shift* in plasma vasopressin levels.

Pathophysiologic effects of vasopressin in heart failure

To assess whether vasopressin is truly a neuroendocrine pathogen in the development and progression of HF, consideration must be given to its potential pathophysiologic role, and its association with long-term outcomes [15,16]. In multivariate analysis, vasopressin levels obtained 1 month after myocardial infarction in patients enrolled in the Survival and Ventricular Enlargement (SAVE) Study correlated independently with severe HF (relative risk [RR] = 1.6), recurrent myocardial infarction (RR = 2.3), and a combined endpoint measure of cardiovascular mortality or HF or myocardial infarction (RR = 1.6) [17]. This suggests that vasopressin levels in this setting have prognostic significance.

Effects on water balance. Elevated plasma vasopressin concentrations seem to be associated with impaired free water excretion in patients who have HF [9,12]. When comparing rats with mild, compensated HF without elevated LV end-diastolic pressure (LVEDP) or reduced plasma sodium concentration, rats with an elevated LVEDP and reduced plasma sodium had a significantly increased expression of AQP-2 mRNA [18]. Although these observations are helpful in explaining the clinical observations of volume expansion and hyponatremia in HF, the role for implicating vasopressin in these processes is strengthened by further experimental observations regarding selective inhibition of V_2 receptors in animals with HF.

VPA-985, a specific and selective nonpeptide V_2 receptor antagonist, is a potent aquaretic compound in dogs and rats [19]. Furthermore, in humans, a randomized, placebo-controlled study administering VPA-985 resulted in a significant, dosage-related increase in water excretion and resulting elevation of serum sodium concentration and serum osmolality in patients who had advanced HF [20]. In this study, an observed reduction in urinary AQP-2 protein levels suggested that the observed aquaresis may have been secondary to a reduction in AQP-2 expression at the level of the renal collecting duct.

Effects on hemodynamics. Under normal physiologic conditions, the vasoconstrictive effects of vasopressin usually are not associated with appreciable changes in arterial blood pressure at plasma levels within physiologic range [21]. When vasopressin is infused intravenously in patients who have HF, however, various hemodynamic effects have been observed [22]. In the setting of stepwise increments in vasopressin infusion, statistically significant and dosage-dependent increases in systemic vascular resistance (SVR) and pulmonary capillary wedge pressure (PCWP) occur, along with decreases in stroke volume (SV) and cardiac output (CO) (Fig. 2).

These hemodynamic effects are believed to be mediated primarily through activation of V_{1a} receptors on vascular smooth muscle cells, which promotes an increase in afterload by means of arteriolar vaso-

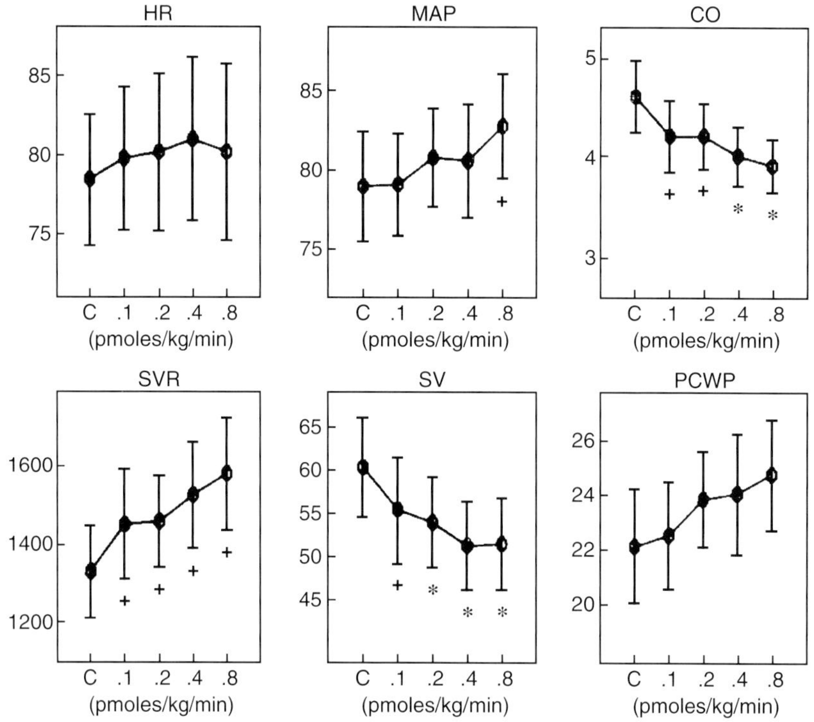

Fig. 2. Overall hemodynamic responses to infused arginine vasopressin. Data are shown as mean ± standard deviation for each infusion rate. The mean basal plasma arginine vasopressin level was 6.4 ± 39 pg/mL at peak infusion rate. During the infusion, heart rate (HR, beats/min) and mean arterial pressure (MAP, mm Hg) did not change, except for a small increase in blood pressure at the highest infusion rate. A statistically significant decline in CO (L/min) and SV (mL) was recorded, as was a statistically significant increase in SVR (dyne.s.cm^{-5}). There was significant overall variation ($P < .01$) in the PCWP (mm Hg), but no individual pairs attained statistical significance. Right atrial pressure and pulmonary artery pressure (not shown) did not change. (+ denotes $P < .05$, * $P < .01$, C denotes control group [no vasopressin].) (*From* Goldsmith SR, Francis GS, Cowley AW, et al. Hemodynamic effects of infused arginine vasopressin in congestive heart failure. J Am Coll Cardiol 1986; 8:779–83; with permission.)

constriction [23,24]. Indirect effects mediated by V_2 receptor agonism may result in increased water retention, however, which increases circulating blood volume and hence preload, with concomitant increases in PCWP and LV filling pressure. At the myocyte level, vasopressin may be positively inotropic, yet when factoring in the effects of vasoconstriction on the coronary arteries resulting in decreased coronary flow, elevated levels of vasopressin may on balance have a negatively inotropic effect on the failing heart, with an attending decline in SV and CO [15].

Supportive evidence for these hypotheses again comes from observational data using selective V_{1a} receptor antagonists in vivo [24], where significant improvements in SVR and CO were recorded when vasopressin levels were elevated (see Fig. 2). In a model of congestive HF (CHF) induced by rapid ventricular pacing in dogs, administration of the nonpeptide vasopressin antagonist OPC-21268 significantly increased CO and reduced total peripheral resistance [25]. A porcine model of CHF revealed improved ventricular loading conditions when the nonpeptide V_1 receptor antagonist SR49059 was administered, with reduced LV end-diastolic dimension and peak wall stress [26].

Effects on the myocardium. Vasopressin has been implicated in cardiac remodeling, and structural changes in myocardium exposed to high levels have been demonstrated in neonatal and adult myocytes [27–29]. In cultured neonatal rat myocardial cells, cellular hypertrophy by means of enhanced protein synthesis has been observed [27,28]. By means of exposure to V_{1a} receptor antagonists, the observed hypertrophy was inhibited significantly [27,28]. Myocardial V_{1a} receptor agonism increases intracellular calcium concentration as well as protein kinase C (PKC) activity [27,28], which is believed to be central in mediating the observed hypertrophic myocardial cell growth, not unlike effects ascribed to angiotensin II. Whether these structural changes translate into clinically significant outcomes in HF, or contribute to progression of the disease, is unknown.

Vasopressin antagonists

More comprehensive neurohormonal antagonism beyond angiotensin-converting enzyme (ACE) inhibition, β-adrenergic receptor-blockade, and aldosterone antagonism holds promise in modulating the long-term effects (and possibly outcome) of HF. In an effort to harness the potentially beneficial effects of decreasing the activity of vasopressin in this syndrome, in recent years selective and potent vasopressin receptor antagonists have been developed, several of which have reached the stage of human clinical trials designed to determine short- and long-term efficacy. Although vasopressin receptor antagonists have been available for several years, early animal studies used peptide analogs that were limited in their potential for long-term use by their relative species specificity in terms of receptor affinity, inadequate oral bioavailability, and short half-lives [5,30]. These characteristics hindered their further advancement to human trials.

Clinical trials of vasopressin receptor antagonists

V_2 receptor antagonists. V_2 receptor antagonism stimulates aquaresis in humans, with net loss of free water. Unlike with the administration of loop diuretics, antagonism of V_2 receptors does not seem to increase activation of the RAAS [31].

Tolvaptan (OPC-41061) is a specific and selective nonpeptide V_2 receptor antagonist without intrinsic agonist properties, and shown to have potent aquaretic properties in an animal model [32]. In cloned human receptors, the V_2:V_{1a} receptor selectivity was 29:1 [32]. Tolvaptan's half-life is between 6 and 8 hours. Dosage-dependent responses demonstrated in rats include markedly increased free water clearance, significantly less urinary loss of sodium than furosemide, and no significant effect on serum creatinine or BUN [31]. In comparison with furosemide, serum sodium increased in a dosage-dependent fashion in animals given tolvaptan [31], highlighting the drug's potential benefit in hyponatremia.

Prospective randomized trials published assessing the clinical usefulness of tolvaptan have focused on its use in chronic HF [33], and more recently in patients admitted with acutely decompensated HF, to evaluate its short- and intermediate-term effects [34].

In a double-blind study conducted in a group of 254 HF patients, three oral dosages of tolvaptan (30 mg, 45 mg, or 60 mg) given daily for 25 days were evaluated [33]. The study enrolled patients irrespective of LVEF. Abnormally elevated plasma concentrations of vasopressin (>8.0 pg/mL) were observed at baseline in only 6.3% of the patient population. Hyponatremia at baseline (defined as serum sodium $\leq$ 136 mEq/L) was encountered in approximately 30% of the population [35].

This study demonstrated a significant decrease in body weight and edema in modestly volume-overloaded CHF patients, increased urinary volume, and normalization of hyponatremia [33]. These effects were sustained over the full course of therapy.

A statistically significant decrease in body weight was observed on the first day when compared with placebo ($P < .001$), which was not dosage-dependent, and was similar in extent in all patients regardless of LVEF. This reduction was maintained until the end of the study period. Although fluid intake was increased in tolvaptan-treated patients compared with placebo, net fluid losses also were greater in these patients ($P < .05$ at each dosage). Urinary findings seemed to be dosage-dependent: urine osmolality decreased significantly in a dosage-dependent fashion at day 1, and mean decreases in urine sodium from baseline were significantly greater in tolvaptan-treated patients ($P < .05$). Serum sodium increased modestly at day 1 in tolvaptan-treated patients ($P < .0001$). In the hyponatremic subgroup, this was greater than in the normonatremic patients, and was sustained in 82% by the end of the treatment period (versus 40% of placebo-treated patients, $P < .05$) (Fig. 3). No significant changes in serum potassium levels or renal function were reported.

In the multicenter, randomized, double-blind, placebo-controlled ACTIV in CHF trial, three oral, daily dosages of tolvaptan (30 mg, 60 mg, or 90 mg) were compared with placebo in patients hospitalized with acute decompensated HF.

Body weight decreased significantly from baseline in all tolvaptan-treated groups on day 1 (a primary endpoint) when compared with placebo, decreased further during the course of hospitalization, and remained stable after discharge. This effect did not seem to be dosage-dependent. Similarly, urine volume on day 1 was significantly higher in all groups treated with tolvaptan than placebo, and this effect was maintained throughout the period of hospitalization. Diuretic use (defined by furosemide equivalents) decreased in all groups after discharge, but the mean dosage reduction was not significant. Hyponatremia (defined as serum sodium concentration < 136 mEq/L) was observed in 16% of patients randomized to tolvaptan. Serum sodium concentrations were observed to rise and often normalize in this cohort.

In the ACTIV in CHF trial, tolvaptan did not cause a decline in renal function, and no changes in serum potassium were noted. The absence of adverse effects on renal function seen in this trial and other preliminary investigations [36] is potentially important because worsening renal function during hospitalization for decompensated HF is common [37] and associated with an unfavorable hospital course and outcome.

Although no significant differences were observed in rates of rehospitalization or outpatient visits for HF, there was a trend toward longer event-free survival in the tolvaptan groups compared with placebo. In post hoc subgroup analysis, patients with elevated serum urea nitrogen (SUN) levels and severe sys-

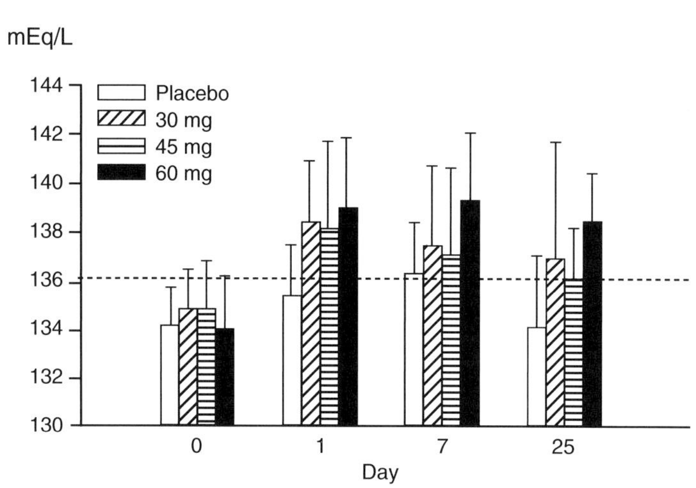

Fig. 3. Mean absolute changes in serum sodium concentration over time in a series of HF patients with hyponatremia (serum sodium < 136 mEq/L) treated with tolvaptan. These patients experienced greater increases in serum sodium than their normonatremic counterparts, and serum sodium concentration remained within normal range during the study. (*From* Gheorghiade M, Niazi I, Ouyang J, et al for the Tolvaptan Investigators. Vasopressin V_2-receptor blockade with tolvaptan in patients with chronic heart failure: results from a double-blind, randomized trial. Circulation 2003;107:2690–6; with permission.)

temic congestion who were treated with tolvaptan experienced lower total mortality rates, although the study was neither sufficiently powered nor prospectively designed to assess mortality.

Importantly, acutely decompensated HF patients with elevated SUN or severe congestion were at high risk for short-term mortality (22.5% and 17.8%, respectively). Whether the possible mortality benefit observed with tolvaptan in these groups is significant requires confirmation in appropriately powered studies.

A randomized, placebo-controlled investigation of 83 New York Heart Association (NYHA) functional Class-II and -III patients who had CHF and congestion who were taken off background diuretic therapy, salt restricted, and given either tolvaptan monotherapy (30 mg/d), furosemide monotherapy (80 mg/d), or a combination for 7 days, aimed at comparing tolvaptan with furosemide for volume reduction [38]. Tolvaptan-treated patients demonstrated a significant decline in body weight and increase in urine output compared with furosemide, whereas serum sodium increased within normal range without a change in serum potassium. These preliminary data suggest that vasopressin receptor antagonism in stable HF patients may reduce or even discontinue loop diuretics in some cases.

In a small open-label, randomized, placebo-controlled, crossover study in patients who had mild to moderate CHF designed to assess the effects of tolvaptan and furosemide on renal function and renal hemodynamics [36], tolvaptan increased urine output, glomerular filtration rate (GFR), and renal blood flow (RBF) to statistical significance. By comparison, furosemide increased urine output to a comparable degree, but at the expense of a decreasing GFR and RBF. This result supports current opinion that V_2 receptor antagonism may help preserve renal function in HF patients while promoting aquaresis.

In summary, the trial data suggest that tolvaptan possesses several properties of significant potential benefit in the treatment of CHF, including decreasing body weight and therefore congestion by increasing urine output, normalizing serum sodium concentration in hyponatremic patients, and possibly preventing a concomitant decline in renal function or significant electrolyte derangement commonly encountered with traditional diuretic regimens. Currently, phase-III studies are underway to assess further the potential benefit of tolvaptan in acute decompensated HF (particularly from a standpoint of mortality and outcome), as well as for the specific treatment of hyponatremia associated with various conditions, including HF.

Lixivaptan (VPA-985) is another specific, nonpeptide, orally active antagonist of the V_2 receptor undergoing evaluation for efficacy in HF and hepatic cirrhosis. Its binding affinity for V_2 receptors is approximately 100 times greater than for V_1 receptors. Dosage-dependent increases in urine output, free water clearance, and serum sodium concentration have been demonstrated in human studies of single dosages of lixivaptan administered to patients with NYHA Class-II and -III HF [20]. Lixivaptan has been evaluated in a multiple-dosage study of 44 patients with hyponatremia (etiologies of which included cirrhosis, CHF, and syndrome of inappropriate secretion of antidiuretic hormone) receiving dosages of 25 mg, 125 mg, or 250 mg orally twice daily for 7 days [39]. The observed effects included a significant overall aquaretic response compared with placebo, with significant dosage-related increases in free water clearance ($P < .05$) and serum sodium ($P < .05$), without significant changes in orthostatic blood pressure or serum creatinine levels. This agent therefore may hold promise in correcting abnormal renal water handling and hyponatremia in conditions associated with water retention. Although safe and effective at lower dosages, the higher dosage (250 mg) resulted in significant dehydration requiring withholding of dosages in 50% of the patients receiving this dosage. Further studies are required to determine the optimal dosage and indication for this new vasopressin antagonist.

V_{1a}/V_2 receptor antagonists. Because of the hemodynamic effects attributed to activation of the V_{1a} receptor in HF, there is a theoretical advantage in antagonizing the V_{1a} and V_2 receptors simultaneously. The result is conceivably a synergistic effect on systemic hemodynamic and renal parameters. The most extensively studied dual receptor vasopressin antagonist is conivaptan.

Conivaptan (YM087) is a nonpeptide vasopressin antagonist with high affinity for V_{1a} and V_2 receptors. Its binding affinities suggest more potent V_2 inhibition than V_{1a} inhibition [30]. Conivaptan may be administered orally and intravenously [40]. The effects of conivaptan on urinary parameters in the rat model, with or without captopril, increase urine volume and sodium concentration compared with placebo [41]. These results were sustained after a 25-day period of administration of conivaptan. Additionally, decreased intracellular free calcium and mitogen-activated protein kinase activity occurred in a dosage-dependent manner [28], suggesting a reduction of intracellular protein synthesis and, by extrapolation, cardiomyocyte hypertrophy. These observations are bolstered by the results of a rat infarct study of ventricular mass after 4 weeks of treatment with conivaptan, captopril, or combination [41], demonstrating a decrease in right ventricular mass compared with placebo, whereas the combination of captopril and conivaptan yielded a greater decrease in left and right ventricular mass, suggesting that vasopressin inhibition may play a role in remodeling after myocyte injury.

Human studies with conivaptan demonstrate that single dosage dual V_{1a}/V_2 antagonism results in significant, positive aquaretic and hemodynamic effects in patients who have HF. In a multicenter study of 142 patients who had severe HF (NYHA Class-III or -IV, LVEF 21%–26%), conivaptan was administered as a single intravenous dosage (10 mg, 20 mg, or 40 mg) and compared with placebo [42].

PCWP and right atrial pressure were reduced significantly after drug administration in the 20-mg ($P < .01$) and 40-mg ($P < .05$) conivaptan groups compared with placebo, without significant change in cardiac index (CI), pulmonary artery pressures, systemic or pulmonary vascular resistance, systemic arterial pressure, or heart rate. The peak effect on PCWP was sustained for approximately 8 hours after administration.

Urine output in the conivaptan-treated group was significantly greater than in the placebo group ($P < .001$), and demonstrated a dosage-dependent response that peaked 2 to 3 hours after the dosage was administered (Fig. 4). Similarly, urine osmolality was reduced significantly by all dosages of conivaptan ($P < .05$), without a significant change in serum osmolality, serum sodium, or serum potassium levels. AVP and serum sodium concentrations were normal on average, and there was no significant correlation between conivaptan effects and baseline levels of either. This suggests that the effects of conivaptan are apparent in a patient population beyond those with hyponatremia or elevated vasopressin levels. A preliminary study of oral conivaptan in relation to potential effects on functional capacity yielded less promising results, and conivaptan did not demonstrate efficacy in terms of improving exercise tolerance or quality of life [43].

In summary, conivaptan has promising properties for the treatment of HF, particularly with regard to increasing urine output and consequently improving hemodynamic parameters of congestion, as well as normalization of serum sodium concentrations in hyponatremic subjects. The intravenous form of conivaptan is undergoing continued development for potential use in hyponatremic states and acute decompensated HF [44]. Recent preliminary data suggest that intravenous administration of conivaptan significantly improves serum sodium in hyponatremic subjects [45].

Summary and future directions

Nonpeptide vasopressin antagonists have been developed that have several beneficial effects on the

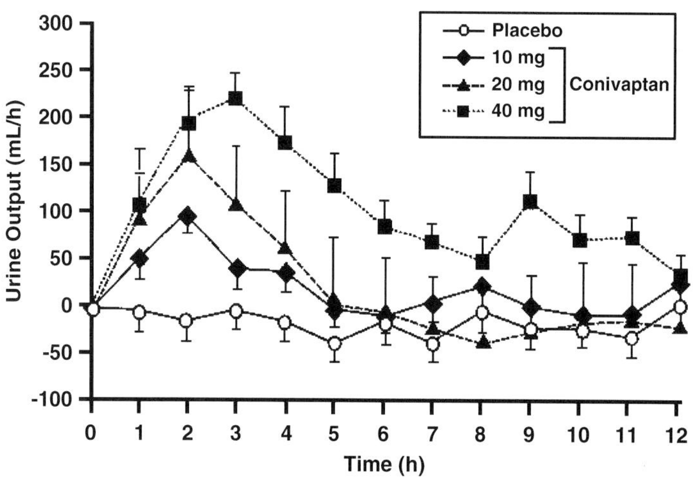

Fig. 4. Urine output rates for the groups randomized to conivaptan or placebo. There was a dosage-dependent increase in urine flow rates with increasing conivaptan dosage ($P < .001$). (*From* Udelson JE, Smith WB, Hendrix GH, et al. Acute hemodynamic effects of conivaptan, a dual V_{1a} and V_2 vasopressin receptor antagonist, in patients with advanced heart failure. Circulation 2001;104:2417–23; with permission.)

Table 3
Properties of vasopressin receptor blockers

Property	Tolvaptan (OPC-41061)	Lixivaptan (VPA-985)	SR-121463	Conivaptan (YM-087)
Receptor	V_2	V_2	V_2	V_{1a}/V_2
Selectivity (K_iV_{1a}:K_iV_2)	29:1	100:1	100:1	10:1
Administration route	Oral	Oral	Oral	IV
Urine volume	Increases	Increases	Increases	Increases
Urine osmality	Decreases	Decreases	Decreases	Decreases
Sodium excretion/24 h	No change (may increase)	No change (no dosage) Increases (high dosage)	No change	No change

Data from Lee CR, Watkins MI, Patterson, JH, et al. Vasopressin: a new target for the treatment of heart failure. Am Heart J 2003;146:9–18.

clinical syndrome of HF. These include a reduction in body fluid volume by promotion of aquaresis with maintenance of electrolyte homeostasis (with consequent symptomatic and hemodynamic improvements) and correction of hyponatremia (in HF as well as other hyponatremic states). The major properties of several vasopressin antagonists under development are summarized in Table 3. Of potentially major importance is that vasopressin antagonism largely maintains renal function in acute decompensated HF while procuring the above effects. Because volume reduction with standard diuretics often is accompanied by hyponatremia and renal function impairment (both of which have been associated with poor outcomes), this property may prove invaluable in managing HF in the future.

The role of cytokines and anticytokine strategies in heart failure

Since the 1990s, studies have examined the role of hormone-like molecules, cytokines, which play important roles in cellular interactions [46]. Cytokines promote inflammation, intravascular coagulation, oxidative stress, cardiac structural and functional abnormalities, endothelial injury, and cardiomyocyte or endothelial cell apoptosis [47,48].

Pathophysiology

Tumor necrosis factor-α

Tumor necrosis factor-α (TNF-α), a hormone-like molecule (157 amino acid polypeptide), exists as two bioactive forms, membrane-bound and secretory [49]. The many sources of TNF-α include activated macrophages (the main source), lymphocytes, fibroblasts, neutrophils, smooth muscle, and mast cells [50,51]. TNF-α acts at the cellular level through two receptors: type I (p55) (TNFRI) and type II (p75) (TNFRII), which are both found in human myocardium [52]. TNF-α seems to have an important role in regulating the nitric oxide metabolism in leukocytes, vascular endothelial cells, and vascular smooth muscle cells [53,54]. At the molecular and cellular levels, this proinflammatory cytokine can stimulate myocyte hypertrophy through the generation of reactive oxygen intermediates in cardiac myocytes, by inducing maladaptive ventricular remodeling. Remodeling may occur through stimulation of the extracellular matrix protein production and increased turnover of matrix by causing cardiomyocyte loss through necrosis and apoptosis [55–58].

The effects of TNF-α on the heart depend on the amount and duration of cytokine expression. Short-term expression of TNF-α may be an adaptive response to various forms of *stress*. Too much stress may create a maladaptive situation whereby TNF-α is overexpressed long term and produces cardiac decompensation [59]. The direct relationship between TNF-α levels and the clinical manifestations and progression of CHF (Fig. 5) has been documented in multiple studies [34,59,60,62,63].

Analysis of cytokines in the Vesnarinone Evaluation of Survival Trial (VEST) [64] included over 1200 patients who had advanced HF, and showed that TNF-α was an independent predictor of mortality. TNF-α levels were increased significantly in patients who had ischemic heart disease compared with patients who had dilated cardiomyopathy [64].

Before human trials, translational studies reported the overexpression of TNF-α in mice models. A landmark study demonstrated that a myopathy attributed to continuous infusion of TNF-α could be reversible with termination of the infusion [65]. Other studies examined overexpression of TNF-α and the

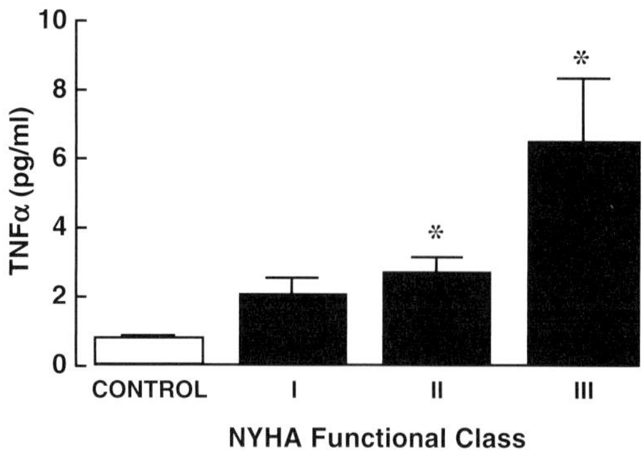

Fig. 5. Levels of TNF-α in normal subjects and patients with NYHA functional class I to III HF. Compared to age-matched normal subjects (*open bar*), the plasma TNF-α levels for patients with HF (*solid bars*) were elevated in direct proportion to the patients in NHYA classes I–III ($P < .001$ by analysis of variance). (* $P < .05$ versus normal subjects.) (*From* Torre-Amione G, Kapadia S, Benedict CR, et al. Proinflammatory cytokine levels in patients with depressed left ventricular ejection fraction: a report from the studies of left ventricular ejection fraction (SOLVD). J Am Coll Cardiol 1996;27:1201–6; with permission.)

cellular effects after adenoviral tranduction of its soluble receptor (sTNFR) or treatment with anti-TNF monoclonal antibody. The increased activity of sTNFR and anti-TNF monoclonal antibody separately ameliorated the biologic harm that TNF-α caused at the cellular level [65–68]. These models established the link between TNF-α and HF and helped fuel the research on anticytokine strategies in HF.

Interleukin-6

Interleukin-6 (IL-6) and other related cytokines play a pivotal role in regulating cardiac myocyte hypertrophy and apoptosis. Several studies have associated high levels of IL-6 in the setting of CHF [61,69–73]. IL-6 has a significant correlation with right heart pressures in human HF [72]. One study has suggested that IL-6 is the most powerful predictor of HF episodes, death, or need for heart transplantation in severe CHF patients [73]. IL-6 levels were more predictive of these events than TNF-α levels, plasma neurohormone levels, and LV systolic function.

Soluble cytokine receptors

The extracellular domain fragments of TNF receptors shed from the cell surfaces, and soluble forms remain in the circulation (sTNFRI and sTNFRII) [74]. The soluble receptors play a role in immunomodulation by binding to TNF-α, to prevent binding to the receptors on the cell surface and also preventing destabilization of TNF-α to inactive monomers [74]. High concentrations of sTNFRI and sTNFRII, as seen in patients who have severe CHF, could inhibit the pathologic increase of TNF-α activity [75–77]. Soluble TNFRs potentially can act like anti-TNF molecules. On one hand, their presence could act as protection to the amplification of TNF-α in HF. On the other hand, these soluble receptors may be a *carrier* protein that merely reflects increases in response to high TNF-α levels [78].

Anticytokine therapeutic strategies

Broad-spectrum anticytokine therapy

Pentoxifylline. **Background:** Pentoxifylline is a xanthine derivative used in the treatment of peripheral vascular disease. Pentoxifylline is believed to increase intracellular levels of cyclic adenosine monophosphate (cAMP) and decrease the level of inflammatory mediators by blocking the translation of inflammatory mediators at the transcription level (Fig. 6) [79]. Pentoxifylline inhibits and reduces production of TNF-α in vitro and in vivo [80,81]. **Clinical studies:** In a single-center, prospective, randomized trial [82], 28 participants were randomized to placebo or treatment with pentoxifylline, 400 mg three times per day. After 6 months, the proportion of patients in NYHA Class I or II was higher in the pentoxifylline group than in the placebo group (14/14 versus 10/14; $P = .01$), and ejection fraction was higher (mean 38.7% [standard deviation 15.0] versus 26.8% [standard deviation 11.0], $P = .04$), and TNF-α plasma concentrations were significantly lower (2.1 pg/mL [standard deviation 1.0] versus 6.5 pg/mL [standard deviation 5.0], $P = .001$) [81]. A second small prospective, randomized, placebo-controlled study involving pentoxifylline showed that, after 6 months, LVEF improved (from 24% ± 9% to 31% ± 13%, $P < .03$) in the treatment group.

Vesnarinone. **Background:** Vesnarinone is a positive inotropic agent that enhances cardiac contractility through multiple mechanisms, including an increase in the inward calcium influx attributable to elevated cAMP levels through phosphodiesterase inhibition [83,84]. In vitro, vesnarinone inhibits the production of proinflammatory cytokines in human cell lines [85–87], and in HF patients whose blood was stimulated from lipopolysaccharide [88]. **Clinical studies:** Initial small-scale studies with vesnarinone reported beneficial effects on quality of life, as well as morbidity and mortality in patients who had advanced HF [89–92]. In the VEST trial, treatment with vesnarinone, 30 mg or 60 mg, had no effect on circulating levels of cytokines (TNF-α, IL-6) or cytokine receptors (sTNFR1, sTNFR2, sIL-6R) in patients who had advanced HF.

Targeting tumor necrosis factor-α

Fig. 6 shows potential molecular targets for antagonizing proinflammatory cytokine expression. The two approaches described below specifically target a single cytokine, TNF-α, unlike the other broad-spectrum anticytokine therapies described above.

Etanercept. **Background:** Etanercept (Enbrel) is recombinant human soluble TNF receptor. This drug acts by binding to soluble (circulating) TNF-α and functionally inactivates TNF-α by preventing it from binding to its receptors on cell surfaces. Etanercept has a long half-life (median approximately 5 days) and is administered by subcutaneous injection. Treatment with etanercept is clinically effective in patients who have rheumatoid arthritis, ankylosing spondylitis, and psoriasis, although it has not been effective in treatment of Crohn's disease or severe sepsis [93–97]. **Clinical studies:** After initial in vivo studies in rats showed that etanercept reversed some deleterious effects of TNF-α [67,98], early human studies showed that a single intravenous infusion of etanercept was tolerable, and seemed to improve functional status, increase LVEF, and decrease LV volume in HF patients [99]. In the ENEBREL study [99], 47 patients with NYHA Class-III to -IV symptoms and LVEF < 35% were administered biweekly injections of etanercept for 3 months in addition to standard background therapy. The 3-month use of etanercept resulted in a significant dosage-related increase in LVEF, decrease in LV volumes, and improved remodeling, and showed a trend toward improvement in functional status [99].

These promising results led to an ambitious pivotal trial program, encompassing two multicenter

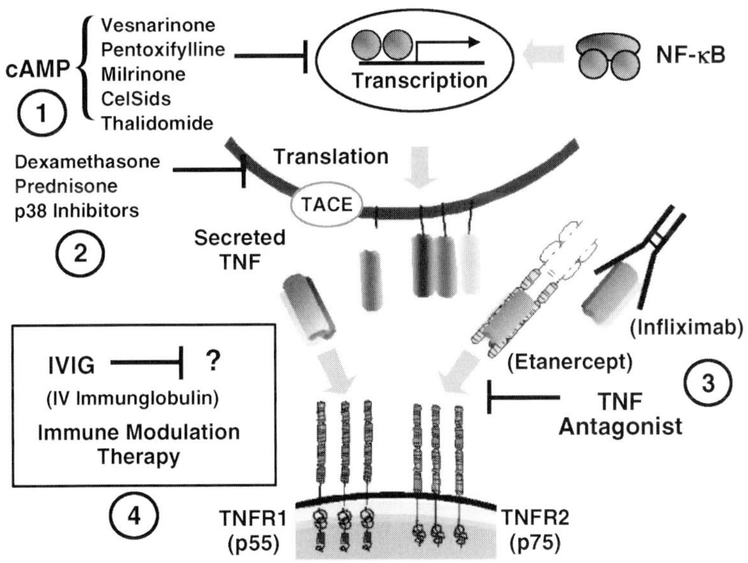

Fig. 6. Therapeutic strategies for antagonizing proinflammatory mediators. TNF gene transcription is mediated, in part, by activation of NF-κB. Agents that increase intracellular levels of cAMP (1), such as vesnarinone, petoxifylline, milrinone, thalidomide, and thalidomide analogues (CelSids), decrease the level of inflammatory mediators through transcriptional blockade of inflammatory gene expression. Agents such as dexamethasone and prednisone and some p38 inhibitors suppress inflammation by blocking the translation of inflammatory mediators (2). Secreted TNF can be neutralized (3) by soluble TNF antagonists (etanercept) or by neutralizing antibodies (infliximab) that prevent TNF from binding to its cognate type 1 (p55) and type 2 (p75) TNF receptors. In addition to these targeted approaches, immunomodulatory strategies with IVIG (4) and IMT with irradiated whole blood have been used. (*From* Mann DL. Inflammatory mediators and the failing heart: past, present, and the foreseeable future. Circ Research 2002;91:988–98; with permission.)

trials, the Research into Etanercept Cytokine Antagonism in Ventricular Dysfunction (RECOVER) and the Randomized Etanercept North American Strategy to Study Antagonism of Cytokines (RENAISSANCE), which together comprised the Randomized Etanercept Worldwide Evaluation (RENEWAL) [100]. The two similar double-blind, randomized, placebo-controlled clinical each enrolled NYHA Class-II to -IV CHF patients with LVEF $\leq$ 30% (1500 combined for RENEWAL). In RECOVER, patients were randomized to one of three groups: (1) placebo, (2) etanercept, 25 mg subcutaneously once a week, (3) and entanercept, 25 mg subcutaneously twice a week. In RENAISSANCE, patients differed in the treatment groups in that they received entanercept, 25 mg subcutaneously, either twice or three times a week. The inclusion criteria also required a 6-minute walk distance of < 375 m (or < 425 m if hospitalized for CHF within the previous 6 months). The primary endpoint findings from RENEWAL, RENAISSANCE, and RECOVER are summarized in Table 4 [84]. On the basis of prespecified stopping rules, both trials were terminated prematurely owing to lack of benefit. Contrary to prior preclinical and clinical studies, etanercept had no effect on clinical status in RENAISSANCE (P = .17) or RECOVER (P = .34) and had no effect on the death or CHF hospitalization endpoint in RENEWAL (etanercept to placebo RR = 1.1%, 95% confidence interval [CI] 0.91–1.33, P = .33) [99]. RENAISSANCE seemed to suggest that etanercept (25 mg, twice a week, 29%) worsened patients compared with placebo (20%). Etanercept-treated patients showed a trend (P = .067) toward more infections in RECOVER but not in RENAISSANCE [100].

Infliximab. **Background:** Infliximab is a recombinant immunoglobulin G1-κ, human-murine chimeric monoclonal antibody that specifically and potently binds to and neutralizes the soluble TNF-α homotrimer and its membrane-bound precursor, as well as lysing TNF-α–expressing cells through complement fixation [101]. This treatment is effective in moderate-to-severe Crohn's disease when conventional therapies are inadequate and for active rheumatoid arthritis refractory to methotrexate [102]. **Clinical studies:** In the Anti-TNF Therapy Against Congestive Heart Failure (ATTACH) trial [103], patients were divided into three groups to receive either placebo; infliximab, 5 mg/kg; or infliximab, 10 mg/kg at 0, 2, and 6 weeks after randomization with a follow-up period of 28 weeks. Neither dosage of infliximab improved clinical status at 14 weeks, the primary endpoint of the study. Inflammatory markers (IL-6 and C-reative protein) were suppressed in dosage-dependent manner at 14 weeks and then gradually returned toward baseline by 28 weeks. Measured serum levels of TNF-α in the infliximab groups also were reduced immediately after each infusion, but were elevated at all other points throughout the 28-week period. Accompanying the reduction of proinflammatory markers was a corresponding modest increase in ejection fraction in the patients receiving infliximab, 5 mg/kg (P = .013). The combined risk for death from any cause or hospitalization for HF through 28 weeks was increased in the patients randomized to infliximab, 10 mg/kg (hazard ratio 2.84, 95% CI 1.01–7.97; nominal P = .043). Thus, based on the ATTACH trial, short-term infliximab administration had no benefit to HF patients and at high dosages (10 mg/kg) may worsen the clinical condition of patients who have moderate-to-severe CHF [103]. In addition to these findings from prospective trials, the US Food and Drug Administration (FDA) made a postmarketing report of 47 cases of new or worsening CHF in patients on anti–TNF-α therapy for those with rheumatoid arthritis or Crohn's disease [104]. After TNF antagonist therapy, 38 patients (26 receiving etanercept and 12 receiving infliximab) developed new-onset CHF,

Table 4
Risk ratios for all-cause mortality/congestive heart failure hospitalizations in the etanercept trials

	Dosage of etanercept			
Trial	25 mg/wk	25 mg/×2 wk	25 mg/×3 wk	25 mg/×2 wk + ×3 wk
RECOVER	1.01 (0.7–1.4)	0.87 (0.61–1.24)	—	—
RENAISSANCE	—	1.21 (0.92–1.58)	1.23 (0.94–1.61)	—
RENEWAL	—	1.08 (0.87–1.33)	—	1.10 (0.91–1.33)

Values represent the risk ratio (95% confidence interval).
Data from Mann DL, McMurray JJ, Packer M, et al. Targeted anticytokine therapy in patients with chronic heart failure: results of the Randomized Etanercept Worldwide Evaluation (RENEWAL). Circulation 2004;109:1594–602.

and nine patients (three receiving etanercept and six receiving infliximab) experienced CHF exacerbation. Nineteen of the 38 patients (50%) with new-onset CHF (12 receiving etanercept and seven receiving infliximab) had no identifiable risk factors. In 10 patients younger than 50 years of age, new-onset HF developed after they received TNF antagonists. These data from the FDA were composed using MedWatch, a passive postmarket surveillance program, which may underestimate events. Explanations as to why the anti-TNF therapies may have been harmful include the possibility that there was excessive TNF suppression or loss of the beneficial aspects of cytokine signaling in these studies. Another theory is that there is a "TNF rebound" and complement fixation. Infliximab can fix to complement located on the surface of the cells expressing TNF-α, and in vitro is directly cytotoxic to myocytes [95]. Failing myocytes especially express TNF-α on their cell surfaces, and have been postulated to be particularly susceptible to infliximab, which could make matters worse in the setting of HF [103].

Immunomodulatory strategies

Intravenous immunoglobulin. **Background:** The exact mechanism of action of intravenous immunoglobulin (IVIG) is unknown. It is believed to act by either Fc receptor blockade, neutralization of autoantibodies, modulation of cytokine activity, or activation of an inhibitory Fc receptor [105]. An initial report by McNamara and colleagues [106] claimed that IVIG was beneficial in acute cardiomyopathy, which led to the hypothesis that IVIG could downregulate inflammatory responses in CHF patients and have potential benefits on LVEF. **Clinical studies:** Gullestad and colleagues [107] performed a randomized, double-blind clinical trial involving 40 patients who had chronic CHF and LVEF < 40%. Patients were randomized to receive IVIG therapy or placebo for 26 weeks. IVIG treatment induced a significant rise compared with placebo in plasma levels of the anti-inflammatory mediators interleukin-10 (IL-10), IL-1 receptor antagonist, and soluble TNFRs. LVEF showed a significant increase from 26% ± 2% to 31% ± 3% ($P < .01$) with IVIG therapy regardless of HF etiology. Levels of N-terminal pro–atrial natriuretic peptide also were decreased significantly once IVIG therapy was started and this trend continued throughout treatment ($P < .001$) [107]. This preliminary study suggested that IVIG therapy could cause a net anti-inflammatory effect in CHF and ultimately improve LV function in addition to conventional cardiovascular care in these patients.

Immune modulation therapy. **Background:** Immune modulation therapy (IMT) uses a medical device (the VC7000 Blood Treatment System, Vasogen, Mississauga, Ontario) to expose a patient's blood sample to a variety of physiochemical stressors ex vivo [79]. That same treated blood sample then is administered intramuscularly back to the patient. The theory is that these stressors will initiate and facilitate apoptotic cell death, and that the apoptotic cells will be taken up by macrophages and ultimately downregulate proinflammatory cytokines and upregulate production of anti-inflamatory cytokines [108–110]. **Clinical studies:** Initial studies showed that IMT decreased production of proinflammatory cytokines in HF patients [100], and may restore the homeostasis between proinflammatory and anti-inflammatory states. Another recent trial enrolled 73 patients with moderate HF and showed that the group receiving IMT experienced fewer hospitalizations (24 versus 41) and deaths (1 versus 7) compared with the placebo groups. The IMT groups also showed increased quality of life and NYHA clinical classification [111,112]. These trials were limited in size but showed some promise, now being explored in larger trials.

Summary and future directions. The role of cytokines in the development and progression of HF is complex. There is substantial evidence to support a role for cytokines as an important influence in the syndrome of HF.

Why were these anticytokine therapies not beneficial and possibly harmful? Of the patients enrolled in RENEWAL and ATTACH, only 3% and 5%, respectively, fell into NYHA Class IV [101,103]. Because there is a known correlation between the level of TNF-α and the severity of HF, the patients with the most cachexia, the greatest degree of exercise impairment, and likely the highest TNF-α levels may have been more ideal candidates. Another important factor could be the pharmacogenomic variability of the HF patients selected.

Another theory suggests that TNF-α blockers are intrinsically cytotoxic to failing myocytes [113,114]. Infliximab is directly cytotoxic to failing myocytes by complement fixation and results in sustained myocarditis and cardiac myocyte lysis mediated by the complement membrane attack complex [115]. Etanercept can act as a carrier protein, which essentially can stabilize TNF-α and in turn will accumulate increased amounts of TNF-α in circulation [116]. TNF-α bound to etanercept does not remain so for long, but dissociates with a fast off rate (approximately 620 ms) [117]. The duration of TNF-α bioactivity becomes extended, which may act as a "stimulating antagonist" and worsen CHF, the opposite of the intended effect [118].

A third explanation as to why TNF-α antagonism failed to benefit and showed detrimental effect in HF is that TNF-α may confer cytoprotective effects in the heart during acute ischemic injury [119–121]. Low physiologic levels likely play a role in tissue remodeling and repair [122]. It is speculated that the current therapies tested disrupt homeostasis and lower the physiologic levels past the minimal amount required to repair the myocardium [122].

Despite the failures of certain anticytokine therapies, especially etanercept and infliximab, other strategies using small molecules with broad-spectrum antiinflammatory properties (pentoxiphylline, thalidomide or its analogs, and statins) and immunomo-

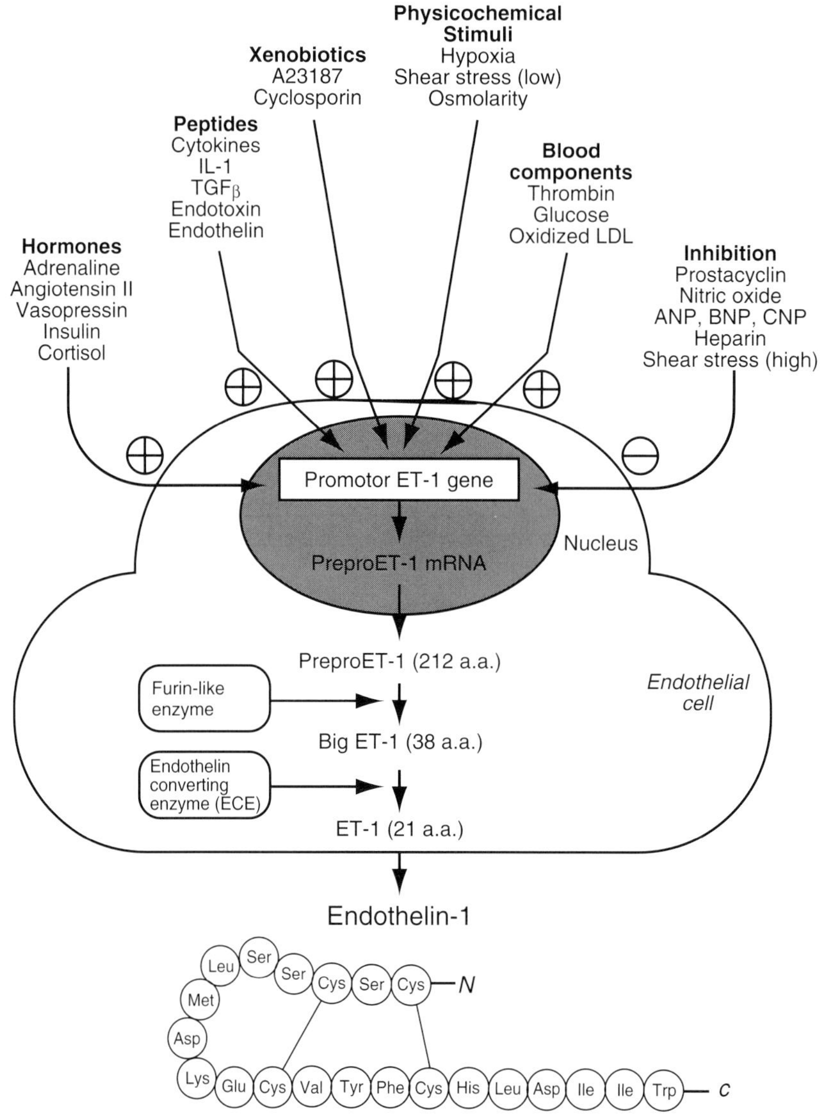

Fig. 7. A schematic summary of endothelin synthesis and regulation. ANP/BNP/CNP, atrial, b-, and c-type natriuretic peptides, respectively; IL-1, interleukin-1; LDL, low-density lipoprotein; TGF-β, transforming growth factor β. (*From* Webb DJ, Strachan FE. Clinical experience with endothelin antagonists. Am J Hypertens 1998;11:71–9S; with permission.)

dulatory strategies (IVIG and IMT) have shown some promise in preliminary clinical trials [79]. Only through future research and large clinical trials will the fate of these therapies ultimately be determined.

The role of endothelin and endothelin antagonists in heart failure

The discovery of endothelin, a novel vasoactive peptide in the medium of cultured porcine endothelial cells by Yanagisawa and colleagues in 1988 [123], prompted the proliferation of considerable scientific data, which has resulted in the definition of the components of the human endothelin system [124].

Pathophysiology: the endothelin system

Synthesis and release of endothelin

Three human isoforms of endothelin have been cloned and sequenced: endothelin-1 (ET-1), endothelin-2 (ET-2), and endothelin-3 (ET-3). ET-1 is the predominant isoform generated in the vasculature, as well as the most potent vasoconstrictor, and as such is of greatest significance in cardiovascular hemodynamic regulation. ET-2 has been identified in the kidney and intestines where it exerts vasoconstrictive effects, but it is not present in human plasma. The major source of ET-3, which has minimal vasoconstrictive properties and is usually present at plasma concentrations probably insufficient to exert a direct influence on vascular tone, is unclear.

ET-1 is synthesized in a paracrine fashion by vascular endothelial cells [123–125], and is secreted abluminally (ie, toward the adjacent vascular smooth muscle). Autocrine synthesis in (and secretion from) cardiac myocytes and fibroblasts also has been described [126,127]. Analagous to the tissue RAAS, it has been hypothesized that such local secretion can result in high local myocardial ET-1 concentrations, which may in turn affect cardiomyocyte structure and function.

Endothelin synthesis is believed to be regulated primarily at the gene transcription level. The product of ET-1 gene transcription is preproendothelin-1, a 212 amino acid peptide, which is cleaved by an endoprotease to generate "big endothelin", a 38 amino acid peptide [123]. Big endothelin undergoes enzymatic conversion to the mature, biologically active ET-1 by intracellular endothelin-converting enzyme (ECE), of which the predominant type (ECE-1) is found in the myocardium, striated muscle, and renal medulla [128]. The half-life of endothelin is less than 5 minutes; it is cleared efficiently in the pulmonary and renal circulation by receptor binding and neutral endopeptidase metabolism [129,130]. Fig. 7 presents a schematic summary of endothelin synthesis and regulation.

Endothelin receptors

Humans have two distinct, high-affinity endothelin receptor subtypes—endothelin receptor type A (ET-A) and type B (ET-B) —through which the biologic functions of ET-1 are mediated (Table 5) [131]. Both receptor subtypes have been identified in various human tissues. ET-A receptor mRNA can be detected ubiquitously, with highest expression in aorta, heart, and kidney. The ET-A receptor is expressed principally on vascular smooth muscle cells [132] and cardiac myocytes [133], but has not been demonstrated on endothelial cells. Stimulation of ET-A and ET-B receptors on vascular smooth muscle cells results in vasoconstriction [134], brought about by an inositol trisphosphate-mediated rapid rise in intracellular [Ca^{2+}], a sustained rise in intracellular [Ca^{2+}] through the opening of membrane calcium channels, and an increase in the calcium-responsiveness of the contractile apparatus mediated by diacylglycerol-activated PKC. The latter mecha-

Table 5
Endothelin receptor subtypes and the cardiovascular system

Receptor	ET-A	ET-B
Agonist affinity	ET-1 > ET-2 > ET-3	ET-1 ≈ ET-2 ≈ ET-3
Tissue distribution	Vascular smooth muscle cells	Vascular smooth muscle cells
	Cardiac myocytes	Endothelial cells
Action	Vasoconstriction	Vasoconstriction
	Inotropy	Vasodilation
	Myocyte hypertrophy	—

nism has been invoked as an explanation for the observed positive inotropic effects of ET-1 [135]. ET-A stimulation by ET-1 further results in myocyte and fibroblast cellular proliferation [136]. ET-B stimulation on endothelial cells brings about vasodilation as a result of the release of nitric oxide, prostacyclin, and thromboxane A_2 [137].

The endothelin system in heart failure

Circulating ET-1 levels, as well as tissue ET-1 levels, are increased in patients who have HF compared with normal subjects [138–141]. Several explanations for this observation have been postulated, among which is the suggestion from animal studies that this rise may be caused in part by the direct action of angiotensin II, which is elevated in HF and seems to stimulate ET-1 production and release from the endothelium. Decreased clearance by the pulmonary vasculature in circumstances of pulmonary hypertension has been demonstrated, and may play an additional role in the elevation of plasma ET-1 concentration [129]. Furthermore, failing myocardium itself may be an important source of ET-1 release in HF [142].

In symptomatic patients who have HF (without regard for etiology), plasma ET-1 achieved levels two to three times those found in normal controls, which correlated with an increase in pulmonary arterial pressures and pulmonary vascular resistance [138]. In univariate analysis, elevated plasma ET-1 levels in HF patients have been correlated positively with clinical severity of HF (increased NYHA functional class, reduced exercise capacity) [141–143].

To the extent that plasma ET-1 (and big endothelin) levels reflect disease severity in HF, correlation also has been shown between endothelin level and prognosis. An elevated plasma ET-1 level (> 5 pg/mL) was the most significant prognostic marker of outcome in a series of 120 patients with ischemic or nonischemic cardiomyopathy: patients with increased plasma ET-1 had a significantly higher 1-year mortality rate than those with normal values [144]. Plasma ET-1 also may have prognostic value in patients suffering an acute ischemic event, irrespective of underlying cardiac function. Plasma ET-1 concentration was determined in 142 patients on day 3 after a documented myocardial infarction and was related to 1-year mortality [145].

Experimental data from human studies of dilated cardiomyopathy show that, beyond the observed increase in ET-1 concentration in plasma and at a local tissue level, there is an up-regulation in number and density of ET-A receptors on cardiac myocytes, without a change in ET-B receptor density (and possibly a down-regulation in ET-B density) [135,141]. The left ventricle seems to be most affected by these changes [141]. There seems to be more of an up-regulation in receptor density in nonischemic than in ischemic cardiomyopathy [135,146].

The endothelin system in HF therefore seems to be activated in a manner similar to other neurohormonal and cytokine systems, suggesting that the endothelin system may play an important role in the progression of HF.

Endothelin receptor antagonists in experimental heart failure

In a rat study of myocardial infarction, the selective ET-A receptor antagonist BQ-123 improved 12-week survival of treated rats and improved hemodynamic indices, suggesting amelioration of cardiac dysfunction and prevention of remodeling [147]. These results suggested that inhibition of an upregulated myocardial endothelin system may be an important therapeutic target in HF.

The nonselective ET-A/ET-B receptor-antagonist bosentan was studied in a dog model of pacing-induced HF [148]. Bosentan decreased systemic arterial pressure significantly in the early and established phases of HF, and also increased stroke volume significantly in late HF with systolic dysfunction.

Enrasentan, another nonselective ET-A/ET-B receptor-antagonist, was evaluated in a rat model of hypertensive cardiac hypertrophy and dysfunction [149]. Sixteen-week survival was significantly better than controls, and improvements in SV and CI, indices of LV mass, and circulating aldosterone were observed, again suggesting that combined ET-A/ET-B receptor antagonism has the potential to attenuate ventricular remodeling in the experimental setting.

Endothelin receptor antagonists in human heart failure

In an early clinical trial involving the short-term intravenous administration of bosentan, in patients withdrawn from ACE inhibitor therapy, increases in CO and decreases in systemic and pulmonary vascular resistance were observed [150]. In the presence of ACE inhibition, similar trends were observed [151]. Darusentan, a selective ET-A receptor antagonist, also has been associated with favorable hemodynamic changes after short-term administration [152].

The nonselective ET-A/ET-B receptor antagonist tezosentan was studied in the RITZ (Randomized Intravenous Tezosentan) Trials, a set of four studies of tezosentan in patients who had acutely decompensated HF requiring hospitalization. RITZ-1 was designed to assess the effect of intravenous tezosentan for 24 to 72 hours on patient assessment of dyspnea (primary endpoint) and time to death or worsening HF (secondary endpoints) [153]. There was no improvement in either the primary or secondary endpoints, and the dosage of tezosentan used resulted in higher than expected rates of hypotension, dizziness, and renal failure in the treatment group.

RITZ-2, designed to assess acute hemodynamic effects of tezosentan in an acute HF population, randomized 285 patients to either placebo or one of two dosages (50 or 100 mg/h intravenously) of tezosentan [154]. Both dosages significantly increased CI, and substantially reduced PCWP. In the multicenter, randomized, double-blind RITZ-4 trial, the effect of a 48-hour infusion of tezosentan was evaluated in 193 patients who had acute HF in association with acute coronary syndromes [155]. There was no significant improvement in the primary endpoint (a composite of death, worsening HF, recurrent ischemia, and recurrent or new myocardial infarction) in the tezosentan group over those receiving placebo. Furthermore, as in RITZ-1, symptomatic hypotension was encountered more frequently in the treatment group, which was believed to have contributed in part to the increased number of adverse events recorded in this group. The investigators concluded that the dosage of tezosentan used was too high. RITZ-5 evaluated tezosentan when added to standard medical therapy for acute pulmonary edema [156]. Eighty-four patients were randomized to receive tezosentan intravenously for up to 48 hours or placebo. There was no significant change in arterial oxygen saturation from baseline, the primary endpoint. Taken together, these trials did not support a major role for tezosentan in the setting of acute decompensated HF.

The REACH-1 Study (Research on Endothelin Antagonism in Chronic Heart Failure) [157] randomized 370 patients with severe HF to bosentan versus placebo. This trial was terminated prematurely because of the incidence of asymptomatic elevation in liver enzymes (15.6% in the bosentan group), and did not record a difference in clinical status between the two groups. The Endothelin Antagonist Bosentan for Lowering Cardiac Events (ENABLE) trials aimed to determine the effect of bosentan on clinical status after prolonged therapy (9 months) in a population with HF [158]. Two parallel trials (ENABLE-I in Europe and Australia and ENABLE-II in the United States and Canada) enrolled 1613 patients with severe HF (NYHA Class IIB/IV; LVEF $< 35\%$). There was no difference between the treatment and placebo groups in death and hospitalization for HF or all-cause mortality after 9 months of follow-up. There was also an early worsening in HF symptoms (within the first 2–4 weeks) in a significant proportion of patients receiving bosentan. It seems likely that significant fluid retention (as exemplified by an increase in body weight, the development of peripheral edema, and a decrease in hemoglobin) was a major contributory factor. Asymptomatic liver enzyme elevations were noted, as previously recorded with bosentan in REACH-1. The investigators believed that further studies using even lower dosages of bosentan (or more aggressive diuretic therapy) may avoid the effect of fluid overload [159].

Results of the Enrasentan Cooperative Randomized Evaluation (ENCOR) trial, were similarly disappointing [160]. Four hundred and nineteen patients were randomized to one of four dosages of enrasentan, high-dosage ACE-inhibition, or placebo over a 9-month period. The primary clinical composite endpoint of NYHA Class or global assessment worsened with enrasentan, withdrawals caused by adverse events with enrasentan (21%) were higher than placebo (8.3%), and outcomes were worse in the treatment group (75% enrasentan group showed survival free from death, HF hospitalization, or withdrawal from worsening HF versus 92.5% in placebo or ACE-inhibitor treated groups, $P = .007$).

Darusentan, a selective ET-A receptor antagonist, was evaluated for hemodynamic and neurohormonal effects in the Heart Failure ETA Receptor Blockade Trial (HEAT) [161]. In this study, 157 patients who had HF were randomized to receive either placebo or one of three dosages of darusentan orally for 3 weeks, in addition to standard therapy. Only CI increased significantly ($P < .0001$) and SVR decreased significantly ($P = .0001$) after 3 weeks of treatment. Perhaps significantly, the improvement in CI and SVR occurred in the absence of neurohormonal stimulation, increase in heart rate, or drop in blood pressure. Higher dosages of darusentan were associated with more frequent adverse events, including death, and particularly early exacerbation of HF without further hemodynamic benefit compared with moderate dosages.

In the Endothelin-A Receptor Antagonist Trial in Heart Failure (EARTH) [162], 642 patients with chronic HF were assigned to one of five dosages of darusentan or placebo over 24 weeks. The change in LVESV (measured by MRI) was not significantly

Table 6
Endothelin receptor antagonists for heart failure: major findings of clinical trials

Study [Ref.]	No. of patients	Drug	Receptor(s) blocked	Duration of administration	Major outcomes	Comments
RITZ-1 [153]	669	Tezosentan	ET-A/ET-B	72 h	No difference in all endpoints	Excess hypotension and renal failure
RITZ-2 [154]	215	Tezosentan	ET-A/ET-B	24 h	Increase in cardiac output and decrease in PCWP	No significant difference in AEs
RITZ-4 [155]	193	Tezosentan	ET-A/ET-B	24–48 h	No difference in all endpoints	Patients with acute coronary syndrome; excess hypotension
RITZ-5 [156]	84	Tezosentan	ET-A/ET-B	24 h	No improvements in endpoints	Patients with pulmonary edema
REACH-1 [157]	370	Bosentan	ET-A/ET-B	6 mo	No improvements in endpoints	Terminated prematurely because of excessive increase in LFTs
ENABLE I/II [158]	1613	Bosentan	ET-A/ET-B	9 mo	No improvements in endpoints	Worsening HF early in treatment of course; increased fluid retention
ENCOR [160]	419	Enrasentan	ET-A/ET-B	9 mo	No improvements in endpoints	Increased AEs; increased mortality
HEAT [161]	157	Darusentan	ET-A	3 wk	Increase in cardiac index and decrease in systemic vascular resistance	Increased AEs at higher dosages
EARTH [162]	642	Darusentan	ET-A	24 wk	No difference in all endpoints	Well-tolerated; high use of contemporary background therapy

Abbreviations: AEs, adverse events; LFT, liver function test.

different from placebo at any dosage. Importantly, patients enrolled in this study had a high prevalence of background therapy. Additionally, because blood pressure was reduced at all dosages (confirming effective receptor blockade) and circulating ET-1 levels increased in a dosage-dependent manner and remained elevated (indicating displacement of endothelin from its receptor), inadequate dosing or tachyphylaxis was believed to be unlikely to account for the neutral effect of the drug. Overall, darusentan did not improve cardiac remodeling, clinical symptoms, or outcomes in this patient population, which may suggest that ET-A blockade is unlikely to be useful as an add-on treatment in such patients.

What is the role of endothelin receptor antagonists in heart failure?

The experimental animal models of HF, as well as several early clinical studies, have supported a potential beneficial effect of ET-1 blockade in HF. It is therefore somewhat surprising that larger clinical trials performed in HF populations (summarized in Table 6) have failed to demonstrate any value of chronic endothelin suppression in reducing symptoms or ameliorating outcomes. Differences between the early and late stages of HF, the impact of concomitant treatments, and the variety of potential effects of any particular agent may play a role in determining the consequences of new therapies, such as endothelin receptor antagonists [163].

Endothelin has a pathophysiologic role in the progression of HF. Variable (mainly neutral or adverse) responses to endothelin receptor antagonism in *classic* HF populations have underscored the complexity of this condition. Further evaluation of the approach to additive therapeutic modalities such as endothelin antagonism will require better understanding of the multifaceted interactions these agents may have with concomitant therapies and the failing heart.

References

[1] Schrier RW, Abraham W. Hormones and hemodynamics in heart failure. N Engl J Med 1999;341:577–85.

[2] Thibonnier M. Vasopressin receptor antagonists in heart failure. Curr Opin Pharmacol 2003;3:683–7.

[3] Penit J, Faure M, Jard S. Vasopressin and angiotensin II receptors in rat aortic arch smooth muscle cells in culture. Am J Physiol 1983;244:E72–82.

[4] Carmichael MC, Kumar R. Molecular biology of vasopressin receptors. Semin Nephrol 1994;14:341–8.

[5] Lee CR, Watkins MI, Patterson JH, et al. Vasopressin: A new target for the treatment of heart failure. Am Heart J 2003;146:9–18.

[6] Nielsen S, Chou CL, Marples D, et al. Vasopressin increases water permeability of kidney collecting duct by inducing translocation of aquaporin-CD water channels to plasma membrane. Proc Natl Acad Sci USA 1995;92:1013–7.

[7] Kalra PR, Anker SD, Coats AJS. Water and sodium regulation in chronic heart failure: the role of natriuretic peptides and vasopressin. Cardiovasc Res 2001;51:495–509.

[8] Goldsmith SR, Francis GS, Cowley AW, et al. Increased plasma arginine vasopressin levels in patients with congestive heart failure. J Am Coll Cardiol 1983;1:1385–90.

[9] Szatalowicz VL, Arnold PE, Chaimovitz C, et al. Radioimmunoassay of plasma arginine vasopressin in hyponatremic patients with congestive heart failure. N Engl J Med 1981;305:263–6.

[10] Francis GS, Benedict C, Johnstone DE, et al. Comparison of neuroendocrine activation in patients with left ventricular dysfunction with and without congestive heart failure. A substudy of the Studies of Left Ventricular Dysfunction (SOLVD). Circulation 1990;82:1724–9.

[11] Kramer BK, Schweda F, Riegger GAJ. Diuretic treatment and diuretic resistance in heart failure. Am J Med 1999;106:90–6.

[12] Goldsmith SR, Cowley AW, Francis GS, et al. Arginine vasopressin and the renal response to water loading in congestive heart failure. Am J Cardiol 1986;58:295–9.

[13] Bichet DG, Kortas C, Mettauer B, et al. Modulation of plasma and platelet vasopressin by cardiac function in patients with heart failure. Kidney Int 1986;29:1188–96.

[14] Uretsky BF, Verbalis JG, Generalovich T, et al. Plasma vasopressin response to osmotic and hemodynamic stimuli in heart failure. Am J Physiol 1985;248:H396–402.

[15] Goldsmith SR. Vasopressin: A therapeutic target in congestive heart failure? J Card Fail 1999;5:347–56.

[16] Francis GS, Tang WHW. Vasopressin receptor antagonists. Will the "vaptans" fulfill their promise? JAMA 2004;291:2017–8.

[17] Rouleau JL, de Champlain J, Klein M, et al. Activation of neurohumoral systems in postinfarction left ventricular dysfunction. J Am Coll Cardiol 1993;22(2):390–8.

[18] Xu DL, Martin PY, Ohara M, St. John J, Pattison T, Hong Y, et al. Upregulation of aquaporin-2 water channel expression in chronic heart failure rat. J Clin Invest 1997;97:1500–5.

[19] Chan PS, Coupet J, Park HC, et al. VPA-985, a nonpeptide orally active and seleactive vasopressin V_2 receptor antagonist. In: Zingg HH, Bourque CW,

Bichet D, editors. Vasopressin and Oxytocin Molecular, Cellular, and Clinical Advances, Vol 449. New York, NY: Plenum Press; 1998. p. 439–43.
[20] Abraham WT, Oren RM, Crisman TS, et al. Effects of an oral, nonpeptide, selective V2 receptor vasopressin antagonist in patients with chronic heart failure [abstract]. J Am Coll Cardiol 1997;29(2 Suppl A):169A.
[21] Goldsmith SR. Vasopressin as vasopressor. Am J Med 1987;82:1213–9.
[22] Goldsmith SR, Francis SG, Cowley AW, et al. Hemodynamic effects of infused arginine vasopressin in congestive heart failure. J Am Coll Cardiol 1986; 8:779–83.
[23] Monos E, Cox RH, Peterson CH. Direct effects of physiologic doses of arginine vasopressin on the arterial wall in vivo. Am J Physiol 1978;243:H167–73.
[24] Creager MA, Faxon DP, Cutler SS, et al. Contribution of vasopressin to vasoconstriction in patients with congestive heart failure: Comparison with the renin-angiotensin system and the sympathetic nervous system. J Am Coll Cardiol 1986;7:758–65.
[25] Naitoh M, Suzuki H, Murakami M, et al. Effects of oral AVP receptor antagonists OPC-21268 and OPC-31260 on congestive heart failure in conscious dogs. Am J Physiol 1994;267:H2245–54.
[26] Clair MJ, King MK, Goldberg AT, et al. Selective vasopressin, angiotensin II, or dual receptor blockade with developing congestive heart failure. J Pharmacol Exp Ther 2000;293:852–60.
[27] Nakamura Y, Haneda T, Osaki J, et al. Hypertrophic growth of cultured neonatal rat heart cells mediated by vasopressin V_{1a} receptor. Eur J Pharmacol 2000; 391:39–48.
[28] Tahara A, Tomura Y, Wada K, et al. Effect of YM087, a potent nonpeptide vasopressin antagonist, on vasopressin-induced protein synthesis in neonatal rat cardiomyocyte. Cardiovasc Res 1998;38:198–205.
[29] Fuzukawa J, Haneda T, Kikuchi K. Arginine vasopressin increases the rate of protein synthesis in isolated perfused adult rat heart via the V_1 receptor. Mol Cell Biochem 1999;195:93–8.
[30] Thibonnier M, Coles P, Thibonnier A, et al. The basic and clinical pharmacology of nonpeptide vasopressin receptor antagonists. Annu Rev Pharmacol Toxicol 2001;41:175–202.
[31] Hirano T, Yamamura Y, Nakamura S, et al. Effects of the V_2-receptor antagonist OPC-41061 and the lop diuretic furosemide alone and in combination in rats. J Pharmacol Exp Ther 2000;292:288–94.
[32] Yamamura Y, Nakamura S, Ito S, et al. OPC-41061, a highly potent human vasopressin V2-receptor antagonist: pharmacological profile and aquaretic effect by single and multiple oral dosing in rats. J Pharmacol Exp Ther 1998;287:860–7.
[33] Gheorghiade M, Niazi I, Ouyang J, et al, Orlandi C for the Tolvaptan Investigators. Vasopressinn V_2-receptor blockade with tolvaptan in patients with chronic heart failure: Results from a double-blind, randomized trial. Circulation 2003;107:2690–6.
[34] Gheorghiade M, Gattis WA, O'Connor CM, et al. Effects of tolvaptan, a vasopressin antagonist, in patients hospitalized with worsening heart failure: a randomized controlled trial. JAMA 2004;291:1963–71.
[35] Gheorghiade M, Konstam MA, Udelson JE, et al. Vasopressin receptor blockade with tolvaptan in chronic heart failure: differential effects in normonatremic and hyponatremic patients [abstract]. J Am Coll Cardiol 2002;39(5 Suppl. A):171A.
[36] Burnett JC, Smith WB, Ouyang J, et al. Tolvaptan (OPC-41061), a V2 vasopressin receptor antagonist, protects against the decline in renal function observed with loop diuretic therapy (Abstract). J Card Fail 2003;9(5 Suppl.):S12.
[37] Forman DE, Butler J, Wang Y, et al. Incidence, predictors at admission, and impact of worsening renal function among patients hospitalized with heart failure. J Am Coll Cardiol 2004;43:61–7.
[38] Udelson JE, Orlandi C, O'Brien T, et al. Vasopressin receptor blockade in patients with congestive heart failure: Results from a placebo-controlled, randomized study comparing the effects of tolvaptan, furosemide and their combination. J Am Coll Cardiol 2002; 39:156A.
[39] Wong F, Blei AT, Blendis LM, Thuluvath PJ. A vasopressin receptor antagonist (VPA-985) improves serum sodium concentration in patients with hyponatremia: A multicenter, randomized, placebo-controlled trial. Hepatology 2003;37:182–91.
[40] Burnier M, Fricker AF, Hayoz D, et al. Pharmacokinetic and pharmacodynamic effects of YM087, a combined V_1/V_2 vasopressin receptor antagonist in normal subjects. Eur J Clin Pharmacol 1999;55: 633–7.
[41] Naitoh M, Risvanis J, Balding LC, et al. Neurohormonal antagonism in heart failure; beneficial effects of vasopressin V_{1a} and V_2 receptor blockade and ACE inhibition. Cardiovasc Res 2002; 54:51–7.
[42] Udelson JE, Smith WB, Hendrix GH, et al. Acute hemodynamic effects of conivaptan, a dual V_{1a} and V_2 vasopressin receptor antagonist, in patients with advanced heart failure. Circulation 2001;104: 2417–23.
[43] Russell SD, Adams KF, Shaw JP, et al. Results of a twelve week double-blind, placebo controlled, multicenter study of oral conivaptan to assess functional capacity in patients with class III chronic heart failure. J Card Fail 2003;9(Suppl.):S60.
[44] Goldsmith SR, Bisaha JG, Smith N. Evaluating the Efficacy and Safety of the Novel Vasopressin V_{1a} and V_2 Receptor Antagonist Conivaptan for the Treatment of Acute Decompensated Chronic Heart Failure. Study Protocol. J Card Fail 2004;10(Suppl.):S85.
[45] Verbalis JG, Bisaha JG, Smith N. Novel Vasopressin V_{1a} and V_2 Antagonist (Conivaptan) Increases Serum Sodium Concentration and Effective Water Clearance in Patients with Hyponatremia. J Card Fail 2004; 10(Suppl.):S27.

[46] Abbas AK, Lichtman A, Pober JS. Cytokines. In: Abbas AK, Lichtman A, Pober JS, editors. Cellular and molecular immunology. Philadelphia: WB Saunders; 1991. p. 225–43.
[47] Dinarello CA. Proinflammatory Cytokines. Chest 2000; 118:503–8.
[48] Mann DL, Young JB. Basic mechanisms in congestive heart failure: recognizing the role of proinflammatory cytokines. Chest 1994;105:897–904.
[49] Old LJ. Tumor Necrosis Factor (TNF). Science 1985;230:630–2.
[50] Vassali P. The pathophysiology of tumor necrosis factors. Annu Rev Immunol 1992;10:411–52.
[51] Porber JS, Cortan RS. Cytokines and endothelial biology. Physiol Rev 1990;70:427–51.
[52] Torre-Amione G, Kapadia S, et al. Expression and functional significance of tumor necrosis factor receptors in human myocardium. Circulation 1995; 92:1487–93.
[53] Yoshizumi M, Perella MA, Burnett JCJ, et al. Tumor necrosis factor downregulates and endothelial nitric oxide synthase mRNA by shortening its half-life. Circ Res 1993;73:205–9.
[54] Kelly RA, Smith TW. Cytokines and cardiac contractile function. Circulation 1997;95:778–81.
[55] Feldman AM, Combes A, Wagner D, et al. The role of tumor necrosis factor in the pathophysiology of heart failure. J Am Coll Cardiol 2000;35:537–44.
[56] Ferrari R. Tumor necrosis factor in CHF: a double facet cytokine. Cardiovasc Res 1998;37:554–9.
[57] Ferrari R, Angolleti L, Comini L, et al. Oxidative stress during myocardial ischemia and heart failure. Eur Heart J 1998;19(Suppl. B):B2–11.
[58] Adams V, Lenk K, Schubert A, et al. Differentially expressed genes in L6 rat skeletal muscle myoblasts after incubation with inflammatory cytokines. Cytokine 2001;13:342–8.
[59] Packer M. Is tumor necrosis factor an important neurohormonal mechanism in chronic heart failure? Circulation 1995;92:1379–82.
[60] Torre-Amione G, Kapadia S, Benedict CR, et al. Proinflammatory cytokine levels in patients with depressed left ventricular ejection fraction: a report from the studies of left ventricular ejection fraction (SOLVD). J Am Coll Cardiol 1996;27:1201–6.
[61] Levine B, Kalman J, Mayer L, et al. Elevated circulating levels of tumor necrosis factor in severe chronic heart failure. N Engl J Med 1990;323: 236–41.
[62] Testa M, Yeh M, Lee P, et al. Circulating levels of cytokines and their endogenous modulators in patients with mild to severe congestive heart failure due to coronary artery disease or hypertension. J Am Coll Cardiol 1996;28:964–71.
[63] Munger MA, Johnson B, Amber IJ, et al. Circulating concentrations of proinflammatory cytokines in mild or moderate heart failure secondary to ischemic or idiopathic dilated cardiomyopathy. J Am Coll Cardiol 1996;77:723–7.
[64] Deswal A, Petersen NJ, Feldman AM, et al. Cytokines and cytokine receptors in advanced heart failure: an analysis of the cytokine database from the vesnarinone trial (VEST). Circulation 2001;103: 2055–9.
[65] Kubota T, McTiernan CF, Frye CS, et al. Dilated cardiomyopathy in transgenic mice with cardiac specific overexpression of tumor-necrosis factor-alpha. Circ Res 1997;81:627–35.
[66] Kolls J, Peppel K, Silva M, et al. Prolonged and effective blockade of tumor necrosis factor activity through adenovirus-mediated gene transfer. Proc Natl Acad Sci USA 1994;91:215–9.
[67] Kapadia S, Torre-Amione G, Yokoyama T, et al. Soluble TNF binding proteins modulate the negative inotropic properties of TNF-alpha in vitro. Am J Physiol 1995;268(2 pt 2):H517–25.
[68] Kadokami T, Frye C, Lemster B, et al. Anti-tumor necrosis factor-alpha antibody limits heart failure in transgenic model. Circulation 2001;104(10): 1094–7.
[69] Roig E, Orus J, Pare C, et al. Serum interleukin-6 in congestive heart failure secondary to idiopathic dilated cardiomyopathy. Am J Cardiol 1998;82: 688–90.
[70] Tsutamoto T, Hisanaga T, Wada A, et al. Interleukin-6 spillover in the peripheral circulation increases with the severity of heart failure, and the high plasma level of interleukin-6 is an important prognostic predictor in patients with congestive heart failure. J Am Coll Cardiol 1998;31:391–8.
[71] Koller-Strametz J, Packer R, Frey B, et al. Circulating tumor necrosis factor-alpha. Levels in chronic heart failure: relation to its soluble receptor II, interleukin-6, and neurohormonal variables. J Heart Lung Transplant 1998;17:356–62.
[72] MacGowan GA, Mann DL, Kormos RL, et al. Circulating interleukin-6 in severe heart failure. Am J Cardiol 1997;79:1128–31.
[73] Orus J, Roig E, Perez-Villa F, et al. Prognostic value of serum cytokines in patients with congestive heart failure. J Heart Lung Transplant 2000;19:419–25.
[74] Aderka D, Engelmann H, Maor Y, et al. Stabilization of the bioactivity of tumor necrosis factor by its soluble receptors. J Exp Med 1992;175:323–9.
[75] Kapadia S, Dibbs Z, Kurrelmeyer K, et al. The role of cytokines in the failing human heart. Cardiol Clin 1998;16(4):645–56.
[76] Torre-Amione G, Kapadia S, Durand JB, et al. Tumor necrosis factor-α and tumor factor receptors in the failing human heart. Circulation 1996;93:704–11.
[77] Van Zee K, Kohno T, Fischer E, et al. Tumor necrosis factor soluble receptors circulate during experimental and clinical inflammation and can protect against excessive tumor necrosis factor in vitro and in vivo. Proc Natl Acad Sci USA 1992;89:4845–9.
[78] Mohler KM, Torrance DS, Smith CA, et al. Soluble tumor necrosis factor (TNF) receptors are effective therpeutic agents in lethal endotoxemia and function

simultaneously as both TNF carriers and TNF antagonists. J Immunol 1993;151:1548–61.
[79] Mann DL. Inflammatory mediators and the failing heart: past, present, and the foreseeable future. Circ Res 2002;91:988–98.
[80] Waage A, Sorensen M, Stordal B. Differential effect of pentoxifylline on tumor necrosis factor and interleukin-6 production. Lancet 1990;335:543.
[81] Zabel P, Schonharting MM, Wolter DT, et al. Pentoxifylline in endotoxemia. Lancet 1989;ii:1474–7.
[82] Sliwa K, Skudicky D, Candy G, et al. Randomised investigation of effects of pentoxifylline on left-ventricular performance in idiopathic dilated cardiomyopathy. Lancet 1998;351:1091–3.
[83] Iijima T, Taira N. Membrane current changes responsible for the positive inotropic effect of OPC-8212, a new positive inotropic agent, in single ventricular cells of the guinea pig heart. J Pharmacol Exp Ther 1987;240:657–62.
[84] Rapundalo ST, Lathrop DA, Harrison SA, et al. Cyclic AMP-dependent and cyclic AMP-independent actions of a novel cardiotonic agent, OPC-8212. Naunyn Schmiedebergs Arch Pharmacol 1988;338: 692–8.
[85] Shioi T, Matsumori A, Matsui S, et al. Inhibition of cytokine production by a new inotropic agent, vesnarinone, in human lymphocytes, t cell line, and monocytic cell line. Life Sci 1993;54:PL11–6.
[86] Matsumori A, Ono K, Sato Y, et al. Differential modulation of cytokine production by drugs: implications for therapy in heart failure. Journal of Molecular Cell Cardiolgy 1996;28:2491–9.
[87] Jiang H, Bielekova B, Okazaki H, et al. The effect of vesnarinone on TNF production in human peripheral blood mononuclear cells and microglia: a preclinical study for the treatment of multiple sclerosis. J Neuroimmunol 1999;97:134–45.
[88] Matsumori A, Shioi T, Yamada T, et al. Vesnarinone, a new inotropic agent, inhibits cytokine production by stimulated human blood from patients with heart failure. Circulation 1994;89:955–8.
[89] Feldman AM, Becker LC, Llewellyn MP, et al. Evaluation of a new inotropic agent, OPC-8212, in patients with dilated cardiomyopathy and heart failure. Am Heart J 1988;116:771–7.
[90] Asanoi H, Sasayama S, Kameyama T, et al. Sustained inotropic effects of a new cardiotonic agent. OPC-8212 in patients with chronic heart failure. Clin Cardiol 1989;12:133–8.
[91] OPC-8212 Multicenter Research Group. A placebo-controlled, randomized, double-blind study of OPC-8212 in patients with mild chronic heart failure. Cardiovascular Drugs Therapeutics 1990;4:419–26.
[92] Feldman AM, Bristow MR, Parmley WW, et al. Effects of vesnarinone on morbidity and mortality in patients with heart failure. N Engl J Med 1993;329: 149–55.
[93] Weinblatt ME, Kremer JM, Bankhurst AD, et al. A trial of etanercept a recombinant tumor necrosis factor receptor: Fc fusion protein, in patients with rheumatoid arthritis receiving methotrexate. N Engl J Med 1999;340:253–9.
[94] Gorman JD, Sack KE, Davis Jr JC. Treatment of ankylosing spondylitis by inhibition of tumor necrosis factor alpha. N Engl J Med 2002;346:1349–56.
[95] Mease PJ, Goffe BS, Metz J, et al. Etanercept in the treatment of psoriatic arthritis and psoriasis: a randomized trial. Lancet 2000;356:385–90.
[96] Sandborn WJ, Hanauer SB, Katz S, et al. Etanercept for active Crohn's disease: a randomized, double-blind, placebo-controlled trial. Gastroenterology 2001; 121:1088–94.
[97] Fisher Jr CJ, Agosti JM, Opal SM, et al. Treatment of septic shock with the tumor necrosis factor receptor: Fc fusion protein. N Engl J Med 1996;334: 1697–702.
[98] Bozkurt B, Kribbs S, Clubb Jr FJ, et al. Pathophysiology relevant concentrations of tumor necrosis factor-α promote progressive left ventricular dysfunction and remodeling in rats. Circulation 1998;97: 1382–91.
[99] Deswal A, Bozkurt B, Seta Y, et al. A phase I trial of tumor necrosis factor receptor (p75) fusion protein (TNFR:Fc) in patients with advanced heart failure. Circulation 1999;99:3224–6.
[100] Mann DL, McMurray JJV, Packer M, et al. Targeted Anticytokine Therapy in Patients with Chronic Heart Failure: Results of the Randomized Etanercept Worldwide evaluation (RENEWAL). Circulation 2004;109:1594–602.
[101] Knight DM, Trinh H, Le J, et al. Construction and initial characterization of a mouse-human chimeric anti-TNF antibody. Mol Immunol 1993;30:1443–53.
[102] Elliott MJ, Maini RN, Feldmann M, et al. Randomized double-blind comparison of chimeric monoclonal antibody to tumor necrosis factor alpha (cA2) versus placebo in rheumatoid arthritis. Lancet 1994; 344:1105–10.
[103] Chung ES, Packer M, Lo KH, et al for the Anti-TNF Therapy Against Congestive Heart Failure Investigators. Randomized, double-blind, placebo-controlled, pilot trial of infliximab, a chimeric monoclonal antibody to tumor necrosis factor-alpha, in patients with moderate-to-severe heart failure: results of the anti-TNF Therapy Against Congestive Heart Failure (ATTACH) trial. Circulation 2003;107: 3133–40.
[104] Kwon HJ, Cote TR, Cuffe MS, et al. Case reports of heart failure after therapy with a tumor necrosis factor antagonist. Ann Intern Med 2003;138:807–11.
[105] Samuelsson A, Towers TL, Ravetch JV. Anti-inflammatory activity of IVIG mediated through the inhibitory Fc receptor. Science 2001;291:484–6.
[106] McNamara DM, Holubkov R, Starling RC, et al. Controlled trial of intravenous immune globulin in recent-onset dilated cardiomyopathy. Circulation 2001;103:220–5.
[107] Gullestad L, Aass H, Fjeld JG, et al. Immunomodu-

lating therapy with intravenous immunoglobulin in patients with chronic heart failure. Circulation 2001;103(2):220–5.

[108] Fadok VA, Bratton DL, Konowal A, et al. Macrophages that have ingested apoptotic cells in vitro inhibit proinflammatory cytokine production through autocrine/paracrine mechanisms involving TGF-α, PGE2, and PAF. J Clin Invest 1998;101:890–8.

[109] Voll RE, Herrmann M, Roth EA, et al. Immunosuppressive effects of apoptotic cells. Nature 1997;390: 350–1.

[110] Babaei S, Stewart DJ, Picard P, et al. Effects of VasoCare therapy on the initiation and progression of atherosclerosis. Atherosclerosis 2002;162:45–53.

[111] Wood S. Immune modulation therapy holds promise for HF patients, company says. HeartWire News, March 1, 2002. Available at: http://www.theheart.org.

[112] Torre-Amione G, Young JB, Sestier F. A double-blind parallel group, randomized, placebo-controlled feasibility study to assess the safety and effectiveness of immune modulation therapy (IMT) in patients with chronic congestive heart failure. Paper presented at: Annual Meeting of the Heart Failure Society of America, September 25, 2002

[113] Wolfe F, Michaud K. Heart failure in rheumatoid arthritis: rates, predictors, and the effect of anti-tumor necrosis factor therapy. Am J Med 2004; 116(5):305–11.

[114] Torre-Amione G, Kapadia S, Lee J, et al. Tumor necrosis factor-α and tumor necrosis factor receptors in the failing human heart. Circulation 1996;93: 704–11.

[115] Hoimeister JW, Lucchesi BR. Complement activation and inhibition in myocardial ischemia and reperfusion injury. Annu Rev Pharmacol Toxicol 1994;34: 17–40.

[116] Scallon BJ, Moore MA, Trinh H, et al. Chimeric anti-TNF-α monoclonal antibody cA2 binds recombinant transmembrane TNF-α and activates immune effector functions. Cytokine 1995;7:251–9.

[117] Frishman JL, Edwards III CK, Sonnenberg MG, et al. Tumor necrosis factor (TNF)-α- induced interleukin-8 in human blood cultures discriminates neutralization by the p55 and p75 TNF soluble receptors. J Infect Dis 2000;182:1722–30.

[118] Klein B, Brailly H. Cytokine-binding proteins: stimulating antagonists. Immunol Today 1995;16:216–20.

[119] Nakano M, Knowlton AA, Dibbs Z, et al. Tumor necrosis factor- α confers resistance to injury induced by hypoxic injury in the adult mammalian cardiac myocyte. Circulation 1998;97:1392–400.

[120] Kurrelmeyer K, Michael L, Baumgarten G, et al. Endogenous myocardial tumor necrosis factor protects the adult cardiac myocyte against ischemic-induced apoptosis in a murine model of acute myocardial infarction. Proc Natl Acad Sci USA 2000; 290:5456–61.

[121] Lecour S, Smith RM, Woodward B, et al. Identification of a novel role for sphingolipid signaling in TNFα and ischemic preconditioning mediated cardioprotection. J Mol Cell Cardiol 2002;34:509–18.

[122] Feldman AM, McTiernan C. Is there any future for tumor necrosis factor antagonists in chronic heart failure? American Journal of Cardiovascular Drugs 2004;4(1):11–9.

[123] Yanagisawa M, Kurihara H, Kimura S, et al. A novel potent vasoconstrictor peptide produced by vascular endothelial cells. Nature 1988;332:411–5.

[124] Inoue A, Yanagisawa M, Kimura S. The human endothelin family: three structurally and pharmacologically distinct isopeptides predicted by three separate genes. Proc Natl Acad Sci USA 1989;86: 2863–7.

[125] Nunez DJ, Brown MJ, Davenport AP, et al. Endothelin-1 mRNA is widely expressed in porcine and human tissues. J Clin Invest 1990;85:1537.

[126] Thomas PB, Liu EC, Webb ML, et al. Exogenous effects and endogenous production of endothelin in cardiac myocytes: Potential significance in heart failure. Am J Physiol 1996;271:H2629.

[127] Fujisaki H, Ito H, Hirata Y, et al. Natriuretic peptides inhibit angiotensin II-induced proliferation of rat cardiac fibroblasts by blocking endothelin-1 gene expression. J Clin Invest 1995;96:1059.

[128] Shimada K, Takahashi M, Nishikawa K, et al. Cloning and functional expression of endothelin-converting enzyme from rat lung. J Biol Chem 1993; 268:21394–8.

[129] Dupuis J, Stewart D, Cernacek P, et al. Human pulmonary circulation is an important site for both clearance and production of endothelin-1. Circulation 1996;94:1578–84.

[130] Abassi ZA, Tate JE, Golomb E, et al. Role of neutral endopeptidase in the metabolism of endothelin. Hypertension 1992;20:89–95.

[131] Rubanyi G, Polokoff M. Endothelins: molecular biology, biochemistry, pharmacology, physiology, and pathophysiology. Pharmacol Rev 1994;46:325–415.

[132] Hosoda K, Nakao K, Arai H, et al. Cloning and expression of human endothelin-1 receptor cDNA. FEBS Lett 1991;287:23–6.

[133] Molenaar P, O'Reilly G, Sharkey A, et al. Characterization and localization of endothelin receptor subtypes in the human atrioventricular conducting system and myocardium. Circulation 1993;72:526–38.

[134] Haynes WG, Strachan FE, Webb DJ. Endothelin ET_A and ET_B receptors mediate vasoconstriction of human resistance and capacitance vessels in vivo. Circulation 1995;92:357–63.

[135] Pieske B, Beyermann B, Breu V, et al. Functional effects of endothelin and regulation of endothelin receptors in isolated human nonfailing and failing myocardium. Circulation 1999;99:1802–9.

[136] Ito H, Hirata Y, Hiroe M, et al. Endothelin-I induces hypertrophy with enhanced expression of muscle-specific genes in cultured neonatal rat cardiomyocytes. Circ Res 1991;69:209–15.

[137] Takayanagi R, Kitazumi C, Takasaki K, et al.

Presence of non-selective type of endothelin receptor on vascular endothelium and its linkage to vasodilation. FEBS Lett 1991;282:103–6.
[138] Cody RJ, Haas GJ, Binkley PF, et al. Plasma endothelin correlates with the extent of pulmonary hypertension in patients with congestive heart failure. Circulation 1992;85:504–9.
[139] Good JM, Nihoyannopoulos P, Ghatel MA, et al. Elevated plasma endothelin concentrations in heart failure: an effect of angiotensin II? Eur Heart J 1994;15:1634.
[140] Galindo-Fraga A, Arrieta O, Castillo-Martnez L, et al. Elevation of plasmatic endothelin in patients with heart failure. Arch Med Res 2003;34:367–72.
[141] Del Ry S, Andreassi MG, Clerico A, et al. Endothelin-1, endothelin-1 receptors and cardiac natriuretic peptides in failing human heart. Life Sci 2001;68: 2715–30.
[142] Sakai S, Miyauchi T, Sakurai T, et al. Endogenous endothelin-1 participates in the maintenance of cardiac function in rats with congestive heart failure: Marked increase in endothelin-1 production in the failing heart. Circulation 1996;93:1214–22.
[143] Krum H, Goldsmith R, Wilshire-Clement M, et al. Role of endothelin in the exercise intolerance of chronic heart failure. Am J Cardiol 1995;75:1282–3.
[144] Pousset F, Isnard R, Lechat P, et al. Prognostic value of plasma endothelin-1 in patients with chronic heart failure. Eur Heart J 1997;18:254–8.
[145] Omland T, Lie RT, Aakvaag A, et al. Unstable angina / myocardial infarction: plasma endothelin determination as a prognostic indicator of 1-year mortality after acute myocardial infarction. Circulation 1994;89: 1573–9.
[146] Pönicke K, Vogelsang M, Heinroth M, et al. Endothelin receptors in the failing and nonfailing human heart. Circulation 1998;97:744.
[147] Sakai S, Miyauchi T, Kobayashi M, et al. Inhibition of myocardial endothelin pathway improves long-term survival in heart failure. Nature 1996;384: 353–5.
[148] Choussat R, Hittinger L, Barbe F, et al. Acute effects of an endothelin-1 receptor antagonist bosentan at different stages of heart failure in conscious dogs. Cardiovasc Res 1998;39:580–8.
[149] Willette RN, Anderson KM, Nelson AH, et al. Enrasentan improves survival, limits left ventricular remodeling and preserves myocardial performance in hypertensive cardiac hypertrophy and dysfunction. J Cardiovasc Pharmacol 2001;38:606–17.
[150] Kiowski W, Sutsch G, Hunziker P, et al. Evidence of endothelin-1-mediated vasoconstriction in severe chronic heart failure. Lancet 1995;346:732–6.
[151] Sutsch G, Kiowski W, Yan XW, et al. Short-term endothelin-receptor antagonist therapy in conventionally treated patients with symptomatic severe chronic heart failure. Circulation 1998;98:2262–8.
[152] Spieker LE, Mitrovic V, Noll G, et al. Acute hemodynamic and neurohumoral effects of selective ETA receptor blockade in patients with congestive heart failure. J Am Coll Cardiol 2000;35: 1745–52.
[153] Coletta AP, Cleland JGF. Clinical trials update: highlights of the Scientific Sessions of the XXIII Congress of the European Society of Cardiology—WARIS II, ESCAMI, PAFAC, RITZ-1 and TIME. Eur J Heart Fail 2001;3:747–50.
[154] Louis A, Cleland JGF, Crabbe S, et al. Clinical trials update: CAPRICORN, COPERNICUS, MIRACL, STAF, RITZ-2, RECOVER and RENAISSANCE-II and cachexia and cholesterol in heart failure. Highlights of the Scientific Sessions of the American College of Cardiology. Eur J Heart Fail 2001;3:381–7.
[155] O'Connor CM, Gattis WA, Adams KF, et al, for the RITZ-4 Investigators. Tezosentan in patients with acute heart failure and acute coronary syndromes. J Am Coll Cardiol 2003;41:1452–7.
[156] Kaluski E, Kobrin I, Zimlichman R, et al. RITZ-5 randomized intravenous tezosentan (an endothelin-A/B antagonist) for the treatment of pulmonary edema. J Am Coll Cardiol 2003;41:204–10.
[157] Packer M, Caspi A, Charlon V, et al. Multicenter, double-blind, placebo-controlled study of long-term endothelin blockade with bosentan in chronic heart failure: results of the REACH-1 trial. Circulation 1998;98(Suppl.):S12.
[158] Packer M. Effects of the endothelin receptor antagonist bosentan on the morbidity and mortality in patients with chronic heart failure: Results of the ENABLE 1 and 2 trial program. Congress of the American College of Cardiology 2002; Late breaking clinical trials: Special Topic #412
[159] Kalra PR, Moon JCC, Coats AJS. Do the results of the ENABLE (Endothelin Antagonist Bosentan for Lowering Cardiac Events in Heart Failure) study spell the end for non-selective endothelin antagonism in heart failure? Int J Cardiol 2002;85:195–7.
[160] Fonarow GC. Oral endothelin antagonist worsens clinical status in chronic heart failure. Best of the ACC Scientific Session. Rev Cardiovasc Med 2001; 2:144–5.
[161] Luscher TF, Enseleit F, Pacher R, et al. Hemodynamic and neurohormonal effects of selective endothelin A (ETA) receptor blockade in chronic heart failure: The Heart Failure ETA Receptor Blockade Trial (HEAT). Circulation 2002;106:2666–72.
[162] Anand I, McMurray J, Cohn JN, et al. Long-term effects of darusentan on left-ventricular remodeling and clinical outcomes in the Endothelin-A Receptor Antagonist Trial in Heart Failure (EARTH): randomized, double-blind, placebo-controlled trial. Lancet 2004;364:347–54.
[163] Konstam MA, DeNofrio D. Endothelin expression and the progression of heart failure: Exemplifying the vagaries of therapeutic development. Circulation 2004;109:143–5.
[164] Nicod P, Waeber B, Bussien JP, et al. Acute hemodynamic effect of a vascular antagonist of

vasopressin in patients with congestive heart failure. Am J Cardiol 1985;55(8):1043–7.
[165] Pruszczynski W, Vahanian A, Ardaillou R, et al. Role of antidiuretic hormone in impaired water excretion of patients with congestive heart failure. J Clin Endocrinol Metab 1984;58(4):599–605.
[166] Goldsmith SR, Francis GS, Levine TB, et al. Impaired response of plasma vasopressin to orthostatic stress in patients with congestive heart failure. J Am Coll Cardiol 1983;2(6):1080–3.
[167] Gavras H, Ribeiro AB, Kohlmann O, et al. Effects of a specific inhibitor of the vascular action of vasopressin in humans. Hypertension 1984;6(2 Pt 2): I156–60.

ELSEVIER
SAUNDERS

Heart Failure Clin 1 (2005) 129 – 139

HEART
FAILURE
CLINICS

Natriuretic Peptides and Remodeling in Heart Failure

John C. Burnett, Jr, MD[a,b,*]

[a]Mayo Clinic College of Medicine, Rochester, MN, USA
[b]Mayo Clinic and Foundation, Rochester, MN, USA

Since the discovery of the cardiac hormone atrial natriuretic peptide (ANP) by DeBold and coworkers in 1981 [1], the field of natriuretic peptides has advanced significantly, with translation of new knowledge to the clinical practice of heart failure (HF). This new knowledge has underscored the importance of cardiorenal mechanisms that contribute to optimal cardiovascular homeostasis. Work has also established direct myocardial actions broadening their therapeutic potential beyond renal mechanisms. Indeed, one such therapeutic target is cardiac remodeling and fibrosis based upon the unique cardiorenal protective properties. The objective of this article is to review new insights into the use of natriuretic peptides as novel therapeutic agents for cardiorenal protection in progressive HF, which serves to limit cardiac remodeling and fibrosis and thus the progression of HF.

Sodium and aldosterone regulating actions of natriuretic peptides

The natriuretic peptide system consists of three known peptides that are distinct gene products: ANP and brain natriuretic peptide (BNP), which are primarily found in cardiomyocytes, and C-type natriuretic peptide (CNP), which is chiefly found in endothelial cells [2–4]. These three peptides function through the second messenger cyclic GMP (cGMP), where ANP and BNP bind to natriuretic peptide receptor A and CNP binds to natriuretic peptide receptor B (Fig. 1) [5]. All three peptides are cleared by a clearance receptor, which is a nonparticulate guanylyl cyclase–linked receptor, termed natriuretic peptide receptor C [6]. All are degraded enzymatically by widely distributed neutral endopeptidase 24.11 (NEP) [7]. Following studies in cell systems, novel mouse models of altered natriuretic peptide production or receptor disruption, integrative studies in pathophysiologic models, and in human subjects, a unifying understanding of the biology of these peptides has emerged. This unique concept of cardiorenal protection by activation of cGMP is a result of biological properties that include natriuresis, vasodilatation, inhibition of the renin–angiotensin–aldosterone system (RAAS), positive lusitropism, and inhibition of fibrosis [8–13]. Based on such an understanding, their therapeutic application has been advanced [14–19].

In HF, BNP is most potent from a therapeutic perspective in augmenting sodium excretion and exerting direct myocardial actions. This contributes to unloading of the heart and improving congestion. Specifically, in a model of severe HF, we have demonstrated that BNP is markedly more potent in augmenting sodium excretion compared with ANP or the renally altered form of ANP, which is Urodilatin [20]. The mechanism of this greater natriuretic action is explained by greater glomerular filtration rate (GFR)-enhancing actions and decrease in terminal nephron sodium reabsorption. We speculate that the

* Cardiorenal Research Laboratory, Division of Cardiovascular Diseases, Department of Internal Medicine, Mayo Clinic and Foundation, 200 First Street SW, Rochester, MN 55905.

E-mail address: burnett.john@mayo.edu

1551-7136/05/$ – see front matter
doi:10.1016/j.hfc.2005.01.002

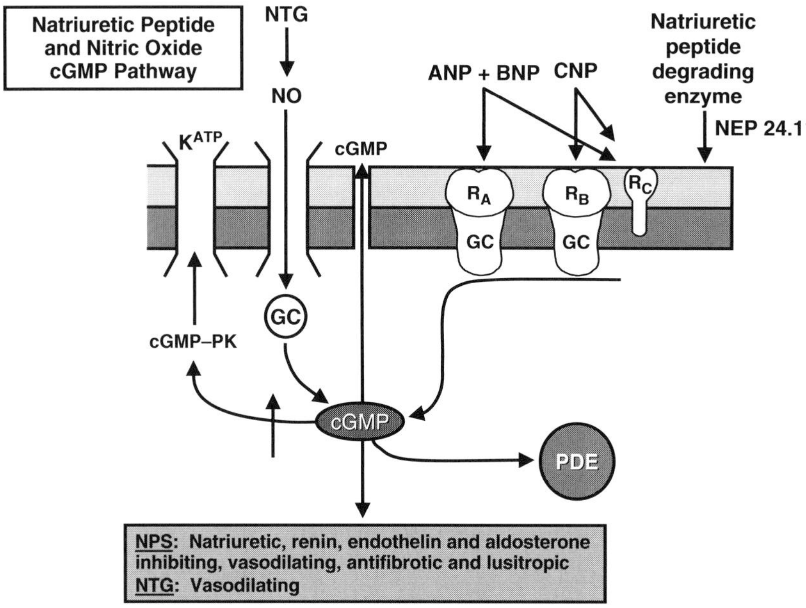

Fig. 1. Natriuretic peptide and nitric oxide cGMP pathway.

more potent renal actions of BNP may be explained by a greater resistance to NEP degradation secondary to its more extended C-terminus as compared with ANP. CNP lacks natriuretic actions [21].

This renal-enhancing action of BNP has understandable importance in developing BNP-based therapies for the treatment of HF. Increasing evidence supports the concept that the kidney plays a key role in HF, because the presence of reduced GFR is the most robust marker for poor survival, more so than even New York Heart Association class or ejection fraction [22]. Indeed, the concept of enhancing renal function in HF has emerged as an important therapeutic strategy to delay disease progression [23]. Furthermore, the development of renal resistance to the natriuretic peptides may be an ominous sign of very high risk for increased mortality [24,25].

Natriuretic peptide receptor A, to which both ANP and BNP bind, is highly expressed in the adrenal gland [26,27]. One of the first demonstrations of the biologic action of ANP was its inhibition of aldosterone (ALDO) synthesis and release and that of angiotensin II stimulated increases in ALDO [28,29]. As a potential therapeutic strategy in HF, with the exception of direct ALDO receptor antagonists, there is no other biologic factor that has such functionally important direct ALDO-suppressing properties. Based on the renal sodium retaining and fibrotic actions of ALDO, the clinical use of the cardiac natriuretic peptides in HF deserves special consideration.

Fig. 2 illustrates the recent findings of Cataliotti and coworkers [30] in which the coadministration of intravenous BNP at a high dose and intravenous furosemide enhanced GFR, which was not observed with furosemide alone in a model of overt HF. Furthermore, low- and high-dose BNP plus furosemide demonstrated a greater diuretic and natriuretic response. Most importantly, there was a lack of activation of ALDO with coadministration of BNP and furosemide, in contrast to marked activation of ALDO with the loop diuretic alone. Not illustrated is the greater unloading of the heart, which occurred with coadministration of both sodium-regulating compounds. This study underscores the potential benefit of chronic BNP therapy in HF to modulate ALDO, enhance renal sodium and water excretion, and maintain GFR. These findings were also supported by our investigations with the natriuretic peptide-based therapeutic agent omapatrilat, which simultaneously inhibits NEP and ACE [31]. Specifically, in a model of early stage HF, we observed that omapatrilat administered with furosemide was superior in enhancing renal function, unloading the heart, and inhibiting activation of ALDO compared with ACE inhibition with a diuretic. Therefore, BNP possesses novel renal and ALDO-regulating properties, and both natriuretic peptide–based therapies

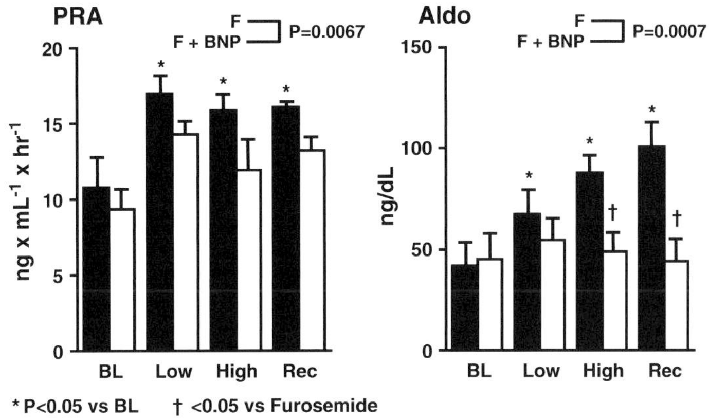

Fig. 2. BNP inhibits furosemide-induced aldosterone activation in experimental CHF.

attenuated furosemide activation of ALDO. In addition, there were greater GFR-enhancing actions of natriuretic peptide–based therapies. Indeed, these data support a rationale for a more physiological approach to enhancing renal function in HF with BNP therapy with the additional benefit of suppressing ALDO. This is most timely, as conventional loop diuretics like furosemide have been associated with adverse actions especially with potassium wasting properties and excessive activation of the RAAS [32–34].

One might ask whether the biologic actions of the natriuretic peptides are specific to particulate guanylyl cyclase (pGC) activation or can be mimicked by direct stimulation of soluble guanylate cyclase (sGC). Regarding this question, we used a novel new molecule BAY 41-2272, which is orally available and directly stimulates the heterodimeric hemeprotein sGC while increasing its sensitivity to its natural stimulator, nitric oxide. Unlike conventional organic nitrates, which are associated with the development of tolerance, direct sGC stimulation with BAY 41-2272 is devoid of tolerance and therefore can be considered an effective therapy for cardiovascular disease (eg, hypertension) as well as a pharmacological tool to understand cGMP-mediating mechanisms in cardiovascular regulation [35]. In these recent studies, direct sGC stimulation demonstrated potent cardiovascular actions with unloading of the heart, particularly pulmonary capillary wedge pressure with enhancement of renal blood flow, at high doses [36]. In contrast to BNP, however, there was no enhancement of GFR or sodium excretion, nor was there suppression of an already-activated RAAS. Thus, pGC activation by BNP is unique and differs from cGMP activation through direct sGC stimulation, again underscoring the novelty of targeting pGC with chronic BNP as a therapeutic strategy for HF.

Direct myocardial actions of brain natriuretic peptide

Acute intravenous BNP in HF enhances ventricular function. The basis for BNP approval as an intravenous agent for the treatment of acute decompensated human HF was its superiority compared with the cGMP-activating drug nitroglycerin in reducing cardiac filling pressures over a 3-hour period in association with improved symptoms compared with placebo [19]. In experimental overt HF, intravenous BNP was more potent than ANP in enhancing diastolic function in this model of systolic dysfunction together with reducing both end-systolic and end-diastolic volume [12]. Furthermore, only BNP, and not ANP or CNP, decreased both end-diastolic volume and end-systolic volume in experimental HF. Moreover, there was a greater improvement in diastolic function in this model of systolic HF with BNP compared with the other two peptides, because Tau was significantly more reduced. This increase in the rate of left ventricular (LV) relaxation may improve LV filling and maintain cardiac output, which are effects that would be beneficial in HF. Importantly, the reduction in both end-systolic pressure and end-systolic volume, as well as the more prominent improvement in end-diastolic volume with BNP compared with ANP, would be therapeutically useful because it would tend to reduce congestion while maintaining cardiac output. Therefore, these data provide additional insight into the potential therapeutic actions of BNP in the treatment of HF.

In normal humans, an additional favorable action of intravenous BNP is to increase myocardial perfusion and reduce oxygen consumption [37]. If one considers that BNP also has the additional characteristics of enhancing renal function and modulating ALDO release, it stands as a highly beneficial agent for the treatment of HF.

Mouse models of disrupted natriuretic peptide system pathways were the first to demonstrate direct myocardial structural actions of the natriuretic peptides independent of renal actions. Most recently, targeted deletion of natriuretic peptide receptor A in cardiomyocytes of a murine model was associated with cardiac hypertrophy and altered ventricular relaxation [38,39]. In addition, disruption of the BNP gene has been associated with marked cardiac fibrosis independent of changes in arterial pressure [40]. In this murine model, increases in afterload produced by aortic constriction also resulted in exaggerated cardiac fibrosis compared with wild-type animals. That BNP could play a key role in the heart as an antifibrotic factor has major clinical ramifications, because cardiac fibrosis is a hallmark of HF and has been one of the therapeutic targets of two landmark clinical trials in human HF [41,42]. The clinical significance of cardiac fibrosis is well recognized and contributes to impaired myocardial contraction and relaxation, cellular hypoxia due to impaired myocardial perfusion secondary to reduced diffusion of oxygen from blood vessels to cardiomyocytes, and a predisposition to atrial and ventricular dysrhythmias with slowing and greater dispersion of the cardiac action potential [43–46]. This is especially important in chronic HF where atrial fibrosis may serve as a participating mechanism of atrial fibrillation [47]. Because we have only limited modalities to target cardiac fibrosis clinically, the significance of the proposed studies is high.

Cardiac fibrosis and the natriuretic peptides

Cardiac fibrosis is a hallmark of HF. As discussed above, the clinical significance of cardiac fibrosis is well recognized and contributes to impaired myocardial contraction and relaxation, cellular hypoxia due to impaired myocardial perfusion secondary to reduced diffusion of oxygen from blood vessels to cardiomyocytes, and a predisposition to atrial and ventricular dysrhythmias with slowing and greater dispersion of the cardiac action potential.

Although cardiomyocytes occupy most of the space in the myocardium, cardiac fibroblasts (CFs) account for two thirds of the total population of cells in the heart and play a key role in the regulation of myocardial structure and function [48]. CFs regulate the production of collagen and, through induction of matrix metalloproteases (MMPs), the degradation of collagen [49,50]. When there is balance of production and degradation of collagen, myocardial structure is maintained to optimally maintain function. With imbalance there is either excessive degradation of collagen with ventricular dilatation and systolic dysfunction or with excessive proliferation of CFs and increased production of collagen cardiac fibrosis and diastolic dysfunction.

Two recent clinical trials have brought renewed focus on the potential importance of cardiac fibrosis as a target for cardiovascular drug therapies. First, the Randomized Aldactone Evaluation Study in congestive HF (CHF) reported that a relatively low dose of the nonselective aldosterone antagonist, spironolactone, in addition to the standard medical regimen, reduced mortality and hospitalization for worsening HF [41]. The mechanism for the beneficial effect of spironolactone remains unknown, but it was speculated that this aldosterone receptor antagonist blocked the profibrotic actions of this hormone. This speculation was supported by the observation that a biomarker for collagen (procollagen type III peptide) decreased in the spironolactone treated subgroup compared with placebo [51]. Recently, the results of the Eplerenone Post-Acute Myocardial Infarction Heart Failure Efficacy and Survival Study (EPHESUS) were reported [42]. Eplerenone is a selective ALDO antagonist that acts as a competitive antagonist of the mineralocorticoid receptor, but has greater selectivity for the mineralocorticoid receptor than spironolactone. EPHESUS showed that eplerenone added to optimal medical therapy reduced morbidity and mortality in patients who had LV dysfunction and HF after an acute myocardial infarction. The investigators speculated that the benefit was related to a favorable impact of therapy on ventricular remodeling and fibrosis.

We have recently focused on cardiotrophin 1 (CT-1) as a profibrotic factor, which in CFs is more potent than endothelin-1 (ET-1) or angiotensin II in promoting CF proliferation and collagen synthesis [52]. CT-1 is a member of the interleukin 6 superfamily, which has growth-promoting properties in cardiomyocytes [53]. CT-1 binds to glycoprotein130 (gp130) and the leukemia inhibitory factor receptor, a component of the gp130 receptor. Two signaling pathways, signal transducer and activator of transcription and mitogen-activated protein kinase, have been identified for CT-1 in cardiomyocytes [54,55] More recently, we have extended studies in cardiomyocytes to CFs and demonstrated that CT-1 in CFs also involves mitogen-activated protein kinase signaling. We have also reported its production in both CFs and in ECs and that CT-1 is also a secretagogue for ET-1 secretion from ECs [56]. In addition, in these in vitro studies in CFs, we speculated that ET-1 and CT-1 could represent a paradigm of humoral cross-talk based on similar signaling pathways. We therefore defined the effect of ET_A receptor antagonism on CT-1–stimulated DNA synthesis. We therefore investigated the actions of BQ123, a specific ET_A receptor antagonist, on ET-1–stimulated DNA synthesis. BQ123 significantly inhibited not only basal (ie, by endogenous ET-1) but also DNA synthesis stimulated by exogenous ET-1. In addition, BQ123 significantly attenuated CT-1–stimulated DNA synthesis. Interestingly, anti-gp130 or leukemia inhibitory factor receptor action inhibited the basal as well as the ET-1–stimulated DNA synthesis. This underscores our suggestion that profibrotic factors function via redundant pathways.

The report that genetic deletion of BNP in mice results in cardiac fibrosis set the stage for considering BNP and the natriuretic peptides as antifibrotic therapies [40]. This report established that genetic deletion of the BNP gene resulted in an increase in ventricular fibrosis independently of increases in arterial pressure. Fujisaki and coworkers [57] determined that the natriuretic peptides inhibited angiotensin II or ET-1–induced increases in DNA synthesis. Interestingly, BNP was approximately twofold more potent than ANP with respect to the inhibition of DNA synthesis. They also confirmed that intracellular cGMP formation plays an important role in the natriuretic peptide–mediated inhibition of DNA synthesis and ppET-1 mRNA expression in CFs. Most recently, Horio and coworkers [58] have reported that adult rat CFs express and secrete CNP and that CNP potentially regulates fibrosis in an autocrine fashion.

While the natriuretic peptides possess antifibrotic and anti-aldosterone actions that are thought to be related to cGMP activation by pGC, an equally important question related to therapy for fibrosis is whether sGC activation—especially by novel orally available molecules—can be considered efficacious. Calderone and colleagues [59] investigated the effect of ANP and the nitric oxide donor S-nitroso-*N*-acetyl-D,L-penicillamine (SNAP) on norepinephrine stimulated neonatal rat cardiomyocytes and CFs and compared SNAP to ANP. Both SNAP and ANP significantly reduced norepinephrine induced hydrogen 3 ([^{3}H])–leucine incorporation in cardiomyocytes and [^{3}H]-thymidine in CFs. Bromo 8–cGMP mimicked this action. These data strongly suggest that sGC can also be a drug target for inhibition of cardiac fibrosis. As discussed above, we have recently reported efficacious cardiorenal actions of a novel orally available sGC stimulator (BAY 41-2272) in experimental severe CHF [36]. The use of this molecule therefore provides the opportunity to determine if the mechanism of cGMP activation is important in determining the antifibrotic actions of NPs and provides an additional potential therapy.

We recently sought to determine if BNP is produced by CFs and to determine the action of BNP on CFs [60]. We specifically investigated whether CFs were a source of BNP, whether BNP and its signaling system contribute to the regulation of collagen production in CFs, and whether BNP modulates MMPs and their enzymatic activity.

Immunohistochemical staining demonstrated that BNP was diffusely present in the cytoplasm of CFs confirming BNP presence and supporting the conclusion that BNP is produced in CFs [60]. Radioimmunoassay further confirmed this with reverse-transcriptase polymerase chain reaction detection of BNP mRNA. CFs secreted BNP into the medium at a rate of 11.2 ± 1.0 pg/10^5 cells per 48 hours, and this secretion was significantly augmented in a time-dependent fashion with TNF-α. BNP was analyzed by way of high-performance liquid chromatography, which revealed one major peak that appeared at an elution position identical to that of synthetic full-length canine BNP_{1-32}.

Our next goal was to determine BNP action on CFs with the specific hypothesis that we could demonstrate antifibrotic properties of BNP. BNP (1 μM) significantly increased intracellular cGMP (Fig. 3). The effect of BNP on de novo collagen synthesis was assessed by measuring [^{3}H]-proline incorporation. BNP significantly inhibited [^{3}H]-proline incorporation by 29%, clearly demonstrating antifibrotic properties in vitro in CFs. To determine if BNP could also degrade collagen, we sought to define its action on several MMPs. We accomplished this by defining zymographic MMP abundance. For detection of MMP and TIMP proteins in CFs, Western blotting was performed.

We also reported that BNP could attenuate the profibrotic actions of ET-1. BNP alone significantly increased zymographic total MMP-2 abundance at 24 hours, but TNF-α (10^{-7} M) alone did not [60]. However, TNF-α in combination with BNP significantly increased BNP-induced MMP-2 abundance.

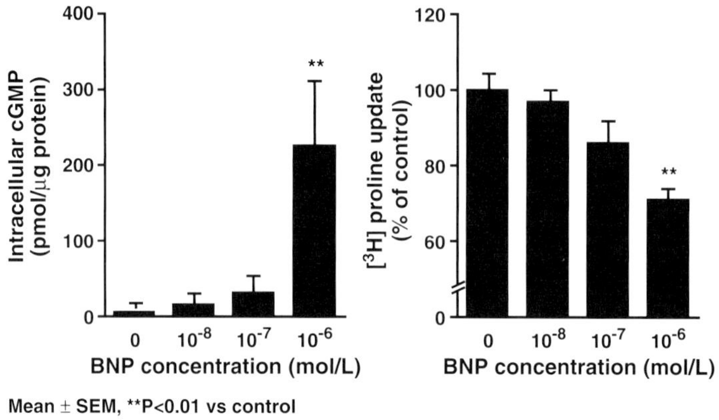

Fig. 3. BNP activates cGMP production in CFs and inhibits collagen synthesis.

ET-1 (10^{-7} M) significantly down-regulated the zymographic MMP-2 abundance after 3 hours of incubation. Coincubation of BNP (10^{-6} M) and ET-1 (10^{-7} M) reversed the action of ET-1, resulting in increased zymographic MMP-2 abundance.

More recently, Kapoun and coworkers [61] have reported further evidence of the potent antifibrotic effects of BNP in CFs. Recognizing the reported properties of BNP in CFs, and because TGF-β is associated with profibrotic processes, they tested whether BNP could inhibit TGF-β–induced effects on primary human CFs. BNP inhibited TGF-β–induced cell proliferation as well as the production of collagen 1 and fibronectin. Complementary DNA microarray analysis revealed that TGF-β but not BNP treatment resulted in a significant change in the RNA profile. However, BNP treatment resulted in an 85% alteration of all TGF-β–regulated mRNA. BNP opposed TGF-β–regulated genes related to fibrosis and inflammation, and these actions were linked to cGMP. These studies therefore importantly demonstrated that BNP has direct effects on CFs to inhibit fibrotic responses by extracellular signal-regulated kinase pathway by way of cGMP-dependent protein kinase signaling suggesting that BNP functions as an antifibrotic factor in the heart to prevent cardiac fibrosis.

How does BNP mediate its antiproliferative actions? First, we recognize that the regulation of cell proliferation involves the production and actions of a variety of proteins that modulate the cell cycle. It is also recognized that an intricate and well-conserved cell cycle controls cell division. Extensive work in the field of cancer research has demonstrated that the cell cycle is regulated by important protein families, whose mutational inactivation or overexpression is an important factor in the pathogenesis of tumors [62]. Indeed, a greater understanding of the cell cycle has led to novel compounds that may restore control of cell division in human cancers. Indeed, the natriuretic peptides and BAY could emerge as novel cell cycle–targeted therapies. This is supported by key reports that cGMP decreases expression of cell cycle–promoting genes such as cyclin D1 in vascular smooth muscle [63]. In addition, cGMP and ANP increase expression of cell cycle inhibitors such as p16 in astrocytes [64]. It should be acknowledged that while in cancer the major pathogenetic characteristic is the loss of control over cell proliferation, the problem in cardiac fibrosis is not a loss of control but rather a pathophysiologic or maladaptive proliferation of CFs induced by profibrotic factors. One could speculate that natriuretic peptides and BAY counteract this maladaptive CF proliferation by enhancing physiologic antifibrotic signaling pathways.

In summary, studies support the concept that the antifibrotic properties of cGMP-activating compounds like the natriuretic peptides have unique multitissue actions that support their therapeutic action in cardiac fibrosis. First, a direct action on CF proliferation and the cell cycle emerges as a seminal action. However, the ability to decrease myocardial load due to vascular and renal actions is an additional mechanism. The ability of the natriuretic peptides to also retard activation of the RAAS and ET-1 are additional humoral actions that complement these other properties.

Chronic brain natriuretic peptide therapy

In human and experimental HF, the increase in circulating ANP and BNP represents increased

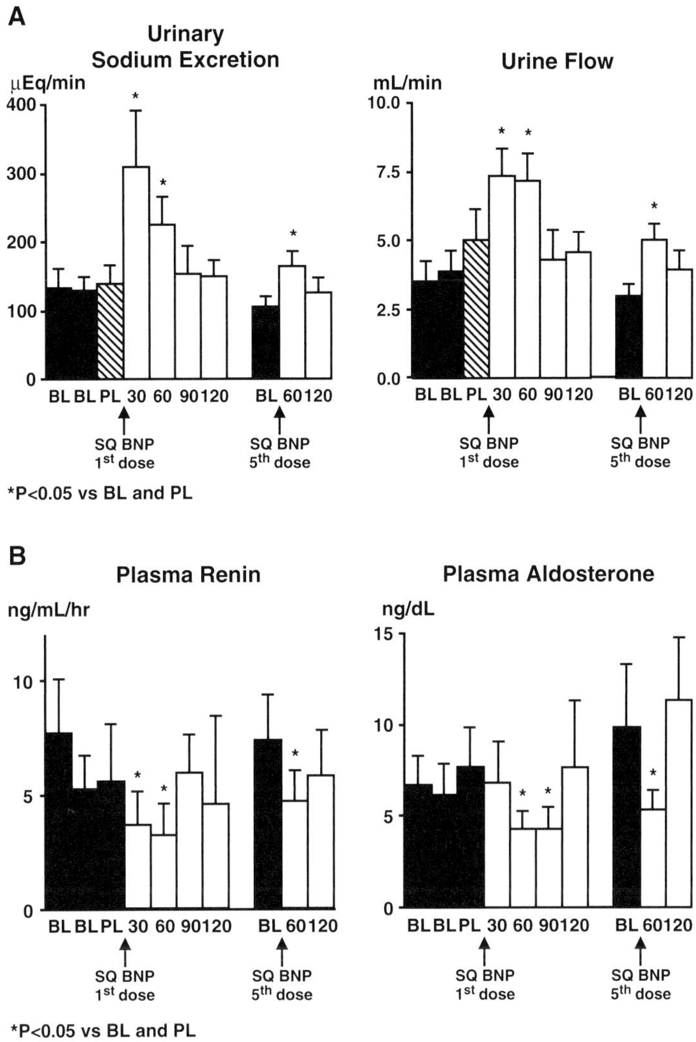

Fig. 4. AQ BNP (*A, B*) in human CHF.

production and release from atrial and ventricular myocardium [65,66]. We have reported that acute administration of a natriuretic peptide receptor antagonist accelerates the onset of sodium retention with premature activation of the RAAS [67,68]. Such findings support the conclusion of a compensatory role of increased ANP and BNP in early stage HF to maintain sodium homeostasis and suppress the RAAS. In late-stage HF, administration of a natriuretic peptide antagonist also is reported to induce further sodium retention to indicate a continued renal protective property of elevated natriuretic peptides even in the terminal phases of HF [69]. However, as suggested in a previous report from our laboratory, plasma BNP has not achieved the peak concentration in experimental early stage HF as in overt CHF, which is partially explained by the lack of recruitment in early stage HF of ventricular production [70]. This underscores the rationale of exogenous chronic BNP therapy in early evolving HF, which we consider a relative deficiency state.

We reported previously that 10-day subcutaneous BNP in experimental HF had beneficial effects to unload the heart without evidence of tolerance [71]. We have extended this concept of chronic subcutaneous BNP (SQ BNP) to human studies and have reported the first demonstration that a 3-day period of SQ BNP increases circulating concentrations of BNP, activates plasma and urinary cGMP, enhances sodium and water excretion (Fig. 4A), and reduces activation of the RAAS (Fig. 4B) [72]. Most importantly, safety studies in humans with severe CHF using intermittent BNP have been reported [73]. This study of over 12 weeks with retrospective analysis indicated a reduction in combined end point of worsening HF and hospitalization with chronic BNP therapy, which has led to a new major clinical trial called FUSION II.

Circulating brain natriuretic peptide: diagnostic and biological significance

A hallmark of HF as well as chronic renal failure is early and sustained elevation of circulating ANP and BNP [74–77]. Others and we have demonstrated the clinical use of measuring these two cardiac peptides to aid in the diagnosis of HF and to guide therapy [78,79]. The potential for BNP for early detection of reduced systolic function in the general community has been enhanced with our finding that N-terminal proBNP is superior to BNP in detecting reduced systolic function in the general population and especially in men over the age of 65 [80]. Of relevance to a possible deficiency of BNP in HF is an association of reduced plasma BNP with obesity and diabetes. As suggested in studies by the Framingham group, BNP is lower in obesity in the general population, and there may be an additive action in diabetes [81].

A major paradox of advanced HF is markedly elevated circulating ANP and BNP, which increases above normal values almost 100-fold. Despite this, there is often marked cardiorenal impairment and, in some subjects, inappropriate low levels of circulating cGMP [82]. Ongoing studies have suggested that there may be altered forms of circulating BNP as well as ANP to explain this paradox [83–86]. The mechanism of altered forms of BNP has not been defined but may be related to impaired processing or enhanced enzymatic degradation [87]. Most importantly, the lack of highly sensitive and specific technologies in the past have prevented detection of such altered forms. In addition, the actual biologic activity of potentially altered forms is unexplored. More state-of-the-art technologies are needed to address this issue.

Clinical relevance of delaying the progression of heart failure

HF is an increasing epidemic worldwide [88]. Projections by the National Institues of Health and other federal agencies have indicated an increase in the prevalence of HF over the next four decades, particularly in the elderly. Studies from Framingham have indicated that the reduction in mortality over the last four decades has been modest, requiring a focus on disease prevention and on the development of novel therapeutic strategies [89]. Others and we have also reported that almost half of subjects with systolic ventricular dysfunction are asymptomatic [88–91]. Furthermore, Framingham has reported a sixfold increase in the risk of developing HF in asymptomatic LV dysfunction and a threefold higher mortality [91]. In addition, the increasing recognition that pharmacologic blockade of ALDO has important clinical benefit also underscores the need to identify novel ALDO opposing strategies. Therefore, the clinical use of the natriuretic peptides addresses a very important need in cardiovascular disease, which is the development of enhanced therapies for HF such as BNP, which may delay disease progression and prevent cardiac remodeling and fibrosis.

References

[1] DeBold A, Borenstein HB, Veress AT, et al. A rapid and potent antriuretic response to intravenous injection of atrial myocardial extract in rats. Life Sci 1981;28: 89–94.

[2] Mukoyama M, Nakao K, Hosoda K, et al. Brain natriuretic peptide as a novel cardiac hormone in humans. Evidence for an exquisite dual natriuretic peptide system, atrial natriuretic peptide and brain natriuretic peptide. J Clin Invest 1991;87:1402–12.

[3] Stingo AJ, Clavell AL, Heublein DM, et al. Presence of C-type natriuretic peptide in cultured human endothelial cells and plasma. Am J Physiol 1992;263: 1318–21.

[4] Suga SI, Nakao K, Itoh H, Komatsu Y, Ogawa Y, Hama N, et al. Endothelial production of C-type natriuretic peptide and its marked augmentation by transforming growth factor-beta. Possible existence of "vascular natriuretic peptide system." J Clin Invest 1992;90:1145–9.

[5] Chinkers M. Regulation of the atrial natriuretic peptide receptor guanylyl cyclase. Proc Soc Exp Biol Med 1996;213:105–8.

[6] Charles CJ, Espiner EA, Nicholls MG, et al. Clearance receptors and endopeptidase 24.11: equal role in natriuretic peptide metabolism in conscious sheep. Am J Physiol 1996;271:R373–80.

[7] Chen HH, Lainchbury JG, Harty GJ, et al. Maximizing the natriuretic peptide system in experimental heart failure. Subcutaneous brain natriuretic peptide and acute vasopeptidase inhibition. Circulation 2002;105: 999–1003.

[8] Burnett Jr JC, Granger JP, Opgenorth TF. Effects of

synthetic atrial natriuretic factor on renal function and renin release. Am J Physiol 1984;247:F863–6.
[9] Kishimoto I, Dubois SK, Garbers DL. The heart communicates with the kidney exclusively through the guanylyl cyclase-A receptor: acute handling of sodium and water in response to volume expansion. Proc Natl Acad Sci U S A 1996;93:6215–9.
[10] Lopez MJ, Wong SKF, Kishimoto I, et al. Salt-resistant hypertension I mice lacking guanylyl cyclase-A receptor for atrial natriuretic peptide. Nature 1995; 378:65–8.
[11] Wright RS, Wei CM, Kim CH, et al. C-type natriuretic peptide-mediated coronary vasodilation: role of the coronary nitric oxide and particulate guanylate cyclase systems. J Am Coll Cardiol 1996;28:1031–8.
[12] Lainchbury JG, Burnett Jr JC, Meyer D, et al. Effects of the natriuretic peptides on load and myocardial function in normal and heart failure dogs. Am J Physiol 2000;278:H33–40.
[13] Yamamoto K, Burnett Jr JC, Redfield MM. Effects of endogenous natriuretic peptide system on ventricular and coronary function in the failing canine heart. Am J Physiol 1997;273:H2406–14.
[14] Hobbs RE, Mills RM, Young JB. An update on nesiritide for treatment of decompensated heart failure. Expert Opin Invest Drugs 2001;10:935–42.
[15] Boerrigter G, Burnett Jr JC. Recent advances in natriuretic peptides in congestive heart failure. Expert Opin Invest Drugs 2004;13:643–52.
[16] Chen HH, Burnett JC. The natriuretic peptides in heart failure: diagnostic and therapeutic potentials. Proc Assoc Am Physicians 1999;111:406–16.
[17] Colucci WS, Elkayam U, Horton DP, et al. The Nesiritide Study Group. Intravenous nesiritide, a natriuretic peptide, in the treatment of decompensated congestive heart failure. N Engl J Med 2000;343:246–53.
[18] Marcus LS, Hart D, Packer Yushak M, et al. Hemodynamic and renal excretory effects of human brain natriuretic peptide infusion in patients with congestive heart failure: a double-blind placebo controlled, randomized crossover trial. Circulation 1996; 94:3184–9.
[19] Publication Committee for the VMAC Investigators. (Vasodilation in the Management of Acute Heart CHF). Intravenous nesiritide versus nitroglycerin for treatment of decompensated congestive heart failure: a randomized controlled trial. J Am Med Assoc 2002; 287:1531–40.
[20] Chen HH, Cataliotti A, Schirger JA, et al. Equimolar doses of atrial and brain natriuretic peptides and urodilatin have differential renal actions in overt experimental heart failure. Am J Physiol 2004 [Epub ahead of print].
[21] Clavell AL, Stingo AJ, Wei C-M, et al. C-type natriuretic peptide: a selective cardiovascular peptide. Am J Physiol 1993;264(Regulatory Integrative Comp Physiol 33):R290–5.
[22] Hillege HL, Girbes AR, de Kam PJ, et al. Renal function, neurohormonal activation, and survival in patients with chronic heart failure. Circulation 2000; 102:203–10.
[23] Dries DL, Exner DV, Domanski MJ, et al. The prognostic implications of renal insufficiency in asymptomatic and symptomatic patients with left ventricular systolic dysfunction. J Am Coll Cardiol 2000; 35:681–9.
[24] Margulies KB, Perrella MA, Heublein DM, et al. ANF-mediated renal cyclic GMP generation in congestive heart failure. Am J Phyiol 1991;260: F562–8.
[25] Wang DJ, Dowling TC, Meadows D, et al. Nesiritide does not improve renal function in patients with chronic heart failure and worsening serum creatinine. Circulation 2004;110:1620–5.
[26] Kudo T, Baird A. Inhibition of aldosterone production in the adrenal glomerulosa by atrial natriuretic factor. Nature 1984;312:756–7.
[27] Higuchi K, Hashiguchi T, Ohashi M, et al. Porcine brain natriuretic peptide receptor in bovine adrenal cortex. Life Sci 1989;44:881–6.
[28] Chartier L, Schiffrin E, Thibault G, et al. Atrial natriuretic factor inhibits the stimulation of aldosterone secretion by angiotensin II, ACTH and potassium in vitro and angiotensin II-induced steroidogenesis in vivo. Endocrinology 1984;115:2026–8.
[29] Nawata H, Ohashi M, Haji M, et al. Atrial and brain natriuretic peptide in adrenal steroidogenesis. J Steroid Biochem Mol Biol 1991;40:367–79.
[30] Cataliotti A, Boerrigter G, Costello-Boerrigter LC, et al. Brain natriuretic peptide enhances renal actions of furosemide and suppresses furosemide-induced aldosterone activation in experimental heart failure. Circulation 2004;109:1680–5.
[31] Cataliotti A, Chen HH, Harty GJ, et al. Differential cardiorenal and humoral actions of a vasopeptidase inhibitor compared to ACE inhibitor and diuretic in experimental mild CHF. Circulation 2002;105: 639–44.
[32] Domanski M, Norman J, Pitt B, et al. Diuretic use, progressive heart failure, and death in patients in the Studies of Left Ventricular Dysfunction (SOLVD). J Am Coll Cardiol 2003;42:705–8.
[33] McCurley JM, Hanlon SU, Wei SK, et al. Furosemide and the progression of left ventricular dysfunction in experimental heart failure. J Am Coll Cardiol 2004; 44:1301–7.
[34] Lopez B, Querejeta R, Gonzalez A, et al. Effects of loop diuretics on myocardial fibrosis and collagen type-1 turnover in chronic heart failure. J Am Coll Cardiol 2004;43:2028–35.
[35] Stasch JP, Becker EM, Alonso-Alija C, et al. NO-independent regulatory site on soluble guanylate cyclase. Nature 2001;410:212–5.
[36] Boerrigter G, Costello-Boerrigter LC, Cataliotti A, et al. Cardiorenal and humoral properties of a novel direct soluble guanylate cyclase stimulator BAY 41–2272 in experimental congestive heart failure. Circulation 2003;107:686–9.

[37] Michaels AD, Klein A, Madden JA, et al. Effects of intravenous nesiritide on human coronary vasomotor regulation and myocardial oxygen uptake. Circulation 2003;107:2697–701.
[38] Molkentin JD. A friend within the heart: natriuretic peptide receptor signaling. J Clin Invest 2003;111: 1275–7.
[39] Holtwick R, van Eickels M, Skryabin BV, et al. Pressure-independent cardiac hypertrophy in mice with cardiomyocyte-restricted inactivation of the atrial natriuretic peptide receptor guanylyl cyclase-A. J Clin Invest 2003;111:1399–407.
[40] Tamura N, Ogawa Y, Chusho H, et al. Cardiac fibrosis in mice lacking brain natriuretic peptide. Proc Natl Acad Sci U S A 2000;97:4239–44.
[41] Pitt B, Zannad F, Remme WJ, et al, for The Randomized Aldactone Evaluation Study Investigators. The effect of spironolactone on morbidity and mortality in patients with severe heart failure. N Engl J Med 2001;341:709–17.
[42] Pitt B, Remme W, Zannad F, et al. Eplerenone Post-Acute Myocardial Infarction Heart Failure Efficacy and Survival Study Investigators. Eplerenone, a selective aldosterone blocker, in patients with left ventricular dysfunction after myocardial infarction. N Engl J Med 2003;348:1309–21.
[43] Burlew B, Weber KT. Cardiac fibrosis as a cause of diastolic dysfunction. Herz 2002;27:92–8.
[44] Frohlich ED, Apstein C, Chobanian AV, et al. The heart in hypertension. N Engl J Med 1992;327: 998–1008.
[45] Manabe I, Shido T, Nagai R. Gene expression in fibroblasts and fibrosis: involvement in cardiac hypertrophy. Circ Res 2002;91:1103–13.
[46] Kohl P. Heterogenous cell coupling in the heart: an electrophysiological role for fibroblasts. Circ Res 2003;93:381–3.
[47] Cha Y-M, Dzeja PP, Shen WK, et al. Failing atrial myocardium: energetic deficits accompany structural remodeling and electrical instability. Am J Physiol Heart Circ Physiol 2003;284:H1313–20.
[48] Frank JS, Langer GA. The myocardial interstitium: its structure and its role in ionic exchange. J Cell Biol 1974;60:586–601.
[49] Spinale FG. Matrix metalloproteinases: regulation and dysregulation in the failing heart. Circ Res 2002;90: 520–30.
[50] Tsuruda T, Costello-Boerrigter LC, Burnett Jr JC. Matrix metalloproteinases: pathways of induction by bioactive molecules. Heart Fail Rev 2004;9:53–60.
[51] Zannad F, Dousset B, Alla F. Treatment of congestive heart failure: interfering the aldosterone-cardiac extracellular matrix relationship. Hypertension 2001;38: 1227–32.
[52] Tsuruda T, Jougasaki M, Boerrigter G, et al. Cardiotrophin-1 stimulation of cardiac fibroblast growth: roles for glycoprotein 130/leukemia inhibitory factor receptor and the endothelin type-A receptor. Circ Res 2002;90:128–34.
[53] Pennica D, King KL, Shaw KJ, et al. Expression cloning of cardiotrophin 1, a cytokine that induces cardiac myocyte hypertrophy. Proc Natl Acad Sci U S A 1995;92:1142–6.
[54] Fukuzawa J, Booz GW, Hunt RA, et al. Cardiotrophin-1 increases angiotensinogen mRNA in rat cardiac myocytes through STAT3: an autocrine loop for hypertrophy. Hypertension 2000;35:1191–6.
[55] Sheng Z, Knowlton K, Chen J, et al. Cardiotrophin-1 (CT-1) inhibition of cardiac myocyte apoptosis via a mitogen-activated protein kinase-dependent pathway: divergence from downstreat CT-1 signals for myocardial cell hypertrophy. J Bio Chem 1997;272:5783–91.
[56] Jougasaki M, Larsen AM, Cataliotti A, et al. Cardiotrophin-1 stimulates endothelin-1 via gp130 in vascular endothelial cells. Peptides 2002;23:1441–7.
[57] Fujisaki H, Itoh H, Hirata Y, et al. Natriuretic peptides inhibit angiotensin II-induced proliferation of rat cardiac fibroblasts by blocking endothelin-1 gene expression. J Clin Invest 1995;96:1059–65.
[58] Horio T, Tokodume T, Maki T, et al. Gene expression, secretion, and autocrine actions of C-type natriuretic peptide in cultured adult rat cardiac fibrosis. Endocrinology 2003;144:2279–84.
[59] Calderone A, Thaik CM, Takahashi N, et al. Nitric oxide, atrial natriuretic peptide, and cyclic GMP inhibit the growth-promoting effects of norepinephrine in cardiac myocytes and fibroblasts. J Clin Invest 1998; 101:812–8.
[60] Tsuruda T, Boerrigter G, Huntley BK, et al. Brain natriuretic peptide is produced in cardiac fibroblasts and induces matrix metalloproteinases. Circ Res 2002; 91:1127–34.
[61] Kapoun A, Liang F, O'Young G, et al. B-type natriuretic peptide exerts broad functional opposition to transforming growth factor-β in primary human cardiac fibroblasts: fibrosis, myofibroblast convsion, proliferation, and inflammation. Circ Res 2004;94: 334–42.
[62] Swanton C. Cell-cycle targeted therapies. Lancet Oncol 2004;5:27–36.
[63] Kronemann N, Nockher WA, Busse R, et al. Growth-inhibitory effect of cyclic GMP- and cyclic AMP-dependent vasodilators on rat vascular smooth muscle cells: effect on cell cycle and cyclin expression. Br J Pharmacol 1999;126:349–57.
[64] Pedram A, Razandi M, Hu R-M, et al. Astrocyte progression from G_1 to S phase of the cell cycle depends upon multiple protein interaction. J Biol Chem 1998;273:13966–72.
[65] Burnett Jr JC, Kao PC, Hu DC, et al. Atrial natriuretic peptide elevation in congestive heart failure in the human. Science 1986;231:1145–7.
[66] Luchner A, Stevens TL, Borgeson DD, et al. Differential atrial and ventricular expression of myocardial BNP during evolution of heart failure. Am J Physiol 1998;274:H1684–9.
[67] Stevens TL, Burnett Jr JC, Kinoshita M, et al. A functional role for endogenous atrial natriuretic peptide in

a canine model of early left ventricular dysfunction. J Clin Inv 1995;95:1101–8.

[68] Stevens TL, Rasmussen TE, Wei C-M, et al. Renal role of the endogenous natriuretic peptide system in acute congestive heart failure. J Card Fail 1996;2:119–25.

[69] Wada A, Tsutamoto T, Matsuda Y, et al. Cardiorenal and neurohumoral effects of endogenous atrial natriuretic peptide in dogs with severe congestive heart failure using a specific antagonist for guanylate cyclase-coupled receptors. Circulation 1994;89:2232–40.

[70] Lee S-C, Stevens TL, Sandberg SM, et al. The potential of brain natriuretic peptide as a biomarker for New York Heart Association Class during the outpatient treatment of heart failure. J Card Fail 2002; 8:149–54.

[71] Chen HH, Grantham A, Schirger J, et al. Subcutaneous administration of BNP in experimental heart failure. J Am Coll Cardio 2000;36:1706–12.

[72] Chen HH, Redfield MM, Nordstrom LJ, et al. Subcutaneous administration of the cardiac hormone BNP in symptomatic human heart failure. J Card Fail 2004;10:115–9.

[73] Yancy CW, Salzberg MT, Berkowitz RL, et al. Safety and feasibility of using serial infusions of nesiritide for heart failure in an outpatient setting (from the FUSION Trial). Am J Cardiol 2004;94:595–601.

[74] Maisel AS, Krisnaswamy P, Nowak RM, et al. Breathing Not Properly Multinational Study Investigators. Rapid measurement of B-type natriuretic peptide in the emergency diagnosis of heart failure. N Engl J Med 2002;347:161–7.

[75] Cataliotti A, Malatino L, Jougasaki M, et al. Circulating natriuretic peptide concentrations in patients with end-stage renal disease: role of brain natriuretic peptide as a biomarker for ventricular remodeling. Mayo Clin Proc 2001;76:1111–9.

[76] Lubien E, DeMaria A, Krishnaswamy P, et al. Utility of B-natriuretic peptide in detecting diastolic dysfunction: comparison with Doppler velocity recordings. Circulation 2002;105:595–601 [erratum: Circulation 2002;106:387].

[77] Troughton RW, Frampton CM, Yandle TG, et al. Treatment of heart failure guided by plasma amino terminal brain natriuretic peptide (N-BNP) concentrations. Lancet 2000;355:1126–30.

[78] McCullough PA, Nowak RM, McCord J, et al. Krishnaswamy P, Kazanegra R, Maisel A, for the BNP Multinational Study Investigators. B-type natriuretic peptide and clinical judgment in emergency diagnosis of heart failure analysis from Breathing Not Properly (BNP) Multinational Study. Circulation 2002;106:416–22.

[79] Yamamoto K, Burnett JC, Bermudez EA, et al. Clinical criteria and biochemical marker for the detection of systolic dysfunction. J Card Fail 2000;6:194–9.

[80] Costello-Boerrigter LC, Redfield MM, Rodeheffer RJ, et al. NT-proBNP is superior to BNP in the detection of left ventricular systolic dysfunction in the community. Circulation 2004;110(Suppl III):368.

[81] Wang TJ, Larson MG, Levy D, et al. Impact of obesity on plasma natriuretic peptide levels. Circulation 2004; 109:594–600.

[82] Tsutamoto T, Wada A, Maeda K, et al. Attenuation of compensation of endogenous cardiac natriuretic peptide system in chronic heart failure: prognostic role of plasma brain natriuretic concentration in patients with chronic symptomatic left ventricular dysfunction. Circulation 1997;96:509–16.

[83] Yandle TG, Richards AM, Gilbert A, et al. Assay of brain natriuretic peptide (BNP) in human plasma: evidence for high molecular weight BNP as a major plasma component in heart failure. J Clin Endocrinol Metab 1993;76:832–8.

[84] Shimizu H, Masuta K, Asada H, et al. Characterization of molecular forms of probrain natriuretic peptide in human plasma. Clin Chim Acta 2003;334:233–9.

[85] Shimizu H, Masuta K, Aono K, et al. Molecular forms of human brain natriuretic peptide in plasma. Clin Chim Acta 2002;316:129–35.

[86] Wei CM, Kao PC, Lin J-T, et al. Heart failure: circulating beta atrial natriuretic factor in congestive heart failure in humans. Circulation 1993;88:1016–20.

[87] Langenickel TH, Pagel I, Buttergereit J, et al. Rat corin gene: molecular cloning and reduced expression in experimental heart failure. Am J Physiol Heart Circ Physiol 2004;287:H1516–21.

[88] Redfield MM, Jacobsen SJ, Burnett Jr JC, et al. Burden of systolic and diastolic ventricular dysfunction in the community. Appreciating the scope of the heart failure epidemic. J Am Med Assoc 2003;289:194–202.

[89] Levy D, Kenchaiah S, Larson MG, et al. Long-term trends in the incidence of and survival with heart failure. N Engl J Med 2002;347:1397–402.

[90] McDonagh TA, Morrison CE, Lawrence A, et al. Symptomatic and asymptomatic left-ventricular systolic dysfunction in an urban population. Lancet 1997; 350:829–33.

[91] Wang TJ, Evans JC, Benjamin EJ, et al. Natural history of asymptomatic left ventricular systolic dysfunction in the community. Circulation 2003;108:977–82.

ELSEVIER
SAUNDERS

Heart Failure Clin 1 (2005) 141 – 150

HEART
FAILURE
CLINICS

Pharmacogenomics for Neurohormonal Intervention in Heart Failure

Dennis M. McNamara, MD*

University of Pittsburgh Medical Center, Pittsburgh, PA, USA

Variations useful to man...have undoubtedly occurred in the great and complex battle of life.
Charles Darwin, *On the Origin of Species* [1].

After an initial myocardial injury, individuals progress to the syndrome of heart failure at markedly different rates, as noted by Sir William Osler over a century ago [2]. The myocardial injury elicits a complex systemic response involving the central nervous system, the kidney, and the vascular endothelium, collectively termed *neurohormonal activation*. The magnitude of this systemic response determines the rate of progression to the clinical syndrome. The advances of the human genome project have led to increased recognition of the inherent variation of important disease modifiers and the potential medical implications [3]. The clinical heterogeneity noted by Osler is to a great extent genetically based, because an individual's genetic background is a major determinant of the degree of neurohormonal activation.

Through modulating the neurohormonal response to injury, genetic background will influence heart failure progression and alter the impact of the pharmacologic therapy. Analysis of the critical genetic loci behind this "background effect" should facilitate individualized treatment decisions. To understand how pharmacogenetic interactions influence the impact of treatment, it is essential to begin with the main targets of current pharmacotherapy: the angiotensin-converting enzyme (ACE) and the cardiac β-adrenergic receptors (βARs).

Angiotensin-converting enzyme deletion/insertion polymorphism

Heart failure outcomes

The ACE deletion/insertion (D/I) biallelic polymorphism of intron 16 is the most extensively studied cardiovascular polymorphism, and has been the subject of hundreds of investigations since its initial discovery [4,5]. Although the clinical implications of this polymorphism have been controversial, the physiologic association of the ACE D/I polymorphism with enzymatic activity has been consistent. The D allele has been linked in nearly every clinical study to increased activity of ACE and higher levels of the product of ACE activity, the peptide mediator angiotensin II (a2) [6]. The cellular mechanism is unknown, but this linkage of genotype with ACE activity is consistent across different clinical paradigms from hypertension to myocardial infarction [7–9] and demonstrates a D allele "dose effect" for a2 levels. Subjects with the DD genotype have the highest levels of a2, heterozygotes are intermediate, and those homozygous for I allele have the lowest levels. For disease states such as heart failure, where a2 facilitates disease progression, the potential implications of this genetically "ordered" ACE activity are apparent.

This article was supported in part by National Institute of Health Grants HL 69912 and HL 075038.

* Heart Failure/Transplantation Program, University of Pittsburgh Medical Center, S-558 Lothrop Street, Pittsburgh, PA 15213.

E-mail address: mcnamaradm@upmc.edu

1551-7136/05/$ – see front matter
doi:10.1016/j.hfc.2004.10.001

Given the role of renin-angiotensin activation in heart failure, it is hypothesized that the ACE D allele functions as a genetic modifier, accelerates disease progression, and worsens survival. This has been demonstrated in three clinical investigations. The first, a study of 193 subjects who had idiopathic dilated cardiomyopathy, demonstrated poorer survival for subjects homozygous for the D allele [10]. Most recently, the adverse impact of the ACE D allele was demonstrated in 978 subjects post–myocardial infarction [11]. The impact in this cohort was primarily in subjects who had lower left ventricular ejections fraction (LVEF) or higher brain naturetic peptide levels. Forty-five percent of the subjects in

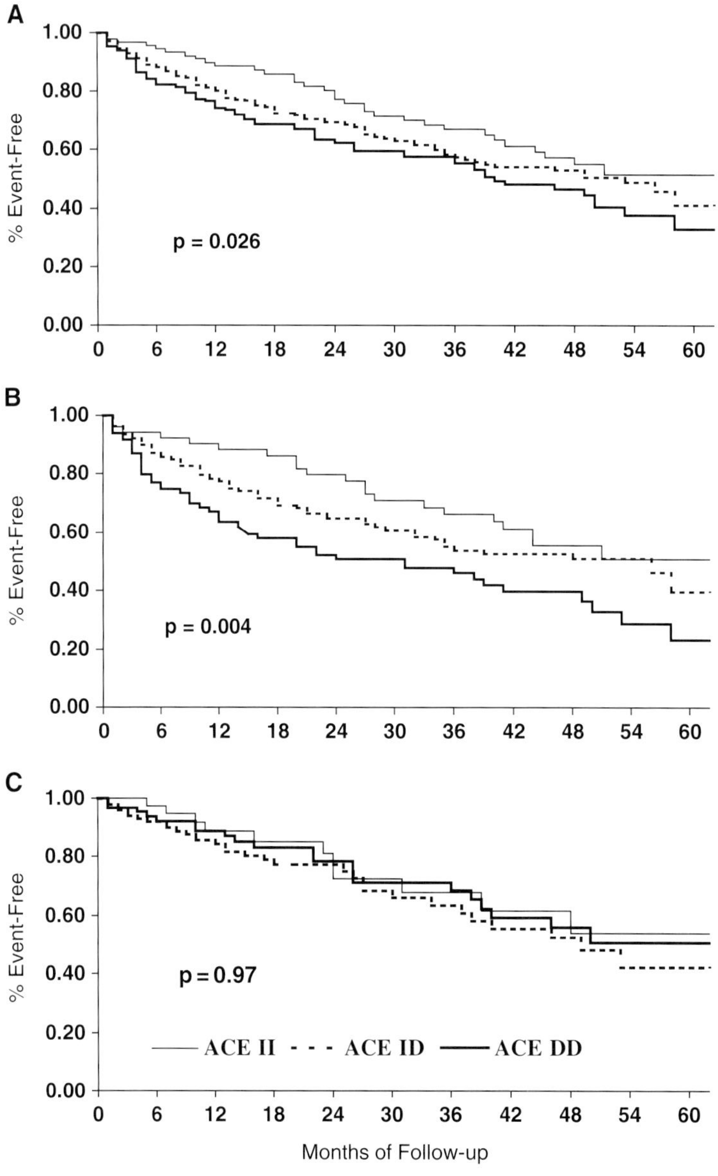

Fig. 1. Transplant-free survival by ACE D/I genotype, GRACE study, University of Pittsburgh. (*A*) Overall cohort, ACE D allele associated with poorer event-free survival (n = 479, *P* = .026). (*B*) Subset with no β-blocker therapy (n = 277, *P* = .004). (*C*) Subset treated with β-blocker therapy (n = 202, *P* = .97). (*From* McNamara DM, Holubkov R, Postava L, et al. Phamacogenetic interactions between ACE inhibitor therapy and the angiotensin-converting enzyme deletion polymorphism in patients with congestive heart failure. J Amer Coll Cardiol 2004;44:2019–26; with permission.)

the post–myocardial infarction study were on ACE inhibitor therapy, compared with only 25% of subjects in the study of idiopathic dilated cardiomyopathy. Neither study addressed the potential pharmacogenetic interactions of the ACE D/I polymorphism with the medical therapy of heart failure.

Pharmacogenetics of the angiotensin-converting enzyme deletion/insertion polymorphism: Genetic Risk Assessment of Cardiac Events

A similar overall impact of the ACE D allele on heart failure outcomes was demonstrated in a study at the University of Pittsburgh, the GRACE study of Genetic Risk Assessment of Cardiac Events. Four hundred seventy-nine subjects who had systolic dysfunction (mean LVEF 0.25 ± 0.08) with ischemic and nonischemic etiologies were followed for a median of 3 years until death or cardiac transplantation. The D allele was associated with poorer transplant-free survival, and demonstrated the same "gene-ordered" effect shown for ACE activity: II homozygotes demonstrated the best survival, DD homozygotes the poorest, and heterozygotes showed the predicted "intermediate" survival between the homozygotes. The adverse impact of the D allele on survival for this cohort first was reported on an analysis of the first 328 subjects [12], and remained evident during analysis of the entire cohort (Fig. 1) [13].

β-Blocker therapy

Genetic background must interact with environment, and for the heart failure patient a critical aspect of the local "environment" is the pharmacologic milieu. GRACE examined how pharmacologic inhibition may alter the effect of genetic modulation of neurohormonal activation on heart failure outcomes. Ninety-five percent of subjects in GRACE were on ACE inhibitors or a2 receptor blockers (ARBs), whereas only 42% were on β-blockers, reflecting the evolution of care when the study began. For β-blockers, analysis by treatment subset demonstrated the effects of ACE D on outcomes to be primarily in subjects not treated with β-blockers [12,13] and that β-blocker therapy eliminates the impact of the polymorphism (see Fig. 1). For subjects not on β-blockers, the 2-year event-free survival for DD subjects was 51%, versus 80% for the II homozygotes. In contrast, for subjects on β-blockers, no effect of the D allele on outcomes was apparent. The elimination of the effect of the D allele by β-blocker therapy likely reflects their role as inhibitors of renin release. Sympathetic activation is an important stimulus to the renin angiotensin activity in heart failure, and β-blockers markedly reduce a2 levels [14].

The potential usefulness of this pharmacogenetic interaction is evident when examining the impact of β-blocker therapy within ACE D/I genetic subsets (Fig. 2). Although β-blockers improved survival overall in the GRACE cohort, much of that benefit is in the DD homozygotes genetically predicted to have the highest levels of ACE activity. The impact of therapy is diminished in the heterozygotes, and in this small cohort is no longer evident for subjects who are II homozygotes. These results suggest the ACE D/I polymorphism delineates genetic subsets of heart failure patients in whom the therapeutic impact of β-blockade on heart failure survival is different. A recent study [15] of the effect of β-blockers in 199 subjects who had chronic heart failure demonstrated similar improvements in LVEF in all three genetic subsets, and suggests the ACE D/I polymorphism does not predict this particular endpoint of β-blocker response.

Angiotensin-converting enzyme inhibitor therapy

Based on ACE activity, it is predicted that the ACE D/I polymorphisms should modulate the effect of ACE inhibitors. Because 95% of the subjects in GRACE were on either an ACE inhibitor or an ARB, this pharmacogenetic interaction was investigated in this cohort using a dose analysis comparing the effect of higher dose ACE therapy (>50% of target daily

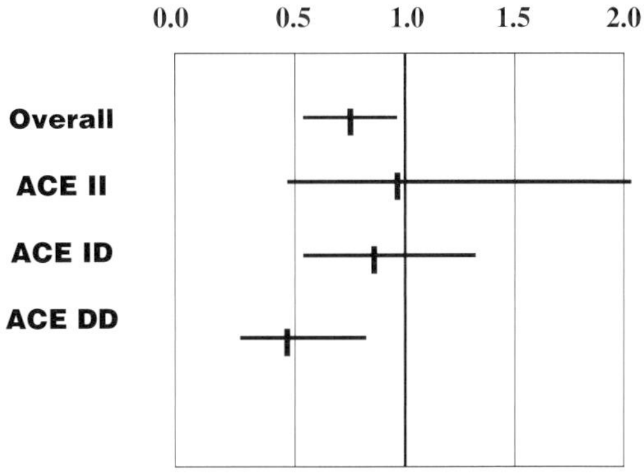

Fig. 2. Relative risk of event (death or transplantation) by β-blocker use, GRACE study: overall cohort and by ACE D/I, DD, DI, and II genotype. (*Data from* McNamara DM, Holubkov R, Postava L, et al. Phamacogenetic interactions between ACE inhibitor therapy and the angiotensin-converting enzyme deletion polymorphism in patients with congestive heart failure. J Amer Coll Cardiol 2004;44: 2019–26.)

dose defined by national guidelines) on transplant-free survival to low-dose therapy (≤ 50%). This resulted in a roughly threefold difference in the mean dose for the high-dose group compared with the low-dose group. In contrast, the multicenter Assessment of Treatment with Lisinopril and Survival (ATLAS) trial [16] evaluated the impact of a 10-fold difference in the mean dose of ACE inhibitor. Analysis by ACE dose treatment subset suggests higher doses of ACE inhibitors limit the adverse impact of the ACE D allele [13], and this effect of high-dose therapy was particularly evident in subjects not treated with β-blockers (Fig. 3).

In overall event-free survival, the benefits of higher dose ACE inhibitors were modest with the relative risk (RR) of high-dose therapy 0.88. This 12% reduction was not statistically significant, but was similar to the trend in survival benefit seen in ATLAS. The RR reduction with higher dose ACE inhibitor therapy within ACE genotype class demonstrated a gene-ordered effect similar to that seen with β-blockers, with the greatest impact within the DD subset, although this failed to reach significance (Fig. 4).

The effect of high-dose therapy in DD homozygotes is consistent with greater resistance to ACE inhibition in this subset. In subjects who have heart failure, the blood pressure response to captopril demonstrates minimal effects in DD subjects, an intermediate response in heterozygotes, and the greatest impact in II patients [17]. A similar interaction was demonstrated for chronic therapy with angiotensin-receptor antagonists in hypertensive subjects [18]. The studies suggest a diminished response to ACE inhibition or blockade with the ACE D allele. The higher ACE activity evident in ACE DD homozygotes is the most likely mechanism of this genetically determined drug "resistance."

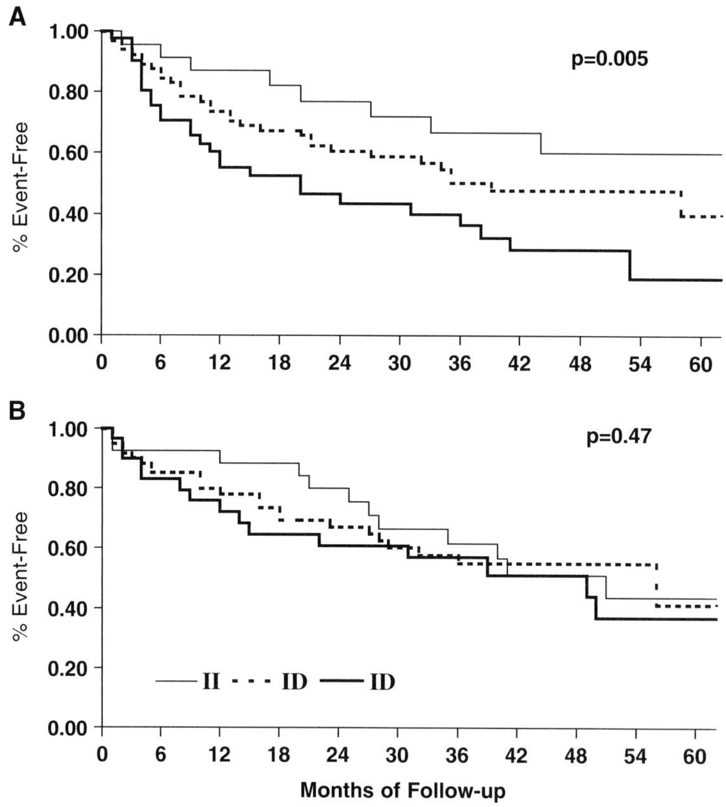

Fig. 3. Transplant-free survival by ACE D/I genotype, GRACE study, University of Pittsburgh. (*A*) Subset on low-dose ACE inhibitors and no β-blockers. ACE D allele was associated with poorer event-free survival (n = 130, *P* = .005). (*B*) Subset with high-dose ACE inhibitor therapy and no β-blockers (n = 117, *P* = .47). (*Data from* McNamara DM, Holubkov R, Postava L, et al. Phamacogenetic interactions between ACE inhibitor therapy and the angiotensin-converting enzyme deletion polymorphism in patients with congestive heart failure. J Amer Coll Cardiol 2004;44:2019–26; with permission.)

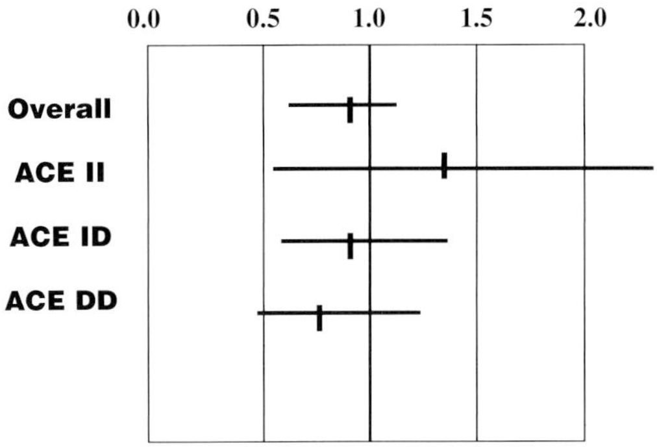

Fig. 4. Relative risk of event (death or transplantation) by ACE inhibitor dose use, GRACE study: overall cohort and by ACE D/I, DD, DI, and II genotype. (*Adapted from* McNamara DM, Holubkov R, Postava L, et al. Phamacogenetic interactions between ACE inhibitor therapy and the angiotensin-converting enzyme deletion polymorphism in patients with congestive heart failure. J Amer Coll Cardiol 2004;44:2019–26; with permission.)

Aldosterone receptor antagonists

The prevalence of "aldosterone escape" on ACE inhibitors is greatest in the ACE DD genotype [19]. The impact of the aldosterone receptor antagonist spironolactone on left ventricular remodeling also is diminished in the ACE DD subset compared with the ID and II subsets [20], closely paralleling the diminished clinical response to ACE inhibitors. The influence of the ACE D/I polymorphism on the effect of aldosterone receptor antagonists on survival remains to be determined.

β-Adrenergic receptor variation

Although the ACE D/I polymorphism is an important component, neurohormonal activation is polygenic and variation at multiple loci will determine the overall impact of genetic background on heart failure treatment. Genetic variation in the cellular targets of pharmacologic therapy predicts several genomic loci as potential major determinants of this "background effect." The impact of β-blockers is mediated through β_1- and β_2-adrenergic receptors, and the functional significance of their common genetic polymorphisms has been researched intensely [21].

Structure and function

Activation of both β receptor subtypes is linked to increased cyclic adenosine monophosphate (cAMP) formation through the interaction with stimulatory guanine nucleotide-binding protein (G_s). In the normal heart, β_1 receptors predominate over β_2 receptors at a ratio of approximately 4:1, whereas in the failing myocardium, sympathetic overactivation leads to selective down-regulation of β_1 receptors to a greater extent than β_2; as a result, the percentage of β_2 receptors may increase up to 40% [22]. In contrast, β_2 receptors do not decrease in receptor number, but become deactivated or less responsive to agonist stimulation.

The β_1-adrenergic receptor (Fig. 5) is encoded for by an intronless gene and consists of a protein with 477 amino acid residues and seven transmembrane domains (TMDs). The first 60 amino acids of the amino terminus comprise the extracellular surface of the receptor, whereas the final 90 amino acids are located in the cytoplasmic domain. The β_2 receptor subtype (Fig. 6) has a similar genomic and protein structure [23] with a coding region of 1239 nucleic acids encoding for 413 amino acids. Between β_1 and β_2 adrenergic receptors, the greatest amino acid identity (71%) is found in the TMDs, and the tertiary structure in the lipid bilayer takes on a ring or barrel shape that allows for multiple ligand contact points [24]. The cytoplasmic regions of the two receptor classes are more distinct, which allows for more diversity in their signaling interactions with other intracellular proteins [25].

Functional variation and heart failure outcomes: β_2

Initial investigations of functional genetic variation focused on the β_2 receptor because of its importance in the pharmacologic treatment of asthma [26]. Population studies have revealed three common polymorphisms resulting in an amino acid substitution—Arg16Gly, Glu27Gln, and Thr164Ile—and in vitro studies have demonstrated significant functional consequences in terms of receptor function or regulation [27]. The substitution of Ile for Thr occurs with allele frequency of approximately 3% to 5%, and the Ile164 receptor has significantly lower binding affinity for isoproterenol, epinephrine, and norepinephrine (Table 1) [28]. Agonist stimulation of the Ile variant produces a lower level of adenylyl cyclase activity with the Thr wild type receptor. Examination of murine models seems consistent with in vitro studies, because transgenic mice that overexpress the Ile164 receptor in the heart have a decrease in resting and (agonist-stimulated) contractile function in vivo compared with transgenic controls overexpressing the wild type Thr164 receptor [29].

The functional significance of the Ile164 variant in vitro and in animal models supports a potential

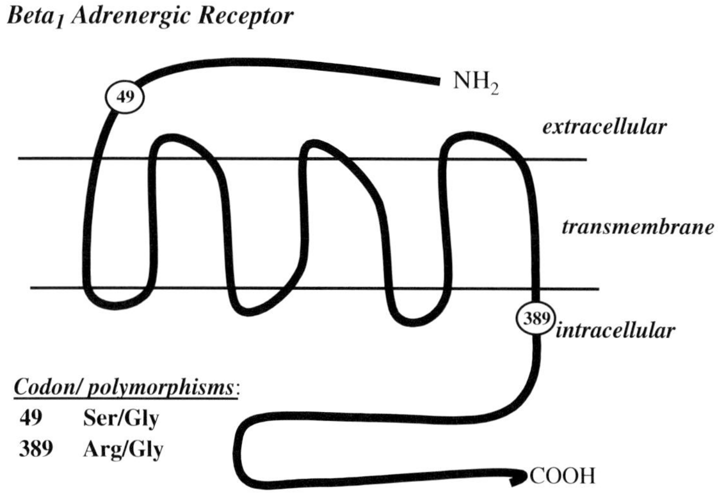

Fig. 5. Structure of the β_1 adrenergic receptor: common polymorphisms. Arg, arginine; COOH, carboxyl terminus; Gly, glycine; NH2, amino terminus; Ser, serine. (*From* McNamara DM, MacGowan GA, London B. Clinical importance of beta adrenoceptor polymorphisms in cardiovascular disease. Am J Pharmacogenomics 2002;2:73–8; with permission.)

clinically significant role in heart failure, which has been demonstrated in clinical outcomes studies. A prospective study at the University of Cincinnati of 259 patients who had class II–IV heart failure found that the presence of the Ile164 receptor polymorphism markedly decreased transplant-free survival with an RR for death or transplant of 4.8 compared with those homozygous for Thr164 [30]. Investigation in this population also revealed a marked reduction in functional capacity, as measured by metabolic stress testing, among patients with the Ile 164 [31]. A study of normal Thr164Ile heterozygotes demonstrated blunted agonist responsiveness compared with subjects homozygous for Thr164 [32,33], which may underlie its adverse impact on heart failure survival.

The effect of the Ile164 variant in these investigations supports the importance of the β_2 receptor in

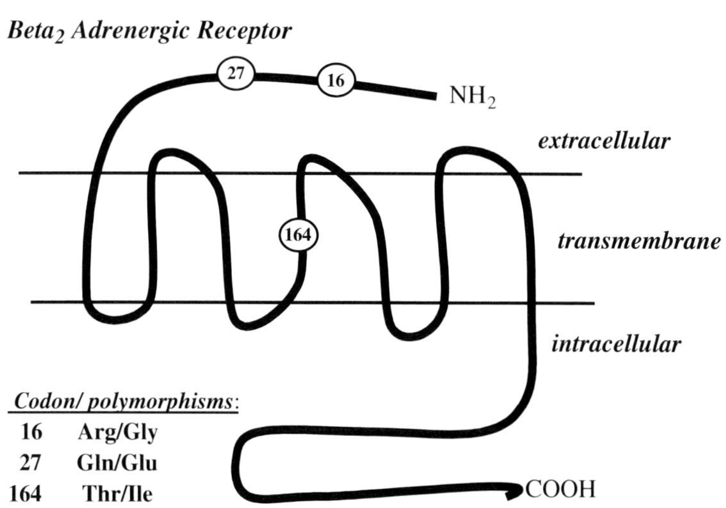

Fig. 6. Structure of the β_2 adrenergic receptor: common polymorphisms. Arg, arginine; COOH, carboxyl terminus; Gln, glutamine; Glu, glutamate; Gly, glycine; Ile, Isoleucine; NH2, amino terminus; Thr, threonine. (*From* McNamara DM, MacGowan GA, London B. Clinical importance of beta adrenoceptor polymorphisms in cardiovascular disease. Am J Pharmacogenomics 2002;2:73–8; with permission.)

Table 1
Frequency and function of β_1 and β_2 polymorphisms

Codon	Region	Polymorphism	Allele frequency (%)	Function in vitro
β_1				
389	Cytoplasmic	Arg/Gly	70/30	Arg: gain of function (increased cAMP)
49	Extracellular	Ser/Gly	85/15	No data
β_2				
16	Extracellular	Arg/Gly	40/60	Gly: enhanced downregulation
27	Extracellular	Gln/Glu	55/45	Glu: resistance to downregulation
164	Transmembrane domain 4	Thr/Ile	95/5	Ile: loss of function, decreased agonist binding, decreased cAMP

Abbreviations: Arg, arginine; Gln, glutamine; Glu, glutamate; Gly, glycine; Ile, isoleucine; Ser, serine; Thr, threonin.
Adapted from McNamara DM, MacGowan GA, London B. Clinical importance of beta adrenoceptor polymorphisms in cardiovascular disease. Am J Pharmacogenomics 2002;2:73–8; with permission.

heart failure progression, although the small number of subjects with the variant limits pharmacogenetic investigations. Several studies have linked the more common Arg16Gly or Glu27Gln polymorphisms to hypertension [34,35], but no influence on heart failure outcomes has been shown [30].

Functional variation and heart failure outcomes: β_1

The two most common polymorphisms for the β_1 receptor are Ser49Gly and Arg389Gl [36], and both seem to be linked to heart failure outcomes. The relative allele frequency for the Arg389Gly variant is approximately 0.70/0.30, and for the Ser49Gly polymorphism 0.85/0.15.

The codon 49 polymorphism is located in the extracellular domain of the receptor (see Fig. 5), and the Gly49 variant is associated in vitro with increased receptor down-regulation [37,38]. In contrast, amino acid 389 is located near the carboxyl-terminus cytoplasmic tail and in vitro demonstrates a higher basal adenylyl cyclase activity with the Arg389 receptor. With agonist stimulation this distinction was magnified greatly, suggesting the Arg389 variant results in a gain of function for G-protein coupling [39].

An examination of more than 1000 normal individuals suggested that the Gly49 variant was associated with lower resting heart rate [40]. A heart failure outcomes study in 184 subjects who had systolic dysfunction suggested the Gly49 variant was associated with improved survival [41]. An examination of the GRACE cohort suggests the Gly49 variant is linked to greater benefit from adrenergic receptor blockade [42]. The Arg389 variant was linked to a greater risk for heart failure in an African-American cohort, but only when co-inherited with a deletion of the α-2C receptor [43]. The genetic substudy of the BEST trial of bucindilol suggests the presence of the 389Arg variant predicts a greater improvement of survival with β-blocker therapy [44], but this linkage of 389Arg to β-blocker benefit was not evident with metoprolol in the MERIT-HF substudy [45]. In a similar fashion, examination of the impact of 389Arg on blood pressure response in hypertensive subjects has led to conflicting results [46,47].

Endothelial nitric oxide synthase

Nitric oxide (NO) plays an important protective role in heart failure [48,49] and endothelial nitric oxide synthase (NOS3) is the predominant source of vascular NO. A common polymorphism (G894T) exists on exon 7 (codon 298: Glu298Asp) for which the wild type glutamate is replaced with aspartic acid [50]. The functional role of this apparently charge-neutral amino acid change is controversial, but the Asp298 variant has a shorter half-life and therefore less NO activity in endothelial cell culture [51]. The Asp298 variant has been linked to the risk for coronary disease, hypertension, and stroke. For subjects who had heart failure, functional assessment by metabolic stress testing demonstrated significantly higher maximum oxygen consumption in subjects who had the Glu298Glu phenotype compared with those homozygous or heterozygous for the Asp298 variant [52]. This modulation of functional capacity by the Asp298Glu polymorphism parallels the impact on survival, because poorer transplant-free survival was evident for subjects with the Asp298 variant compared with individuals homozygous for Glu298 (Fig. 7) [52]. Although the Asp298 variant has been investigated as a risk factor for coronary disease, the impact in GRACE reflects a role as a modulator of heart failure, and was more apparent in the non-ischemic cohort.

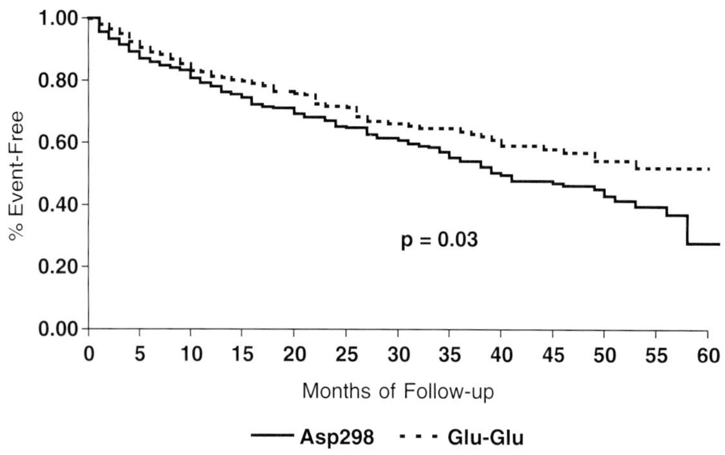

Fig. 7. Transplant-free survival by NOS3 codon 298 polymorphism, GRACE study, University of Pittsburgh. Overall cohort (n = 469): Asp^{298} variant (*solid line*), n = 266; Glu^{298} homozygotes (*dashed line*), n = 203. Event-free survival was significantly poorer in subjects with the Asp^{298} variant (P = .03). (*From* McNamara DM, Holubkov R, Postava L, et al. The Asp^{298} variant of endothelial nitric oxide synthase: effect on survival for patients with congestive heart failure. Circulation 2003;107:1598–602; with permission.)

Pharmacogenetic interactions with endothelial nitric oxide synthase and angiotensin-converting enzyme inhibitors

Clinical and animal studies demonstrate that NOS3 plays a central role in the therapeutic effects of ACE inhibitors. Murine knockout models have demonstrated that the postinfarction benefit of ACE inhibitors on remodeling depends on NOS3 [53]. In clinical studies of vascular reactivity, the effects of ACE inhibitors are diminished by pretreatment with NOS inhibitors. In GRACE, the examination of high-dose versus low-dose ACE inhibitor suggests a pharmacogenetic interaction with the NOS3 Glu298Asp polymorphism, because the impact of Asp298 was primarily in subjects on low-dose ACE inhibitor, and was not evident in those receiving high-dose therapy [54]. Analysis of the impact of ACE inhibitor dose by genetic subset suggests the variable benefit of ACE inhibitors may be explained partially by variation at the NOS3 locus, but this will need additional investigation in larger cohorts.

Summary

For the ACE D/I polymorphism, linkage of the D allele to higher ACE activity results in a predictable impact for therapies inhibiting a2 production: ACE inhibitors and β-receptor antagonists. Both therapies seem to have their greatest impact on the 30% of the population who are homozygous for the D allele, genetically predicted to have the highest levels of neurohormonal activation. Several independent groups of investigators have demonstrated the adverse impact of the ACE D allele in heart failure, which is consistent with the role of renin-angiotensin activation in clinical progression. Genotyping of the ACE locus may identify large subsets of patients who receive maximal benefit for aggressive neurohormonal blockade.

Predictably, genetic influences on heart failure therapy are polygenic. In addition to ACE, the therapeutic impact of β-receptor antagonists is influenced by variation at the β_1 receptor locus. The effectiveness of ACE inhibitor therapy may be influenced by variation of ACE and NOS3. Pharmacogenetic investigations have not integrated more than one genetic loci into a clinical outcomes model, and larger cohorts will be required for adequate statistical power to address polygenic "background" effects. Analysis of genetic background has become a potential clinical tool for predicting heart failure outcomes and targeting therapeutic intervention. Prospective validation of the predictive impact of genetic variants will be required before the routine implementation of genetically individualized treatments.

References

[1] Darwin C. Natural selection. In: On the origin of species. London: J. Murray; 1859. p. 80.

[2] Osler W. Diseases of the circulatory system. In: The

principles and practice of medicine. New York: D. Appleton and Co.; 1892. p. 623–40.

[3] Ligget SB. Pharmacogenetic applications of the human genome project. Nat Med 2001;7:281–3.

[4] Rigat B, Hubert C, Alhenc-Gelas F, et al. An insertion/deletion polymorphism in the angiotensin I-converting enzyme gene accounting for half the variance of serum enzyme levels. J Clin Invest 1990;86:1343–6.

[5] Rigat B, Hubert C, Corvol P, et al. PCR detection of the insertion/deletion polymorphism of the human angiotensin converting enzyme gene (DCP) (dipeptidyl carboxypeptidase 1). Nucleic Acids Res 1992; 20:1433.

[6] Tiret L, Rigat B, Visvikis S, et al. Evidence, from combined segregation and linkage analysis, that a variant of the angiotensin I-converting enzyme (ACE) gene controls plasma ACE levels. Am J Hum Genet 1992;51:197–205.

[7] Danser AH, Derkx FH, Hense HW, et al. Angiotensinogen (M235T) and angiotensin-converting enzyme (I/D) polymorphisms in association with plasma renin and prorenin levels. J Hypertens 1998;16:1879–83.

[8] Cambien F, Poirier O, Lecerf L, et al. Deletion polymorphism in the gene for angiotensin-converting enzyme is a potent risk factor for myocardial infarction. Nature 1992;359:641–4.

[9] Ihnken R, Verho K, Gross M, et al. Deletion polymorphism of the angiotensin I-converting enzyme gene is associated with increased plasma angiotensin-converting enzyme activity but not with increased risk for myocardial infarction and coronary artery disease. Ann Intern Med 1996;125(1):19–25.

[10] Andersson B, Sylven C. The DD genotype of the angiotensin-converting enzyme gene is associated with increased mortality in idiopathic heart failure. J Am Coll Cardiol 1996;28:162–7.

[11] Palmer BR, Pilbrow AP, Yandle TG, et al. Angiotensin-converting enzyme gene polymorphism interacts with left ventricular ejection fraction and brain natriuretic peptide levels to predict mortality after myocardial infarction. J Am Coll Cardiol 2003;41:729–36.

[12] McNamara DM, Holubkov R, Janosko K, et al. Pharmacogenetic interactions between β-blocker therapy and the angiotensin-converting enzyme deletion polymorphism in patients with congestive heart failure. Circulation 2001;103:1644–8.

[13] McNamara DM, Holubkov R, Postava L, et al. Phamacogenetic interactions between ACE inhibitor therapy and the angiotensin-converting enzyme deletion polymorphism in patients with congestive heart failure. J Amer Coll Cardiol 2004;44:2019–26.

[14] Campbell D, Aggrarwal A, Esler M, et al. Beta blockers, angiotenisn II, and ACE inhibitors in patients with heart failure. Lancet 2001;358:1609–10.

[15] de Groote P, Helbecque N, Lamblin N, et al. Beta-adrenergic receptor blockade and the angiotensin-converting enzyme deletion polymorphism in patients with chronic heart failure. Eur J Heart Fail 2004;6: 17–21.

[16] Packer M, Poole-Wilson PA, Armstrong PW, et al. Comparative effects of low and high doses of the angiotensin-converting enzyme inhibitor, lisinopril, on morbidity and mortality in chronic heart failure. Circulation 1999;100:2312–8.

[17] O'Toole L, Stewart M, Padfield P, et al. Effect of the insertion/deletion polymorphism of the angiotensin-converting enzyme gene on the response to angiotensin-converting inhibitors in patients with heart failure. J Cardiovasc Pharmacol 1998;32:988–94.

[18] Kurland L, Melhus H, Karlsson J, et al. Angiotensin-converting enzyme gene polymorphism predicts blood pressure response to angiotensin II receptor type 1 antagonist treatment in hypertensive patients. J Hypertens 2001;19:1783–7.

[19] Cicoira M, Zanolla L, Rossi A, et al. Failure of aldosterone suppression despite angiotensin-converting enzyme (ACE) inhibitor administration in chronic heart failure associated with the ACE DD genotype. J Am Coll Cardiol 2001;37:1808–12.

[20] Ciocoira M, Rossi A, Bonapace S, et al. Effects of ACE gene insertion/deletion polymorphism on response to sprironolactone in patients with chronic heart failure. Am J Med 2004;116:657–61.

[21] McNamara DM, MacGowan GA, London B. Clinical importance of beta adrenoceptor polymorphisms in cardiovascular disease. Am J Pharmacogenomics 2002; 2:73–8.

[22] Bristow MR. Beta adrenergic receptor blockade in the failing heart. Circulation 2000;101:558–69.

[23] Buscher R, Herrmann V, Insel PA. Human adrenoceptor polymorphisms: evolving recognition of clinical importance. Trends Pharmacol Sci 1999;20:94–9.

[24] Steinberg SF. The molecular basis for distinct beta adrenergic receptor subtype action in cardiomyocytes. Circ Res 1999;85:1101–11.

[25] Lefkowitz RF, Rockman HA, Koch WJ. Catecholamines, cardiac beta adrenergic receptors and heart failure. Circulation 2000;101:1634–7.

[26] Liggett SB. Pharmacogenetics of relevant targets in asthma. Clin Exp Allergy 1998;28:77–9.

[27] Liggett SB. β_2 adrenergic receptor pharmacogenetics. Am J Respir Crit Care Med 2000;161:S197–201.

[28] Green SA, Cole G, Jacinto M, et al. A polymorphism of the beta 2-adrenergic receptor within the fourth membrane domain alters ligand binding and functional properties of the receptor. J Biol Chem 1993;268: 23116–21.

[29] Turki J, Lorenz JN, Green SA, et al. Myocardial signaling defects and impaired cardiac function of human beta 2-adrenergic receptor polymorphism expressed in transgenic mice. Proc Natl Acad Sci USA 1996;93:10483–8.

[30] Liggett SB, Wagoner LE, Craft LL, et al. The Ile164 β_2 adrenergic receptor polymorphism adversely affects the outcome of congestive heart failure. J Clin Invest 1998;102:1534–9.

[31] Wagoner LE, Craft LL, Singh B, et al. Polymorphisms of the β_2 adrenergic receptor determine exercise ca-

pacity in patients with heart failure. Circ Res 2000;86: 834–40.

[32] Brodde OE, Busher R, Tellkamp R, et al. Blunted cardiac responses to receptor activation in subjects with Thr164Ile β_2 adrenoceptors. Circulation 2001; 103:1048–50.

[33] Feldman RD. Adrenergic receptor polymorphisms in cardiac function (and dysfunction): a failure to communicate? Circulation 2001;1003:1042–3.

[34] Timmermann B, Mo R, Luft FC, et al. β_2 adrenoceptor genetic variation is associated with genetic predisposition to essential hypertension: the Bergen blood pressure study. Kidney Int 1998;53:1455–60.

[35] Busjahn A, Li GH, Faulhaber HD, et al. β_2 adrenergic receptor gene variations, blood pressure, and heart size in normal twins. Hypertension 2000;35: 555–62.

[36] Maqbool A, Hall AS, Paul SG, et al. Common polymorphisms of β_1 adrenoceptor: identification and rapid screening assay. Lancet 1999;353:897–9.

[37] Levin MC, Marullo S, Muntaner O, et al. The myocardium protective variant of the Gly-49 variant of the beta 1 adrenergic receptor exhibits constitutive activity and increased desensitization and down-regulation. J Biol Chem 2002;34:30429–35.

[38] Rathz DA, Brown KM, Kramer LA, et al. Amino acid 49 polymorphisms of the human beta 1 adrenergic receptor affect agonist promoted trafficking. J Cardiovasc Pharmacol 2002;39:155–260.

[39] Mason DA, Moore JD, Green SA, et al. A gain of function polymorphism in a g-protein coupling domain of the human β_1 adrenergic receptor. J Biol Chem 1999;274:12670–4.

[40] Ranade K, Jorgenson E, Sheu WH, et al. A polymorphism in the beta 1 receptor is associated with resting heart rate. Am J Hum Genet 2002;70:935–42.

[41] Borjesson M, Magnusson Y, Hjalmarson A, et al. A novel polymorphism in the gene coding for the β_1 adrenergic receptor associated with survival in patients with heart failure. Eur Heart J 2000;21: 1810–2.

[42] Postava L, Mahlab D, Holubkov R, et al. $\beta 1$ and $\beta 2$ Adrenergic receptor polymorphisms and heart failure survival: interaction with beta blockade [abstract]. Circulation 2002;19(Suppl):II–611.

[43] Liggett SB, Wagoner LE, Levin AM, et al. Synergistic polymorphisms of beta 1 and alpha 2c adrenergic receptors and the risk of congestive heart failure. N Engl J Med 2002;347:1135–42.

[44] Liggett SB. Late Breaking Clinical Trials. Presented at the Heart Failure Society of America. Toronto, September, 2004.

[45] White HL, de Boar RA, Maqbool A, et al. An evaluation of the beta-1 adrenergic receptor Arg389Gly polymorphism in individuals with heart failure: a MERIT-HF sub-study. Eur J Heart Fail 2003;5:463–8.

[46] Johnson JA, Zineh I, Puckett BJ, et al. Beta-1 adrenergic receptor polymorphisms and antihypertensive response to metoprolol. Clin Pharmacol Ther 2003;74:44–52.

[47] Brodde OR, Stein CM. The Gly389Arg beta 1 adrenergic receptor polymorphism: a predictor of response to beta-blocker treatment? Clin Pharmacol Ther 2003; 74:299–302.

[48] Kelly RA, Balligand JL, Smith TW. Nitric oxide and cardiac function. Circ Res 1996;79:363–80.

[49] Drexler H. Nitric oxide synthases in the failing human heart: a double-edged sword? Circulation 1999;99: 2972–5.

[50] Philip I, Plantefeve G, Vuillaumier-Barrot S, et al. G894T polymorphism in the endothelial nitric oxide synthase gene is associated with an enhanced vascular responsiveness to phenylephrine. Circulation 1999;99: 3096–8.

[51] Tesauro M, Thompson WC, Rogliani P, et al. Intracellular processing of endothelial nitric oxide synthase isoforms associated with differences in severity of cardiopulmonary diseases: cleavage of proteins with aspartate vs. glutamate at position 298. Proc Natl Acad Sci USA 2000;97:2832–5.

[52] McNamara DM, Holubkov R, Postava L, et al. The Asp^{298} variant of endothelial nitric oxide synthase: effect on survival for patients with congestive heart failure. Circulation 2003;107:1598–602.

[53] Yang XP, Liu YH, Sheseley EG, et al. Endothelial nitric oxide gene knockout mice cardiac phenotypes and the effect of angiotensin-converting enzyme inhibitor on myocardial ischemia/reperfusion injury. Hypertension 1999;34:24–30.

[54] Bedi M, Murali S, MacGowan G, et al. High dose ACE inhibitors reduces the impact of the NOS3 Asp298 variant on heart failure survival. Circulation 2003; 1085:IV–444.

ELSEVIER
SAUNDERS

Heart Failure Clin 1 (2005) 151–156

HEART
FAILURE
CLINICS

Index

Note: Page numbers of article titles are in **boldface** type.

A

1551-7136/05/$ – see front matter
doi:10.1016/S1551-7136(05)00011-5

I

L

M

N

O

P

Q

R

Changing Your Address?

Make sure your subscription changes too! When you notify us of your new address, you can help make our job easier by including an exact copy of your Clinics label number with your old address (see illustration below.) This number identifies you to our computer system and will speed the processing of your address change. Please be sure this label number accompanies your old address and your corrected address—you can send an old Clinics label with your number on it or just copy it exactly and send it to the address listed below.

We appreciate your help in our attempt to give you continuous coverage. Thank you.

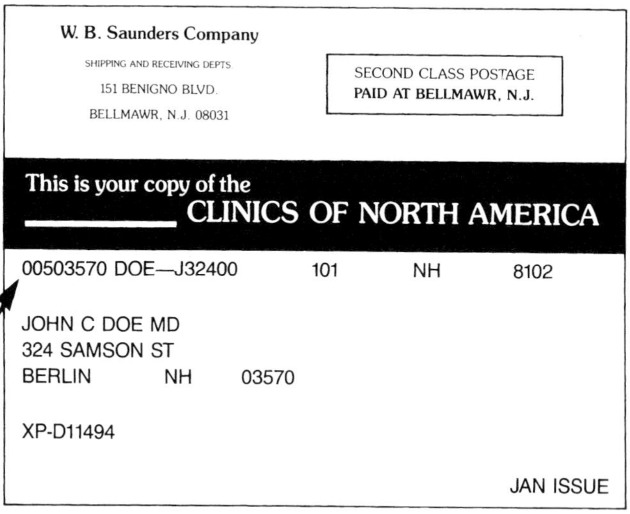
W. B. Saunders Company
SHIPPING AND RECEIVING DEPTS
151 BENIGNO BLVD.
BELLMAWR, N.J. 08031

SECOND CLASS POSTAGE
PAID AT BELLMAWR, N.J.

This is your copy of the
________ CLINICS OF NORTH AMERICA

00503570 DOE—J32400 101 NH 8102

JOHN C DOE MD
324 SAMSON ST
BERLIN NH 03570

XP-D11494

JAN ISSUE

Your Clinics Label Number

Copy it exactly or send your label along with your address to:
W.B. Saunders Company, Customer Service
Orlando, FL 32887-4800
Call Toll Free 1-800-654-2452

Please allow four to six weeks for delivery of new subscriptions and for processing address changes.